Environmental health in emergencies and disasters

A PRACTICAL GUIDE

Edited by
B. Wisner
J. Adams

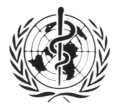

WHO Library Cataloguing-in-Publication Data

Environmental health in emergencies and disasters: a practical
guide.
Edited by B. Wisner, J. Adams.

1.Environmental health.   2.Disasters.   3.Disaster planning.   4.Risk
management.   5.Safety management.   6.Manuals.   I.Wisner, Ben.
II.Adams, John.
ISBN 92 4 154541 0   (NLM/LC classification: WX 185).

Cover photos: Pan-American Health Organization
The named editors alone are responsible for the views expressed in
this publication.
Typeset in Hong Kong
Printed in Malta.

Contents

List of illustrations

Figures

Preface

The WHO *Guide to sanitation in natural disasters* (Assar, 1971) summarized the essential aspects of environmental health management in disasters. These included the provision of emergency water and sanitation services; the burial or cremation of the dead; vector and pest control; food hygiene; and the assessment of the danger of epidemics following emergencies and disasters, etc. Thirty years later these aspects remain essential, though the needs, challenges and opportunities are greater.

This new book deals not only with emergency response, but also with measures designed to reduce the impact of disasters on environmental health infrastructure, such as water supply and sanitation facilities. It also aims to strengthen the ability of people to withstand the disruption of their accustomed infrastructure and systems for environmental health (e.g. shelter, water supply, sanitation, vector control etc.) and to recover rapidly.

What has not changed since the earlier guide was published are the high social and financial costs of emergencies and disasters, and the associated human tragedy, as well as the need for a rapid, efficient, well-prepared response to save life and to restore and maintain a healthy environment. As in previous emergencies, these realities and imperatives remained the same for the earthquakes in Mexico City and Gujarat, the eruption of Mount Pinatubo, the floods in Mozambique and the siege of Sarajevo.

The physical nature of the extreme natural events that can trigger disaster also has not changed. Hagman et al. (1984) and other researchers in the 1980s concluded that the cause of the increase in loss and suffering due to disasters was not that nature had become more violent, but that people had become more vulnerable. Nearly 20 years later, socioeconomic and political factors, such as mass migrations, urbanization, the destruction of natural resources and war continue to account for growing losses from disasters.

There is no evidence that the physical processes causing geological hazards such as earthquakes and volcanoes have altered. However, evidence increasingly indicates that global climatic change related to human activities is affecting human well-being and health (McMichael et al., 1996). And because more people live in exposed places with fewer resources to fall back on, climatic hazards such as floods, hurricanes, wildfires and droughts have a greater impact than in the past. The 1997–1998 El Niño event was the strongest ever recorded and the number of hydrometeorological disasters since 1996 has more than doubled (International Federation of Red Cross and Red Crescent Societies, 2001). If these trends continue, the rise in sea-level will soon have to be added to the factors making many people's lives more hazardous.

While it is too early to judge the full impact of global environmental changes, it is clear that people's vulnerability to disasters has changed. A commitment to economic growth at any cost has brought with it serious health consequences due to increasing poverty and declining living standards for many (Cooper Weil et al., 1990; Warford, 1995) and degradation of the built and natural environments (Cruz & Repetto, 1992). Poverty has often resulted in the misuse of natural resources, causing land degradation (deforestation, destruction of wetlands and desertification) and decreasing food security. In certain parts of the world, high rates of population growth, sometimes combined with ethnic strife, have increased the pressure on urban and rural livelihood systems already weakened by the negative spiral of increasing poverty and decreasing environmental quality.

In a growing number of mega-cities, environmental health conditions are poor at the best of times and catastrophic at times of emergencies. As people try to find places to live in these crowded cities, they occupy increasingly dangerous places—for example, on steep, unstable slopes, in flood plains and near hazardous factories (Mitchell, 1996).

Rapid industrialization and new technologies have produced new hazards. The severity and frequency of technological emergencies have increased. With the proliferation of nuclear power and chemical plants over the last few decades, disasters on the scale of Chernobyl or Bhopal cannot be ruled out.

Political turbulence in many regions of the world has also increased the numbers of refugees and displaced persons fleeing complex emergencies and disasters, who often congregate in large camps where environmental health measures are insufficient. Their vital needs are urgent and massive. As a result, aid agencies are increasingly forced to challenge the orthodox distinctions between development and relief in the attribution of roles among government and nongovernmental organizations (Roche, 1994). In addition, global changes (environmental, economic and political) make an integrated approach to emergency management necessary.

The early 1970s were a watershed in international relief. Within a short period, international agencies had to deal with three large-scale disasters: civil war, causing famine in Biafra; an earthquake in Peru; and a cyclone in Bangladesh (East Pakistan at the time). Lessons were learned about planning and organization that began a new era in the scientific study of emergencies and disaster management. It is now possible to summarize this extensive experience and draw lessons for the environmental health management of emergencies.

During this period of rapid accumulation of international experience with emergency relief and recovery, new management processes were created and scientific and technological advances have begun to aid emergency management. Examples include the use of satellite images, positioning systems and communication aids to warn of disasters early and to coordinate relief. While many of the environmental health principles and actions discussed in this book are old and well established, some technologies such as prefabricated, portable water systems have come into use more recently.

In addition, more professionals are now aware of the links between emergencies, the environment and development. The distribution of goods and the reestablishment of services essential for human survival are no longer considered adequate responses to an emergency. Today, greater care is taken to avoid creating unnecessary dependence among affected communities and there is greater emphasis on supporting people to rebuild and recover by their own efforts after a disaster.

Over the past decade, a consensus has developed concerning the potential effectiveness of citizen and community participation in emergency management. It is easier now to mobilize such participation because of changes in the development models of the past 30 years. Rapid urban growth has brought a new generation of citizen-based organizations and more professional and responsive municipal governments. Citizen environmental and health activism has provided the basis for community participation in risk reduction. In a related development, women have taken on more public roles in society and their vital contributions at all stages of the disaster-management cycle have begun to be recognized.

Because of the experience with emergencies over the last 30 years, there exists today a greater political will to plan and to act strategically to prevent or reduce the impact of disasters and to meet humanitarian needs. A milestone in disaster management was reached with the declaration in 1990 of the International Decade for Natural Hazard Reduction. Also significant for preventing disasters and reducing their impact was the work of the United Nations Conference on Environment and Development (held in Rio de Janeiro in 1992) and the United Nations Conference on Human Settlements (Habitat II, held in Istanbul in 1996).

On the other hand, there still is a large gap between policy commitment and implementation. Many donors still provide far too little support for strengthening emergency preparedness and for preventing disasters. Far worse is the "humanitarian gap." During the 1980s, development assistance to less-developed countries actually decreased (International Federation of Red Cross and Red Crescent Societies, 1993a) and fell by a further 11% in real terms between 1991–2000 (International Federation of Red Cross and Red Crescent Societies, 2001). Since there is a clear connection between successful development and increased protection from hazards, much more needs to be done.

While the number of people affected by disasters, excluding war, varies tremendously from year to year, the general trend is upwards. An average of 147 million people per year were affected by disasters between 1981–1990, but this increased to an average of 211 million people per year between 1991–2000 (though fewer deaths were recorded). The last 30 years' work with disasters demonstrates that much of the resulting suffering is preventable (International Federation of Red Cross and Red Crescent Societies, 1996). This book shows how, in a technical area like environmental health, even small efforts in planning and preparedness can yield great benefits in terms of preventing needless loss.

This book is intended to serve as a practical guide, calling attention to the need to link emergencies, disasters and development, not only in policy statements, but in practical ways. The book identifies physical and social factors and processes determining disaster vulnerability and offers the reader a range of vulnerability-reduction options in development and disaster mitigation. The book covers the main relief and response technologies for a range of natural and technological disasters, and deals with community participation, health education, training and other social aspects relevant to the protection of health and the environment in emergencies and disasters.

Acknowledgments

The World Health Organization (WHO), through its departments of Protection of the Human Environment (PHE) and Emergency and Humanitarian Action (EHA), the International Federation of Red Cross and Red Crescent Societies (IFRC), and the United Nations High Commissioner for Refugees (UNHCR) would like to thank Ben Wisner, Chief editor of this publication, former director of International Studies at California State University at Long Beach, USA, and the Co-editor John Adams, Bioforce, France, for their excellent work. Rudy Slooff, retired staff member of the Environmental Health Division, WHO and short-term policy consultant at the International Decade for Natural Disaster Reduction, should be especially thanked for chairing this project from 1991–1998 and for helping to make this publication a reality. Without his strong leadership, great commitment and effective contribution during the preparation of this book, and his efforts to involve the agencies and experts that contributed to this process over more than a decade, this publication would not have been possible.

José Hueb from WHO should be thanked for his technical inputs and for coordinating the final phases of technical revision and preparation of the book.

The sponsor organizations and editors would like to thank the following: the Directorate-General for International Cooperation of the Netherlands government and the German Fund for Technical Cooperation for their financial and material support in the early days of work on this book.

Although it would not be possible to list all the people who have been involved, the following should be thanked for their contributions:

For sustained guidance and support as members of the WHO/UNHCR/IFRC Review Panel and the Steering Committee: M. Assar, Teheran, Islamic Republic of Iran; S. Ben Yahmed, Geneva, Switzerland; J. Cliff, Maputo, Mozambique; I. Davis, Oxford, England; D. Deboutte, Geneva, Switzerland; N. Domeisen, Geneva, Switzerland; M.W. Dualeh, Geneva, Switzerland; O. Elo, Geneva, Switzerland; H. Farrer Crespo, San José, Costa Rica; E. Giroult, Geneva, Switzerland; A. Holloway, Geneva, Switzerland; W. Kreisel, Geneva, Switzerland; T. Lusty, Oxford, England; S. Nugroho, Jakarta, Indonesia; P. Okoye, Dar es Salaam, United Republic of Tanzania; E. Potts, Wirral, England; C. Rakotomalala, Geneva, Switzerland; G.B. Senador, Manila, Philippines; O. Sperandio, Geneva, Switzerland; Dr M. Toole, Atlanta, GA, USA; Lt. Col. B.A.O. Ward, Bangkok, Thailand; A. Wilson, Geneva, Switzerland.

For significant text contributions: R. Bos, Geneva, Switzerland; A. Cantanhede, Lima, Peru; Gary Coleman, Cardiff, UK; J. Escudero, Buenos Aires, Argentina; J. Falcón, Lima, Peru; A. Girling, Harlestone, England; K. Gutschmidt, Geneva, Switzerland; L. Kheifets, Geneva, Switzerland; C. Osorio, Lima, Peru; S. Palmer, Cardiff, UK; M. Repacholi, Geneva, Switzerland; C. Roy, Melbourne, Australia; L. Sandoval, Lima Peru; M. Simpson-Hebert, Colorado, USA; R. Sloof, Geneva; W. Solecki, Monclair, NJ, USA; R. Stephenson, London England; S. Tharratt, Sacramento, CA, USA; and D. Warner, Washington, DC, USA.

For other text contributions: L. van Drunen, Geneva, Switzerland; B. Kriz, Prague, Czech Republic; and R. Ockwell, Ferney-Voltaire, France.

For substantial review comments: A. Abastable, Oxford, England; H. Abouzaid, Cairo, Egypt; E. Anikpo, Brazzaville, Republic of the Congo; H. Bakir, Jordan; J. Bartram, Geneva, Switzerland; M. Birley, Liverpool, England; S. Cairncross, London, England; M. Courvallet, San José, Costa Rica; P. Deverill, New Delhi, India; M. Gerber, Atlanta, GA, USA; K. Khosh-Chashm, Cairo; J. V. Kreysler, Geneva, Switzerland; P.R. Leger, Wheaton, MD, USA; E. Lohman, Enschede, Netherlands; E. K. Noji, Atlanta, GA, USA; F. M. Reiff, Washington, DC, USA; L. Roberts, Atlanta, GA, USA; H. Sandbladh, Geneva, Switzerland; D. Sharp, Suva, Fiji; G. Shook, San Bernardino, CA, USA; F. Solsona, Lima, Peru; P. Tester, Beaufort, NC, USA; and P. Walker, Boston, USA.

For substantial material support and encouragement: A. Basaran, Manila, Philippines; F. Cuny, Dallas, TX, USA; B. Fawcett, Oxford, England; P. R. Garcia, Quito, Ecuador; K. Kresse, San José, Costa Rica; A. Loretti, Geneva, Switzerland; J. McCusker, Amherst, MA, USA; A. Oliver-Smith, Gainsville, FL, USA; M. Tegegne, Geneva, Switzerland; S. van Voorst tot Voorst, the Hague, Netherlands; and E. Williams, Conway, MA, USA.

Sarah Balance and Kevin Farrell should be thanked for the editorial work which improved considerably the structure and coherence of the book and made it according to the editorial rules of WHO. A. Kofahi and M. Malkawi, Amman, Jordan, should be thanked for their help in preparing the illustrations used in this book.

This has been a long and rich process of updating and compiling the experience of many scientists and practitioners. It is hoped that this sequel to Assar's 1971 guide is worthy of all the effort, energy and support received throughout this process.

1. About this book

1.1 Objectives

Emergencies and disasters can occur anywhere in the world, affecting human health, people's lives and the infrastructure built to support them. Environmental health problems arising from emergencies and disasters are connected to their effects on the physical, biological and social environment that pose a threat to human health, well-being and survival: shelter, water, sanitation, disease vectors, pollution, etc. This book deals with the management of such problems, particularly from the standpoint of the individual with environmental health responsibilities before, during and after emergencies and disasters. It is therefore concerned with:

- Reducing the vulnerability of communities to hazards and increasing their ability to withstand disruption and to recover rapidly.
- Strengthening routine services so that the potential health effects of emergencies and disasters are minimized.
- Responding to emergencies and disasters with appropriate environmental health activities (water supply and sanitation, vector control, etc.).

The book does the following in pursuit of these objectives:

- It emphasizes the importance of setting priorities, and provides an overview of the immediate and long-term health priorities in emergencies and disasters, within the context of overall health plans and multisectoral disaster management.
- It considers environmental health needs in emergencies and disasters in terms of a set of interventions aimed at reducing community vulnerability.
- It provides guidance on environmental health actions in the prevention, preparedness, response and recovery stages of the disaster-management cycle.
- It outlines approaches to decision-making.
- It describes simple, practical, technical interventions which will meet the priority environmental health needs of communities.
- It describes related aspects of primary health care, including training programmes, information systems and community involvement.
- It outlines the need for, and approaches to, coordination and collaboration between all sectors.

The fundamental goals of this book are to provide programme managers and field staff with a framework for thinking about and planning for disasters and emergencies, and with an overview of the technical aspects of environmental health management.

1.2 Target audiences

This book was written mainly for two groups of readers: emergency planners/administrators and environmental technical staff. For the first category, it serves as an introduction to environmental health needs for disaster management. For the second, it provides an insight into environmental health within the overall disaster-management system.

This book will also be of interest to anyone who plans and supervises environmental health activities on a day-to-day basis and to front-line staff working on public health inspection and improvement, such as health officers, sanitarians and employees of water and sanitation companies; community-level workers who may play a leading role in emergency preparedness, such as teachers or Red Cross/Red Crescent workers; and primary health-care workers who may be called upon to respond to an emergency. The book should also be useful to staff and volunteers in nongovernmental organizations who, through their activities in community development, contribute to the long-range management goals of environmental health in emergencies and disasters.

1.3 Organization of the chapters

This book deals with environmental health during the disaster-management cycle, described in Section 1.5. Part I answers the questions: what, where, when, why and who? Part II answers the question: how?

Part I (Chapters 2–5) takes up each element in the disaster-management cycle and shows how appropriate planning and organization can enable those concerned with environmental health to meet the challenge of emergencies, and then how they can help promote disaster prevention as a developmental activity. Chapter 2 gives an overview of emergencies and disasters and presents an integrated approach to managing them, based on the phases of the disaster-management cycle. This is discussed from the point of view of environmental health management in the rest of Part I. Chapter 3 concerns planning, prevention, preparedness and mitigation; Chapter 4 addresses emergency response; and Chapter 5 outlines rehabilitation, recovery and progress towards sustainable development.

Part II (Chapters 6–14) deals with the practical implementation of technical measures, according to the priorities identified in Part I. It is devoted to the environmental health measures necessary to effectively manage and implement emergency relief and recovery. It covers shelter; water supply; sanitation; food safety; vector and pest control; the prevention of epidemics; chemical and radiation incidents; handling of the dead; and health education and community participation.

1.4 Scope

Because this book is intended to be of use in any part of the world, it is general in character and provides guidance on the application of basic principles. Each emergency has its own characteristics and presents specific constraints and opportunities, so recommendations need to be adapted to each context. The book may be useful as a basis for regional- or country-specific guides and training materials in local languages. However, it is not designed as a training course or textbook.

Essentially, the measures recommended are adaptations of environmental health measures appropriate in normal conditions and are neither exclusive nor exhaustive. The special knowledge and initiative of the individual will always be of major importance in emergencies.

The book does not deal directly with complex emergencies (those with a strong military and political dimension), although it does address some of the health consequences of conflict-related disasters, particularly those involving mass population displacements. Complex emergencies are discussed briefly in Chapter 2.

1.5 Approach

As a result of changes in the field of disaster management over the past 30 years, this book takes an integrated approach that follows the phases of the disaster-management cycle. This integrated approach to disaster management has been quite successful in many countries. Together with overall health planning, it provides the context for environmental health management in emergencies and disasters. According to this view, disaster management requires a continuous chain of activities that includes hazard prevention, preparedness, emergency response, relief and recovery, including activities to reconstruct infrastructure and rehabilitate shattered lives and livelihoods. Although there is some variation in terminology for the different phases of disaster management, and numerous typologies have been developed (e.g. Alexander, 1993; Berke, Kartez & Wenger, 1993), they all describe a disaster-management cycle that consists of connected activities and phases, some of which occur simultaneously. For the purposes of this book, the following three major phases have been chosen (see also Figure 1.1):

— planning, prevention, preparedness and mitigation;
— emergency response;
— recovery, rehabilitation and reconstruction to promote sustainable development.

Possible actions for preventing future disasters include early warnings to reduce the effects of extreme events before they happen (usually referred to as mitigation), to reduce potential losses and to increase the level of preparedness in society. Learning from disasters as they occur provides opportunities to increase the effectiveness of disaster preparedness by improving risk assessment and by mapping risk more completely.

Within each phase of the disaster-management cycle, short-range goals can simultaneously contribute to long-range ones, such as strengthening people's capacities to withstand disasters. For example, the reconstruction of water supplies should merge naturally into on-going development activities (such as community mobilization) to further improve the water-supply systems (or other agreed environmental health goals). During "normal" times, these health development activities should aim to reduce the vulnerability of people and infrastructure to future emergencies and disasters. Thus, the routine construction of water works should, for example, incorporate design features that protect them from known hazards. Community participation in each phase strengthens

Figure. 1.1 **The disaster-management cycle**

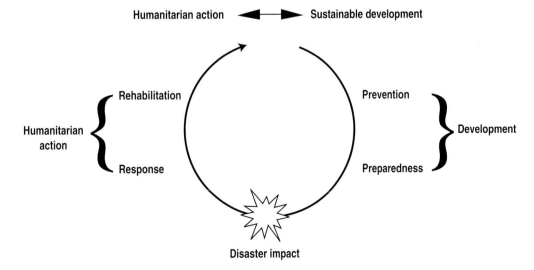

the organizational structure of neighbourhoods and localities, and improves methods of providing early warnings of hazards, of planning emergency responses, etc.

The concept of integration is central to current thinking and practices of disaster management. There are at least four ways in which the integration of efforts is important:

1. *It is necessary for different sectors to work together.* In environmental health management, this often means combining the efforts of the public sector (e.g. health, public works, housing) with those of the private sector (construction, engineering, etc.). This is true for all phases of the disaster-management cycle. Close coordination among sectors is vital, not only for effective emergency response, but also for long-term disaster prevention and emergency preparedness planning.

2. *Environmental health planning must be viewed as part of overall health planning.* Health planning, in turn, should not be conducted in isolation from comprehensive social and economic planning.

3. *Rural and urban communities must participate fully in all phases of emergency relief and development.* The community role in emergency response is obvious, since the community is immediately affected and on the scene when disaster strikes. However, communities can make valuable contributions to planning, as well. Community members know the local circumstances in both rural and urban environments, and understand what makes some people more vulnerable to hazards than others.

4. *A responsive and accountable system of professionals and volunteers is needed.* These personnel can mediate between national counter-disaster agencies and grassroots communities at intermediate administrative levels, including provinces, districts and municipalities.

An integrated approach, defined in this manner and promoted throughout this book, will result in action that is responsive to local needs. It will provide a supportive framework for improvisation by front-line workers in meeting those needs, and will allow all phases of the emergency-management cycle to be improved as lessons are learned.

1.6 Glossary of terms

Many terms used in the field of emergencies and disasters are interpreted in a number of ways, which can lead to confusion. The definitions given here refer to terms frequently used in Part I of this book. Most are drawn from the World Health Organization (1999a).

Community is the smallest social grouping in a country with an effective social structure and potential administrative capacity.

Complex emergencies are situations of disrupted livelihoods and threats to life produced by warfare, civil disturbance and large-scale movements of people, in which any emergency response has to be conducted in a difficult political and security environment.

Disasters are events that occur when significant numbers of people are exposed to hazards to which they are vulnerable, with resulting injury and loss of life, often combined with damage to property and livelihoods.

Emergencies are situations that arise out of disasters, in which the affected community's ability to cope has been overwhelmed, and where rapid and effective action is required to prevent further loss of life and livelihood.

Emergency planning is a process that consists of: determining the response and recovery strategies to be implemented during and after emergencies (based on assessment of vulnerability); responsibility for the strategies; the management structure required for an emergency; the resource management requirements.

Emergency preparedness is a programme of long-term development activities whose goals are to strengthen the overall capacity and capability of a country to manage efficiently all types of emergency and to bring about an orderly transition from relief through recovery and back to sustained development.

Emergency prevention is based on vulnerability assessment and concerns the technical and organizational means of reducing the probability or consequences of disasters and the community's vulnerability.

Environmental health management is the intentional modification of the natural and built environment in order to reduce risks to human health or to provide opportunities to improve health.

Extreme events are known natural or manmade events that occur outside their normal range of intensity, energy or size, which often produce life-threatening hazards.

Hazards are phenomena or substances that have the potential to cause disruption or damage to humans and their environment. The words **threat** and **hazard** are often used in the same way.

Mitigation and prevention are actions aimed at reducing or eliminating the impact of future hazard events, by avoiding the hazard or strengthening resistance to it.

Mitigation comprises measures taken in advance of a disaster aimed at decreasing or eliminating its impact on society and the environment.

Preparedness comprises activities designed to minimize loss of life and damage, to organize the temporary removal of people and property from a threatened location, and facilitate timely and effective rescue, relief and rehabilitation.

Prevention involves activities designed to provide permanent protection from disasters.

Resilience is a community's ability to withstand the damage caused by emergencies and disasters; it is a function of the various factors that allow a community to recover from emergencies.

Susceptibility concerns the factors operating in a community that allow a hazard to cause an emergency (disaster), e.g., proximity to hazard, or level of development.

Vulnerability is the degree to which a population or an individual is unable to anticipate, cope with, resist and recover from the impacts of disasters. It is a function of susceptibility and resilience.

Vulnerability assessment makes it possible to anticipate problems that specific groups will face in the event of a disaster and during the period of recovery. This is also known as hazard assessment, risk assessment or threat assessment.

Vulnerability reduction comprises the steps taken to reduce people's exposure to hazards and increase their capacity to survive and to recover from disasters.

PART I

General aspects

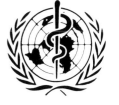

2. The nature of emergencies and disasters

2.1 Environmental health and disasters

Environmental health hazards—threats to human health from exposure to disease-causing agents—are closely associated with disasters and emergencies in a variety of ways. A broad range of activities can be designed to enable the health sector to prevent, mitigate and respond to such hazards.

Disasters and development are connected in ways that necessarily involve the contributions of environmental health professionals. Through better education and higher incomes, development can improve people's capacity to cope with environmental health hazards. On the other hand, certain types of development can create new hazards or new groups of people vulnerable to them. Disasters can set back development, but they can also provide new development opportunities. Strategic planning to increase the capacity of people to withstand disaster hazards must therefore include concerns for environmental health.

Environmental health activities are interdisciplinary, involving engineering, health sciences, chemistry and biology, together with a variety of social, management and information sciences. In times of disaster and recovery, people from many backgrounds engage in activities designed to monitor, restore and maintain public health. Likewise, health workers find themselves cooperating with others to help with non-health-related work, such as search-and-rescue, or work that is only indirectly related to health, such as public education.

2.2 Disasters and emergencies

2.2.1 Hazards and extreme events

A hazard is any phenomenon that has the potential to cause disruption or damage to humans and their environment. Hazards are the potential for an event, not the event itself. Extreme events are natural or man-made processes operating at the extremes of their range of energy, productivity, etc. For example, mudslides, floods, coastal storms, locust or rat invasions are all natural, but extreme events, and to some extent the likelihood of them occurring, may be estimated. Many extreme events, such as severe floods, have been monitored and recorded over many years and have a known probability of occurrence. Man-made hazards, such as the potential for leaks of dangerous chemicals or radiation, also exist and many so-called natural hazards become events or are exacerbated by human activity. For instance, flooding in Bangladesh during the 1990s was made worse because large numbers of discarded plastic bags blocked drainage systems.

Extreme events create stress in human systems and structures because the forces involved are greater than those with which the systems and structures normally cope. For instance, all houses will withstand some wind, but beyond a certain wind speed all will fail. Many farming communities are able to cope with mild and occasional drought, but are overwhelmed by severe and repeated drought.

Extreme events often occur in complex "cascades". Earthquakes may trigger mud or rock slides. Debris may dam a river, producing an artificial lake that threatens downstream settlements with flooding if the dam is breached. Forest fires can produce barren slopes more prone to erosion and flash flooding. Earthquakes may cause electrical fires or explosions of natural gas. Where urban water supplies are stored in reservoirs, earthquakes can damage them, causing flooding and reducing the quantity of water available to fight fires.

The statistical probabilities of such extreme events occurring can be estimated with different degrees of confidence. Some events, such as floods and cyclones, are clustered seasonally. The recurrence of major rainfall and floods can be calculated, but specific floods are harder to predict. Worldwide, the numbers of people affected by natural disasters are strongly associated with the El Niño Southern Oscillation (Bouma et al., 1997). For reasons that are not yet understood, volcanic eruptions seem to be associated with El Niño events (Berlage, 1966; Nicholls, 1988), but it is currently impossible to predict accurately the occurrence of earthquakes.

Some natural events, such as the emergence of a fatal cloud of carbon dioxide and hydrogen sulfide from the depths of Lake Nyos in Cameroon in August 1986, are unexpected and are not amenable to preparedness measures.

2.2.2 Disasters

Disasters are events that occur when significant numbers of people are exposed to extreme events to which they are vulnerable, with resulting injury and loss of life, often combined with damage to property and livelihoods.

Disasters, commonly leading to emergency situations, occur in diverse situations in all parts of the world, in both sparsely populated rural and densely populated urban regions, as well as in situations involving natural and man-made hazards. Disasters are often classified according to their speed of onset (sudden or slow), their cause (natural or man-made), or their scale (major or minor). Various international and national agencies that keep track of disasters employ definitions that involve the minimum number of casualties, the monetary value of property lost, etc. Other definitions are used by countries for legal or diplomatic purposes, e.g. in deciding when to officially declare a region a "disaster area". The terminology used here is less precise so as to cover a broad range of situations. The forces that bring vulnerable people and natural hazards together are often man-made (conflict, economic development, overpopulation, etc.).

An example of natural and technological hazards combining in surprising ways was seen in Egypt in 1994. Heavy rain near the town of Dronka weakened railway lines. A train carrying fuel was derailed and leaking fuel was ignited by electrical cables, causing an explosion. Finally, burning fuel was carried by flood waters through the town, killing hundreds of people (Parker & Mitchell, 1995).

2.2.3 Conflict

Conflict is not considered in detail in this book. However, some of the most serious disasters and emergencies are created or further complicated by conflict and the forced movement of large numbers of people. Conflict is a major cause of direct and indirect land degradation, leading to greater risk of environmental disasters, and also consumes resources that could be used by society to reduce vulnerability to extremes in natural and technological hazards. Conflict also imposes the greatest demands on environmental health personnel, equipment, supplies and supporting services, thus calling for the most skilful use of relief resources. The secondary impact of conflict, in terms of the public health problems it creates and the disruption of environmental health services it causes, are of major importance.

2.2.4 The effects of disasters on environmental health facilities and services

One way in which disasters may cause, or worsen, emergency situations is through the damage they do to environmental health facilities and services. Table 2.1 summarizes the common effects of various natural disasters on environmental health services (Pan American Health Organization, 1982, 1995; Hanna, 1995). Flooding, power failures, broken pipes and blocked roads can all disrupt water, waste and food-handling services

Table 2.1 **Common levels of impact of natural disasters on environmental health services[1]**

	Most common effects on environmental health	Earthquake	Cyclone	Flood	Tsunami	Volcanic eruption
Water supply and wastewater disposal	Damage to civil engineering structures	1	1	1	3	1
	Broken mains	1	2	2	1	1
	Damage to water sources	1	2	2	3	1
	Power outages	1	1	2	2	1
	Contamination (biological or chemical)	2	1	1	1	1
	Transportation failures	1	1	1	2	1
	Personnel shortages	1	2	2	3	1
	System overload (due to population shifts)	3	1	1	3	1
	Equipment, parts, and supply shortages	1	1	1	2	1
Solid waste handling	Damage to civil engineering structures	1	2	2	3	1
	Transportation failures	1	1	1	2	1
	Equipment shortages	1	1	1	2	1
	Personnel shortages	1	1	1	3	1
	Water, soil, and air pollution	1	1	1	2	1
Food handling	Spoilage of refrigerated foods	1	1	2	2	1
	Damage to food preparation facilities	1	1	2	3	1
	Transportation failures	1	1	1	2	1
	Power outages	1	1	1	3	1
	Flooding of facilities	3	1	1	1	3
	Contamination/degradation of relief supplies	2	1	1	2	1
Vector control	Proliferation of vector breeding sites	1	1	1	1	3
	Increase in human/vector contacts	1	1	1	2	1
	Disruption of vector-borne disease control programmes	1	1	1	1	1
Home sanitation	Destruction or damage to structures	1	1	1	1	1
	Contamination of water and food	2	2	1	2	1
	Disruption of power, heating fuel, water supply or waste disposal services	1	1	1	2	1
	Overcrowding	3	3	3	3	2

[1] Source: Pan American Health Organization (2000).
1 - Severe possible effect.
2 - Less severe possible effect.
3 - Least or no possible effect.

for hours or days. More severe damage to civil engineering structures, from bridges to water mains, can cause disruptions lasting days or weeks. In all such cases, contingency plans for temporary repairs and, when necessary, alternative water supplies and sanitation arrangements, are required.

Transportation difficulties and shortage of personnel may cause disruption of vector-control programmes. Some conditions, such as flooding, may result in the proliferation of vector breeding sites which local vector-control programmes cannot deal with.

Droughts may produce a series of problems for water-supply and sewage-treatment systems as a result of low flow from intakes and clogging of intakes; and electricity supplies may be unreliable if power generation is affected.

2.2.5 Emergencies

An emergency is a situation or state characterized by a clear and marked reduction in the abilities of people to sustain their normal living conditions, with resulting damage or risks to health, life and livelihoods. Disasters commonly cause emergency situations, both directly and indirectly. Evacuation or other necessary steps taken to avoid or flee from a disaster, for example, can cause disruption of normal life on a scale calling for emergency action. Sudden, large-scale movements of people within and between countries often produce emergency conditions. Dramatic loss of livelihoods and increased spending needs due to drought or flooding may place people in a very vulnerable situation. A cholera epidemic may overwhelm the capacity of a city's under-resourced health service, creating an urgent need for support. In such emergency situations, local coping mechanisms are overwhelmed and so collective, specialized and often external action is required.

During an emergency, it is common to see primary effects of the disaster followed by secondary effects. For instance, the primary effect of a mudslide might be that many people are injured and need urgent medical attention. A secondary effect might be that blocked sewers and broken water mains lead to an outbreak of water- and sanitation-related disease some weeks later, or that the loss of livelihoods through the destruction of vegetable gardens and workshops leads to reduced food intake and a nutrition emergency some months later. Human needs for non-material things, such as security and cultural identity can also be affected, and the psychological and social impacts of a disaster may be felt many years after the event.

Emergency situations are often described in public health terms, with the crude mortality rate (CMR) being widely accepted as a global measure of their severity. A CMR which is significantly higher than the rate in the affected population before the disaster, or which is above 1 death per 10 000 population per day (or 3 deaths per 1000 population per month) indicates an emergency situation (Centers for Disease Control and Prevention, 1992; Sphere Project, 2000). CMRs in the emergency phase following various types of disaster may be many times the background rate for the region or the affected population. Many more deaths may occur during the post-disaster emergency phase than as a direct result of the disaster itself. However, mortality rates are trailing indicators, that is they do not indicate problems before people die as a result of them, and do not indicate the nature of the problems. Therefore, other indicators concerning health, environmental, social and economic factors are important for understanding the nature of the emergency and how it is likely to change over time, and for understanding how to react effectively.

The term complex emergencies is used to describe situations of disrupted livelihoods and threats to life produced by warfare, civil disturbance and large-scale movements of people, in which any emergency response has to be conducted in a difficult political and security environment. A combination of complex disasters and natural hazards (e.g. military and political problems combined with severe winter weather, coastal storms and flooding, drought and a cholera epidemic) was particularly devastating in the 1990s in such countries as Bosnia and Herzegovina, Iraq, Myanmar, Peru and Somalia.

2.3 Vulnerability to disasters and emergencies

2.3.1 The concept of vulnerability

Vulnerability is the degree to which a population, individual or organization is unable to anticipate, cope with, resist and recover from the impacts of disasters (Blaikie et al. 1994).

Some disasters may involve extreme events that affect a vulnerable population directly, such that their livelihoods and lifelines that support their basic needs are disrupted for a significant period of time. However, the disruption of livelihoods may also be indirect and, even though an emergency situation may not develop, people's vulnerability to future disasters can be increased. An explosion and fire in an industrial quarter of a city might not kill or injure anyone directly, but the employment and income of large numbers of workers and their families may be interrupted. Indirectly, then, there may be an additional threat to the satisfaction of basic needs, since the unemployed workers may not be able to afford an adequate diet, pay rent or pay for health care. These are precisely the kinds of circumstances that can increase a family's vulnerability to future disasters.

Vulnerability is a function of susceptibility (the factors that allow a hazard to cause a disaster) and resilience (the ability to withstand the damage caused by emergencies and disasters and then to recover). See the glossary in Section 1.6 for definitions of terms.

The concept of vulnerability helps to identify those members of a population who are most likely to suffer directly and indirectly from a hazard. It is also useful in identifying those who are more likely to suffer longer-term disruptions of livelihoods and lifelines, as well as those who will find it more difficult to re-establish their accustomed patterns of living. Poverty (and its common consequences, malnutrition, homelessness or poor housing, and destitution) is a major contributor to vulnerability. In many situations, women and children are most vulnerable to disaster emergencies. This has important implications in defining priorities for vulnerability reduction. Some of the main indicators of vulnerability are discussed below.

2.3.2 High susceptibility

Residence or employment in or near a known hazard zone is easy to map. Communities covered would include those living on flood plains, on unprotected coasts or low-lying islands prone to severe storms, on the slopes of an active volcano, or near industries that use or discharge radioactive substances or dangerous chemicals. In urban areas where spontaneous settlement has occurred, self-built housing may be sited on steep, unstable slopes (as in Rio de Janeiro) or in ravines in zones subject to earthquakes (as in San Salvador). In December 2000, heavy rainfall caused mudslides that killed 30 000 people in Venezuela, largely due to unplanned settlements on steep slopes, combined with deforestation.

Some occupations carry a heightened susceptibility to certain extreme events. For instance, those employed in forest industries (in both the formal and informal sectors) may be more susceptible to large fires. Populations that rely on fishing may be more susceptible to storms. Landless and land-poor people are sometimes forced by circumstances to inhabit hazardous zones in order to find arable land, as in Bangladesh.

2.3.3 Low resilience

Communities with a high prevalence of environmental health-related disease may be more at risk to a disaster than others. Malnutrition, which commonly has a seasonal pattern, predisposes people to disease and reduces their resilience. People with disabilities and frail elderly people are less mobile and harder to evacuate. Children and pregnant women are more prone to serious illness from exposure to some industrial chemicals. People in the lowest socioeconomic groups in a population may be the most difficult to warn of dangers because they do not own radios.

In the longer term, people with few financial and social resources, such as recent migrants to cities, elderly people living alone and homeless children, are likely to find it more difficult to recover from a disaster. An increasing number of homeless urban children also fall into this category.

Anderson & Woodrow (1989) identified the following capacities that determine resilience to disasters and which themselves can be diminished by disasters:

— physical/material capacity—command over physical and financial resources;
— social/organizational capacity—support networks in the community and extended family, and access to support by social and political institutions, such as churches and the government;
— attitudinal/motivational/psychological capacity—how people feel about their ability to cope (e.g. whether they feel isolated, connected to others, capable or weak).

Figure 2.1 shows disaster vulnerability as a function of hazards and threats (susceptibility), and capacity to cope and recover (resilience).

2.3.4 The impact of disasters at national level

At a national level, repeated major disasters have a significant effect on development, through their economic and social costs, and may create a vicious cycle as underdevel-

Figure. 2.1 **Disaster vulnerability as a function of exposure to hazards and threats, and reduced capacity to cope and recover**

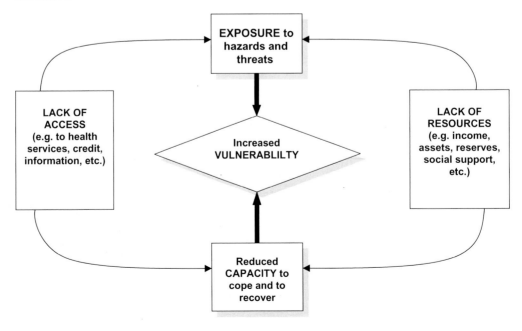

opment increases the vulnerability of people and society to disasters. Box 2.1 illustrates this.

2.4 Human actions that increase vulnerability to disasters

2.4.1 Improper resource management

There are important links between the physical and social processes that determine vulnerability to disasters. Improper land use and land development can increase the physical magnitude of hazards. Deforestation provides a classic example. Many rural people with low incomes convert trees into charcoal. Denuded of vegetation, the land is less able to absorb rainfall, becomes increasingly prone to drought and, because of the increased run-off of water and soil erosion, flooding may be increased downstream. Reservoirs may be silted up more quickly, so that water storage for the next period of drought is reduced, thus increasing the same people's vulnerability.

Disposal of solid wastes in the steep hillside *favelas* (squatter settlements) of Rio de Janeiro provides a similar example in an urban setting. Run-off from rain can build up behind "dams" created by such wastes, and the resulting saturated soil becomes unstable and subject to landslides.

Even self-help initiatives can have tragic, unintended results. Inadequate drainage of self-built water supplies and poorly maintained septic tanks may have contributed to reducing the stability of a hill in Mameyes, Puerto Rico, where a mudslide buried hundreds of people in 1986.

2.4.2 Urbanization and vulnerability to disasters

One of the most striking features of the last few decades has been the rapid rate of urbanization. Currently, more than half of the world's people live in cities and, by the year 2025, almost two-thirds may be urban dwellers (World Health Organization, 2000a). Not only do an increasing percentage of all people live in cities, but the number of so-called mega-cities is increasing. This rapid urbanization poses a challenge to environmental health because it creates conditions that increase human vulnerability to disaster. Table 2.2 lists some of the major agglomerations and cities known to be sited in hazard zones.

Many people live in these cities in spontaneous or informal settlements with little or no access to municipal services. Sometimes there are not even fire lanes for use by emergency services. Refuse collection is sporadic, if it occurs at all, while the provision of water and sanitation facilities generally lags far behind urban population growth.

Informal settlement often takes place in highly dangerous locations, such as steep hillsides, urban flood plains and near dangerous factories. People often live in these

---

Box 2.1 The disaster–development connection[1]

The economic and human costs of disasters continue to retard economic and social development. For example, in the Philippines in 1986–1991, an average of 2377 people died annually from both natural and technological disasters. For the same period, the estimated annual cost of damage from these disasters averaged more than P10.78 billion. Natural disasters included the 1990 earthquake in Northern Luzon that killed 1283 and displaced over a million people, and flash floods and landslides that killed 8000 in Ormoc City in 1991.

In 1990 alone, disasters resulted in direct damage equal to about 3% of the country's GNP. Such losses reduce economic growth, aggravate the country's underdevelopment and increase the vulnerability of the people and society to disasters.

[1] Source: The Citizen Disaster Response Centre (1992).

Table 2.2 **Selected cities exposed to natural hazards[1]**

City	Estimated population in 2002 (millions)	Principal hazards
Beijing	9.2	Earthquake, dust storm
Cairo/Al-Jiza/Shubra al-Khayma	15.1	Flooding
Calcutta/Haora	14.6	Cyclone, flooding
Delhi/Faridabad/Ghaziabad	17.2	Flooding
Dhaka	10.4	Flooding, cyclone
Jakarta/Bekasi/Bogor/Depak	15.9	Earthquake, volcano
Lagos	9.3	Flooding
Los Angeles/Riverside/Anaheim	16.8	Earthquake, wildfire
Manila/Kalookan/Quezon City	13.5	Earthquake, flooding
Mexico City incl. Nezahualcóyotl, Ecatepec, Naucalpan	20.8	Earthquake
Moscow	13.2	Blizzard
New York/Newark/Paterson	21.6	Blizzard, flooding
Rio de Janeiro/Nova Iguaçu/Sao Gonçalo	12.3	Landslide, flooding
São Paulo/Guarulhos	20.3	Landslide, flooding
Shanghai	12.2	Flooding, typhoon
Tehran/Karaj	11.1	Earthquake
Tianjin	5.6	Earthquake
Tokyo/Kawasaki/Yokohama	34.9	Earthquake

[1] Sources: Angotti (1993); Brinkhoff: Principal agglomerations and cities of the world, http://www.citypopulation.de, 11.05.2002.

areas because of poverty, and low income and lack of tenure may prevent them from improving the safety of their homes or the sanitary conditions of their environment. Such families experience stress during "normal" times and therefore have few physiological or financial resources to sustain themselves in a disaster. Urban areas also contain large numbers of homeless people—families who live on the streets and street children, who are among the most vulnerable of all.

Even in wealthy countries with well-designed and constructed infrastructure, the high population density in cities means that large numbers of people may be vulnerable to hazards that would have little impact in a scattered rural community.

Countries and cities are also running out of water. According to one estimate presented to the United Nations Conference on Human Settlement (Habitat II) conference in Istanbul in 1996, most cities in developing countries will face severe water shortages by 2010.

2.4.3 Rural/urban connections

Disaster vulnerabilities in rural and urban areas are connected in an important way. A sizeable proportion of recent urban migrants report leaving rural areas because of disasters from which they have been unable to recover. This emphasizes the importance of including the process of recovery (or failure of recovery) within the concept of the disaster cycle, as survivors of one disaster who do not recover are less resilient and more vulnerable to the next disaster. The converse also appears to be true, providing a unique opportunity to planners and policy-makers. Disasters can offer an opportunity to improve housing, locate housing more safely and lay the foundations for later improvements in environmental health through community mobilization.

2.4.4 Global environmental change

In addition to the local changes in ecosystems previously discussed, there is increasing evidence of global climatic change (e.g. Watson et al., 1996). Although the long-range consequences are hard to predict, more severe cyclonic storms, an increase in both flooding and drought, and a trend towards desertification cannot be ruled out.

The secondary consequences of global climatic change could well result in new hazards. Wildfires and mudslides may become more frequent in the wake of increased drought and flooding. The genetic diversity of food plants may be reduced as climatic zones shift more rapidly than plants can move or adapt. Primary productivity in the oceans may be affected. New disease habitats may be produced; for example, algal blooms are now appearing more frequently in many coastal waters and have been found to harbor *Vibrio cholerae*, the causative organism of cholera. Because of stratospheric ozone depletion—another global environmental change that humans have brought about—the immune systems of people and animals may be weakened by additional ultraviolet radiation.

All of these hazards—some well established and others less so—need to be on the long-term planning agenda of national counter-disaster planners and others concerned with environmental health.

For the possible health effects of global environmental change, see Box 2.2.

2.5 The disaster-management cycle

2.5.1 Disaster management—a developmental approach

As indicated in Chapter 1, the disaster-management cycle is a core concept in environmental health management in disasters and emergencies, and several variations of the cycle have been used effectively (Carter, 1991; United Nations Office of the Disaster Relief Coordinator, 1991; Natural Disasters Organization, 1992; World Health Organization, 1999a).

Appropriate actions at all points in the cycle lead to greater preparedness, better warnings, reduced vulnerability or the prevention of disasters during the next iteration of the cycle. The objectives of such a development-oriented approach are to reduce hazards, prevent disasters and prepare for emergencies. Inappropriate humanitarian action and development processes can lead to increased vulnerability to disasters and loss of preparedness for emergency situations.

Although the disaster-management cycle can be entered at any point, many governments and institutions focus their attention on the steps to take when disaster strikes. As shown in Figure 2.1 (see section 2.3.3), the disaster impact is often followed by an emer-

---

Box 2.2 Health effects of global environmental change[1]

Global warming may cause increased heat-wave-related illness and death, the spread of vector-borne infections, and more frequent cyclones, floods, landslides and fires. The resulting rise in sea levels may lead to health problems associated with deteriorating water supply and sanitation, loss of agricultural land and fishing grounds, and flooding.

Increased ultraviolet radiation resulting from stratospheric ozone depletion will lead to greater risks of skin cancer, ocular effects such as cataracts, and suppression of the immune system with the consequent increased risk of infection. Increased ultraviolet radiation may also cause indirect effects on human health through deleterious effects at lower levels of the food chain, particularly in marine ecosystems.

[1] Sources: McMichael (1993), McMichael et al. (1996).

gency situation calling for a series of immediate and rapid responses. These include initial rapid assessment, search and rescue, and emergency relief to stabilize the situation, followed swiftly by more detailed damage, needs and capacities assessment, leading to short-term interventions to safeguard life, health and livelihoods in the medium term. In the postemergency recovery phase, people's livelihoods should be restored and the infrastructure and housing repaired through rehabilitation and reconstruction. Ideally, there should be a smooth transition from recovery to on-going development, as represented by the common thread that runs through Figure 2.2, uniting its elements. The result should be the enhancement of people's capacity to withstand and recover from future disasters. Enhanced capacity on the part of individuals, communities and institutions is the focus of prevention and mitigation. Preparedness on the part of the emergency services and society as a whole, including better warning systems, completes the cycle. Figure 2.3 adds more detail and provides a sense of timing.

A central message of this book is that the lessons of disasters should be remembered even if complete recovery takes years. Only in this way can the full potential for preparedness, prevention and mitigation be achieved. For an example of the relief–development transition, see Box 2.3.

Box 2.3 The relief–development transition following drought and floods in the Sudan[1]

Operations by the Sudanese Red Crescent Society (SRCS) following drought in 1984–1985 and the flooding of Khartoum in 1988 are a good example of planning a smooth transition from emergency response through relief and recovery to normal development activities. Many people fleeing drought and war settled themselves spontaneously around Khartoum beginning in 1984–1985. In this period, at least 120 000 refugees arrived from drought-affected rural areas, adding nearly 10% to Greater Khartoum's 1983 population of 1.5 million. At first, 60 000 people were supplied by tanker trucks with water on a daily basis. These people were later affected by floods in 1988, further complicating attempts to satisfy their needs. A second phase called for the rehabilitation of existing boreholes and the construction of new public water points. Finally, commercial well-drilling contractors were engaged to increase the capacity of Khartoum's urban water system while fitting in with the long-term water resource development plans of Greater Khartoum, using equipment that was within the Government's ability to maintain and to operate. IFRC provided general management and technical support and coordinated input from member societies, while the SRCS supervised operations on the ground in liaison with the Government.

[1] Sources: Acheson (1993); International Federation of Red Cross and Red Crescent Societies (1993a).

2.5.2 Sustainable livelihoods and disaster management

One of the major goals of disaster management, and one of its strongest links with development, is the promotion of sustainable livelihoods and their protection and recovery during disasters and emergencies. Where this goal is achieved, people have a greater capacity to deal with disasters and their recovery is more rapid and more durable.

2.5.3 Limitations in complex emergencies

Large-scale movements of people often create emergency situations. The disaster-management cycle may apply to such cases, but with limitations. Although there may be some warning of refugee movements, it is often so little that a handful of care-providers are confronted by a large number of people with urgent needs and the care-providers

have insufficient resources to respond promptly and appropriately to prevent or mitigate secondary disasters, such as outbreaks of disease, famine and the dispersal of families. Repatriation of the refugees, their integration within the host community, or asylum
in a third country provide the conditions for long-term recovery and development.

Figure. 2.2 **Developmental considerations contributing to all elements of the disaster-management cycle**

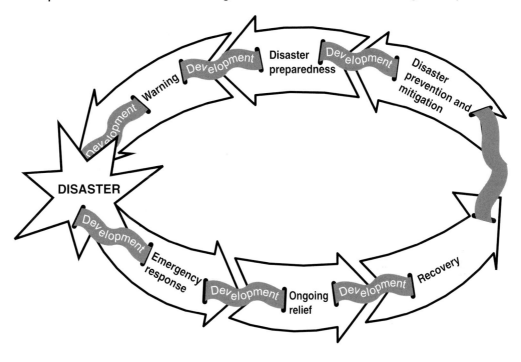

Figure. 2.3 **Development temporarily interrupted by sudden disaster**

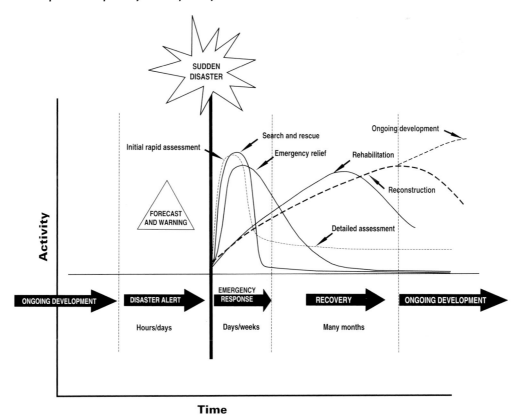

However, refugees and displaced people may spend years away from their homes, in situations where opportunities for development are limited and complete recovery is postponed.

In long-term conflicts people may suffer repeated violence and displacement, so that getting back onto any sort of development path becomes virtually impossible. However, people's ability to learn from every experience increases their capacity to deal with new disasters. Rwandan refugees on the move in eastern Democratic Republic of the Congo in 1996 and 1997 were able to organize basic environmental health services partly because of their experience of doing so in camps for two years since leaving Rwanda in 1994.

2.6 Steps in disaster management

2.6.1 Vulnerability assessment

Using the disaster-management approach involves carrying out a number of pro-active steps—as well as reacting to disasters and emergencies when they occur—the first of which is vulnerability assessment. This provides the basis for reducing vulnerability through work in two areas: disaster prevention/mitigation (to reduce susceptibility) and emergency preparedness (to increase resilience).

Vulnerability assessment makes it possible to anticipate problems that specific groups will face in the event of a disaster and during the period of recovery. The process of vulnerability assessment involves determining the spatial proximity of population subgroups to potential hazards (an assessment of susceptibility), according to personal and socioeconomic characteristics that may influence the immediate and long-term impact of hazards on them (an assessment of resilience).

See Section 3.3 for more detail on vulnerability assessment.

2.6.2 Prevention and mitigation

Complete prevention of disasters is feasible only if it is possible to eliminate people's susceptibility to hazards by moving populations away from hazard zones, providing complete protection from hazards, or preventing the physical hazard altogether. This has occasionally been achieved, e.g. the virus responsible for smallpox was eradicated, and cities have been protected from flooding by diverting rivers to alternative courses. However, to survive or improve well-being, humans are prepared to take risks and will even resettle in areas previously affected by natural disasters.

The best that can usually be done is therefore to reduce the potential impact of emergencies and disasters. Mitigation—actions aimed at reducing (but not eliminating) the impact of future hazard events—and reduction of the susceptibility of high-risk groups are then the goals. The construction of riverbank levees and upstream storage reservoirs are examples of measures for mitigating and reducing the hazard of flooding by rivers.

Efforts to reduce the impact of emergencies or disasters may focus on the extreme event, the humans who are at risk of being affected, or both. For instance, the impact of flooding can also be mitigated by preserving wetlands that can absorb and spread flood waters. On the other hand, improved urban land tenure allows urban residents to invest in making their houses more secure in earthquakes or high winds.

For further detail on disaster prevention and mitigation, see section 3.4.

2.6.3 Emergency preparedness

Emergency preparedness is "a programme of long-term development activities whose goals are to strengthen the overall capacity and capability of a country to manage efficiently all types of emergency and bring about a transition from relief through recovery, and back to sustained development" (World Health Organization, 1995a).

The goal of emergency-preparedness programmes is to achieve a satisfactory level of readiness to respond to any emergency situation through programmes that strengthen the technical and managerial capacity of governments, organizations, institutions and communities. Such programmes are concerned with:

- National legislation and national policy for disaster management.
- Plans and procedures for disaster management and the coordination of emergency response at international, national and subnational levels.
- The strengthening of institutional and human resources for disaster management.
- The establishment and management of stocks of relief supplies and equipment and the identification of transportation options.
- Public education, public awareness and community participation in disaster management.
- The collection, analysis and dissemination of information related to emergencies and disasters that are likely to occur in the region.

Activities in each of these areas will be needed to achieve emergency preparedness.

For further information on emergency preparedness, see section 3.5.

2.6.4 Planning, policy and capacity building

Planning is required at all levels, from the community level to national and international levels, to ensure that programmes for disaster prevention and mitigation are carried out according to clear objectives, with adequate resources and management arrangements, and to ensure that strategies, resources, management structures, roles and resources for emergency response and recovery are determined and understood by key actors. Effective emergency planning can only take place once roles and responsibilities have been agreed.

Emergency and disaster prevention, mitigation, preparedness and response will depend on the incorporation of appropriate measures in national development planning and in the sectoral plans and programmes of the various ministries. They will also depend on the availability of information on hazards, emergency risks and the countermeasures to be taken and on the degree to which government agencies, nongovernmental organizations and the general public are able to make use of this information. The complete disaster-management cycle includes the shaping of public policies and plans that either modify the causes of disasters or mitigate their effects on people, property, assets and infrastructure. Institutional capacity should also be increased through organizational innovation and training. Experience has shown that the result can be a more resilient, less vulnerable population, with fewer disruptions of essential services, such as water and power supplies, improved early warning ability, and better advance planning for evacuations and emergency response.

Health managers, as well as front-line community-based professionals and volunteers who deal with environmental health, can contribute to these longer-term efforts.

For further discussion of emergency planning, see Section 3.5.

2.6.5 Emergency response

The appropriate response will depend on the nature of the emergency or disaster and the effectiveness of mitigation measures, but is also very much conditioned by the degree of preparedness achieved.

In a crisis, the environmental health agencies are usually called upon to deal with the immediate problems. To be able to respond effectively, these agencies must have experienced leaders, trained personnel, adequate transport and logistic support, appropriate communications, and rules and guidelines for working in emergencies. If the necessary preparations have not been made, the agencies concerned will not be able to meet the immediate environmental health needs of the people. It is completely unrealistic to expect an effective response to take place spontaneously, without planning or preparation. It calls for foresight, anticipation and prior effort.

The aim of emergency response is to provide immediate assistance to maintain life, improve health and support the morale of the affected population. Such assistance may range from providing specific but limited aid, such as assisting refugees with transport, temporary shelter, and food, to establishing semipermanent settlement in camps and other locations. It also may involve initial repairs to damaged infrastructure, e.g. flooded sanitation systems, and the control of chemical hazards. Much of the technical literature devoted to emergencies and disasters deals with the actions to be taken in the relief phase.

The emphasis in the relief phase is on removing the immediate environmental hazards to health and meeting the basic needs of the people until more permanent and sustainable solutions to their problems can be found. The philosophy advocated in this book is one of incremental, but continuous, improvement. Over time, the relief phase often merges with long-term recovery and development.

For further information on emergency response, see Chapter 4.

2.6.6 Rehabilitation, reconstruction and recovery

As the emergency is brought under control, the affected population is capable of undertaking a growing number of activities aimed at restoring their lives and the infrastructure that supports them. This may be a slow process and one in which the capacity for such efforts must be carefully nurtured and built up over a period of time, but the process should start early in the emergency phase.

There is no distinct point at which immediate relief changes into recovery and then into long-term sustainable development. Progress in some areas will probably be quicker than in others. Physical rehabilitation and reconstruction can sometimes take place more quickly than social or psychological rehabilitation. Both are necessary, however, if full recovery is to be attained. This phase therefore involves a maturing process in which all of the key elements of environmental health may be involved. Essentially, the process includes the restoration of community life, the participation of the people in the recovery and development activities, and provision of the appropriate environmental health infrastructure (shelter, water supply, sanitation, etc.). There will be many opportunities during the recovery period to enhance prevention and increase preparedness, thus reducing vulnerability. Environmental health activities have an important role in recovery. They can contribute to the long-term reduction of people's vulnerability to hazards by increasing their capacity to cope with, and recover from, future disasters. Examples include the reconstruction of housing with improved local drainage and built-in roof water-catchment systems, the reconstruction of markets with adequate facilities for personal and food hygiene, and the repair and deepening of rural wells and boreholes. There will be many such opportunities for long-term improvements in environmental health during the recovery period, depending on the local situation.

For further information on rehabilitation, reconstruction, and recovery, see Chapter 5.

2.7 Further information

For further information on:

— development, environment and disasters, see: Chen (1973), Kanji, Kanji & Manji (1991), Kreimer & Munasinghe (1991);

— women in disasters, see: Jiggins (1986), Rivers (1987), Drèze & Sen (1989), Agarwal (1990), Gibbs (1990), International Federation of Red Cross and Red Crescent Societies (1991), Martin (1992), Begum (1993), Walker (1994), Ikeda (1995), and Bari (1998);

— reducing vulnerability, see: Anderson & Woodrow (1989), Maskrey (1989), Carter (1991), International Federation of Red Cross and Red Crescent Societies (1993b), Blaikie et al. (1994), Anderson (1995), von Kotze & Holloway (1996), and Pan American Health Organization (1998);

— urban hazards, see: Richards & Thomson (1984), Hardoy & Satterthwaite (1989), Hardoy et al. (1990), and Black (1994);

— disaster management and disaster definitions, see: United Nations Department of Humanitarian Affairs (1992), Neal & Phillips (1995), World Health Organization (1999a), International Federation of Red Cross and Red Crescent Societies (2000), and International Federation of Red Cross and Red Crescent Societies (2001).

3. Predisaster activities

3.1 Introduction

Work done in advance of possible emergencies and disasters is an essential aspect of disaster management. It enables a reduction in the number and severity of disasters, through prevention and mitigation, as well as improved emergency response, through preparation and planning. A number of models have been developed to promote a programmed approach to predisaster activities, based on a systematic assessment of vulnerability, followed by vulnerability reduction through prevention and preparedness activities that are planned, managed, monitored and evaluated. The model presented here is illustrated in Figure 3.1.

Although prevention/mitigation and planning/preparedness are presented separately here, in practice they have many activities in common and should be regarded as interdependent and often overlapping aspects of the overall goal of vulnerability reduction.

The pre-condition for systematic vulnerability reduction is policy development, which ensures that disaster management activities are developed within a favourable policy framework.

3.2 Institutional arrangements

3.2.1 Policy development

Policy development is needed at national, provincial/district and local levels to ensure that common goals are set and common approaches are used. Without a shared disaster management policy that applies to all relevant sectors and all levels, prevention, preparedness and response are likely to be fragmented, badly coordinated and ineffective (World Health Organization, 1999a). Developing and monitoring policies for disaster management requires an active process of analysis, consultation and negotiation. This process should involve consultation among a wide variety of institutions, groups and individuals. These will include nongovernmental organizations, such as the national societies of the Red Cross or Red Crescent, and several governmental bodies, such as the ministries responsible for health, security, welfare, public works, etc. The resultant policies should reflect society's definition of the limits of acceptable risk and its commitment to protecting vulnerable populations. They should also result in a clear definition of the roles and responsibilities of all the partners in emergency management. Table 3.1 illustrates the range of issues in disaster-management policy development and gives recommended options for addressing them.

Certain aspects of policy development depend on learning lessons from previous disasters and emergencies. See Section 3.6.

3.2.2 National and subnational disaster organizations

Predisaster activities should be coordinated in each country at different levels by bodies that are concerned with all stages of the disaster, so that the overall goal of vulnerability reduction is pursued.

Figure 3.1 **Vulnerability reduction**[1]

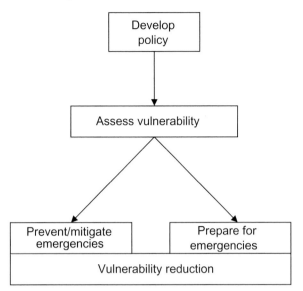

[1] Source: World Health Organization (1999a).

At national level, national disaster organizations (that may have a variety of names and that may be constituted in a variety of ways) should have the following features (Carter, 1991):

They do:

— provide a coherent approach to disaster management;
— serve as a common reference point for departmental activities;
— clearly allocate responsibilities;
— provide a basis for coordinated action;
— provide a setting within which to review and evaluate needs.

They do not:

— duplicate the normal government organization;
— act independently of government;
— seek to control other agencies;
— act outside its legal authority.

National disaster organizations are often composed of representatives from a range of government ministries and nongovernmental organizations that have a role to play in predisaster activities, disaster response and recovery.

At various subnational levels, similar coordination and response bodies may also exist. They require resources, access to information, and authority to be able to operate effectively.

3.3 Vulnerability and capacity assessment

3.3.1 The purpose and process of vulnerability and capacity assessment

The purpose of vulnerability and capacity assessment (VCA)—also commonly called risk analysis or threat assessment—is to identify hazards and their possible effects on communities, activities or organizations, and their capacity to prevent and respond to disasters. This is a vital early stage in the disaster-management process. Vulnerability assessment informs strategies for reducing the vulnerability of development programmes to disruption; it enables emergency prevention, mitigation and preparedness measures

Table 3.1 **Policy issues and recommended options**[1]

Policy issue	Recommended option
1. Emergency preparedness and development planning	Emergency preparedness should be incorporated into all sustainable development objectives and projects.
2. National emergency law and other relevant, enabling legislation	A national emergency law is required with references to emergency management in other laws. Definition of "emergency" should be broad and the language of the law should be as simple as possible.
3. National emergency management organization	A national emergency management organization that is separate from other government agencies is preferable. Responsibility should also be decentralized to provincial government.
4. Responsibility and major mission of national emergency management organization	The mandate of the national organization and its provincial counterparts should cover all aspects of emergency management, including health.
5. Tasks of the emergency management organization	The organization should institutionalize emergency management in other organizations, rather than attempt to undertake all emergency management work itself. It should undertake a number of tasks, but maintain a generalist approach.
6. Community and provincial emergency preparedness	The national level should develop policy and standards for emergency preparedness at all levels of government. Provincial and community-level emergency preparedness should be developed according to the policy and standards.
7. Health sector emergency preparedness	Health sector emergency preparedness should be coordinated with other sectors, the national level developing policy and standards, and the provincial and community levels implementing programmes. Public, private, military and NGO health-service providers should be part of the same preparedness programme, as should each discipline within the health sector.
8. Involving other groups, management and citizens in emergency	All citizens should be involved in emergency management in some way, ranging from active participation in vulnerability assessment and emergency planning, to receiving information on emergency preparedness.
9. Managing resources	Resources for emergency management should be based on existing resources. Emphasis should be on training and information-sharing in emergency management in all sectors and at all levels.
10. Evaluating an emergency preparedness and response programme	Performance indicators for emergency management should be developed to suit the national, provincial and community environments.
11. Priorities in implementing emergency preparedness	Priorities should be based on either expressed or actual needs. This will require at least basic research into vulnerability and immediate needs.

[1] Source: World Health Organization (1999a).

to be carried out effectively; it facilitates rapid and relevant emergency response, based on an understanding of gaps in resources that need to be filled with external support; it provides information on likely damage and operating difficulties; and it provides a picture of the predisaster situation, to enable appropriate objectives to be set for recovery programmes.

The process of VCA may be carried out in a number of ways. The essential steps involved include the following (adapted from World Health Organization, 1999a):

- The *project definition* determines the aim, objectives, scope and context of the VCA, the tasks to be performed, and the resources needed to perform them.
- The formation of a representative *planning group* is essential to VCA and emergency planning. Without this group it will be difficult to gather the required information, obtain the commitment of key individuals, and allow the communities and organizations to participate.
- *Hazard identification and description* reveals and describes the hazards that exist in the community (although it is unlikely that all of the hazards will be discovered). The same hazards may manifest themselves differently in different areas and communities because there is an interaction between hazards, the particular community, and the environment.
- A *community and environment description* outlines the relevant information about the people, property or environment that may affect or be affected by the hazards. More hazards may be identified at this stage. Key aspects of communities' capacity to deal with disasters are identified at this stage.
- A description of *effects* is an account of community vulnerability—what is likely to happen in an accident, incident, emergency or disaster involving a single hazard or multiple hazards.
- *Hazard prioritization* determines the hazards that should be dealt with first, and those that can be dealt with later or ignored, on the basis of their likely effects and community vulnerability.
- *Recommendations for action* are the link between vulnerability assessment and other emergency management activities. Planning, training and education, and monitoring and evaluation should be based firmly on the results of the vulnerability assessment.
- *Documentation* of all results and decisions is necessary to justify the recommendations and any further emergency prevention and preparedness work.

Two key steps in this process—the identification and description of hazards and the assessment of community and organizational resilience—are described below.

3.3.2 Hazard mapping

The average frequency of occurrence and location of most extreme events can be determined with some degree of accuracy. While global maps of hazards, such as potential desertification, severe storms, and earthquake and volcanic activity, do exist, a more detailed approach is of more use to environmental health and disaster planners. Historical records, physical data and computer simulations allow the production of detailed city, subnational or national maps overlaid with zones of probable physical damage from such extreme events as landslides, floods, earthquakes, volcanic eruptions, storm surges and tsunamis.

The same approach can be taken with industrial accidents. Maps of the zones surrounding hazardous factories and the routes used to transport hazardous materials, plus data on seasonal wind velocity and direction, can be used to predict the scale of possible hazards and determine the method of evacuation or other emergency response if leaks or explosions occur. Public and private records of past industrial activity can be a valuable resource for identifying the presence of physical hazards. For instance, Foster (1980) reported that officials in Warsaw, Poland used records to find 2 tons of cyanide in rotting barrels in an abandoned basement workshop. If it had leaked into the water supply, it could have killed most of the city's population.

3.3.3 Vulnerability analysis of water-supply systems

One set of management goals suggested for water-supply systems facing hazard risks (American Water Works Association, 1984) are as follows:

— to provide water for fire fighting;
— to prevent unnecessary loss of stored treated water;
— to develop and maintain adequate amounts of potable water;
— to restore the entire system as soon as possible.

To decide whether a water-supply system will be able to achieve these goals in an emergency, vulnerability analysis must also take into account the effect of a disaster on sources such as surface water (in the case of wildfires) and groundwater (in the case of industrial spills). The vulnerability analysis should be carried out systematically from the source, through the collection works, the transmission and treatment facilities, and finally the distribution system. The analysis should include possible damage to reservoirs and water mains. The effects of power failures, personnel shortages due to lack of transport or injury, and communications difficulties need to be considered.

3.3.4 Assessment of environmental health vulnerability

First, environmental health must be covered in the initial baseline survey of all the hazards and patterns of vulnerability affecting the society. This survey should be organized by geographical region and should also profile the vulnerability of different ethnic and socioeconomic groups. Disparities and priority needs in such areas as water supply, drainage, sanitation, refuse and waste disposal, housing, and food hygiene should be documented. The prevalence of vector-borne and contagious diseases by region and by socioeconomic group should also be integrated into comprehensive risk planning. Finally, the location and safety of industrial facilities in relation to settlements should be reviewed from the point of view of air, soil and water contamination, as well as the risk of radiation, fire, explosion and accidental poisonous emissions.

Such baseline surveys can reveal who is more likely to suffer from an emergency directly related to environmental health as well as where this is most likely to occur. Such emergencies are not randomly distributed in social or spatial terms. For example, the population living near the chemical factory in Bhopal, India and the residents surrounding the Chernobyl, Ukraine and Three Mile Island, USA nuclear reactors were obviously at greater risk than people living further away. In Peru, the densely populated, poor neighbourhoods of the port city of Chimbote and of Lima were more likely to be affected by large numbers of cholera cases than sparsely settled areas in the mountains. Information on the use of survey data to avoid secondary hazards is given in Box 3.1.

3.3.5 Describing communities, their environment and the effects of hazards

The purpose of describing communities is to be able to understand their vulnerability to the hazards identified and mapped, and the likely effects of those hazards. These two factors depend to a great extent on the environment in which the community lives and works. The capacity of communities and local services and organizations to resist and survive disasters is a key determinant of their vulnerability.

Box 3.1 **Using survey data to avoid secondary hazards**

The environmental health baseline survey of hazards and vulnerability provides insight into who and which areas may be affected by secondary environmental health hazards that follow another disaster, such as an earthquake.

For instance, the survey might reveal that a zone of a city has only one water source and that this source is at risk of disruption by an earthquake. It is thus highly likely that residents of this zone could be in danger of water-related diseases or water shortages in the event of an earthquake.

Discussion at community level could then focus on: (1) the possibility of a back-up water supply; (2) strengthening and protecting the existing supply; (3) pre-positioning water tankers in such a way that this high-risk zone is the first to receive emergency water supplies.

Table 3.2 **Principal community characteristics determined in vulnerability analysis**[1]

Demography	Culture	Economy	Infrastructure	Environment
Population and age distribution	Traditions	Trade	Communication networks	Landforms
Mobility	Ethnicity	Agriculture/livestock	Transportation networks	Geology
Useful skills	Social values	Investments	Essential services	Waterways
Hazard awareness	Religion	Industries	Community assets	Climate
Vulnerable groups	Attitudes to hazards	Wealth	Government structures	Flora and fauna
Health level	Normal food types		Resource base	
Education level	Eating habits			
Sex distribution	Power structures			

[1] Source: World Health Organization (1999a).

Table 3.2 Shows the principle community characteristics that determine vulnerability to a given hazard.

Information that describes the community and its environment is gathered in a number of ways, including government and commercial records, maps, academic publications and field studies, which may include surveys, observation and participatory techniques. One important aspect of community assessment is identifying marginalized groups to ensure that their voices are heard and their vulnerabilities and capacities are recognized. These groups are often the most affected by disasters.

Where the community is involved in describing itself for a vulnerability assessment, it is far more likely that participation in planning and emergency preparedness will be successful. A variety of assessment and planning tools may be used for participatory assessment and planning, including rapid rural appraisal, participatory rural appraisal, and participatory learning and action. They differ in important ways, including the degree of participation they enable, and the information, ideas and understanding they produce. Staff carrying out community-based VCA should be familiar with these tools and be able to choose and use the most appropriate one for the context and purpose of their work. For further information on VCA and participatory techniques in vulnerability reduction, see International Federation of Red Cross and Red Crescent Societies (1994) and von Kotze & Holloway (1996).

The information gathered may be mapped, together with information on hazards, to build up a picture of effects and vulnerability. Geographical information systems (GIS) are useful for spatial hazard analysis and mapping. These computer-based information systems allow several types of information from various sources—for instance, the location of settlements and industrial hazards, the contact details for emergency staff, and short-range wind direction forecasts—to be combined and presented to give a complete and up-to-date picture of hazards, their possible effects and response protocols.

3.3.6 Ongoing monitoring of vulnerability

The distribution of hazards and people's vulnerability to them are affected by many economic and political decisions on development projects and investments, urban growth, rural-to-rural migration, and refugee influx, to name only a few. The work of comprehensive vulnerability assessment and reduction can never end. The possible impact on vulnerability of all such policy and project decisions should be monitored. Such vigilance should be the responsibility of national, regional and local emergency-management agencies. Project planners, urban designers and other professionals should systematically include vulnerability analysis in their routine work.

3.3.7 Environmental health review of development policies and projects

Human health has an important place in the environmental impact assessment of policies, plans and project proposals. Environmental health surveillance can contribute to the analysis of change by keeping track of the shifting spatial and seasonal patterns of human population in relation to disease vector habitats and industrial pollutant sources.

The provision of water, drainage, sanitation and other services often lags behind the spontaneous creation of new settlements (e.g. around new mines, forest settlements and logging camps, and refugee facilities). Timely identification of the hazards facing the populations of such settlements and possible measures for dealing with them should also be the work of environmental health personnel working in collaboration with the emergency agency.

For more complete information on hazard identification, community description, and hazard prioritization, see World Health Organization (1999a).

3.4 Prevention and mitigation

3.4.1 Reducing community vulnerability through long-term environmental health improvements

In poorer rural and urban areas of many countries, improvements in water supply and sanitation systems are connected with vulnerability reduction in several ways. First, they reduce the risk of epidemics of diseases such as cholera. Second, they improve the general health status of the population, making people more resilient when they have to face the additional stress of disasters. Third, water and sanitation projects organized on a self-help basis often strengthen cooperation within communities that can be used as the basis of other vulnerability-reduction activities, e.g. the community-based organizations responsible for water improvements may become the core of a community safety committee.

An additional degree of safety can be provided if those responsible for local water or sanitation initiatives are aware of hazards and engage in a discussion of vulnerability with community members as a routine part of planning new works. Many of the same problems arise as those faced by planners of large-scale water-supply systems, including watershed protection and alternative water sources for emergencies.

Traditional means of water purification and traditional rules for segregating water uses (stock watering, bathing, drinking) may assist in reducing vulnerability. They can often provide the key to low-cost improvements and the basis for local level emergency planning.

On-going public education in household water treatment (filtration, chlorination, boiling, storage, etc.), oral rehydration therapy, breastfeeding, food hygiene, hand-washing, the use of latrines, waste disposal, drainage and vermin control will all strengthen the community before any emergencies occur and also play an important role in an emergency.

In unplanned, unserved or underserved urban neighbourhoods, refuse and waste management is also important, as is storm drainage. Such activities provide opportunities for self-help, especially in communities where money and labour are in short supply because of the struggle to make ends meet. Environmental health staff may assist by providing technical advice or preparing and promoting proposals for improvement.

Where water is provided by water vendors, it is important to identify the source of this water and to determine how vulnerable to damage or contamination it is. Where possible, community discussions with water vendors about their own plans in the event of an emergency can considerably reduce vulnerability.

Where a nearby industrial plant contaminates an urban neighbourhood or poses a risk of accidents, an even more difficult process of negotiation will be necessary. Intervention by the municipal authorities or other legally authorized governmental bodies is then necessary. Data collected by environmental health personnel can be vital to the successful resolution of such a conflict of interests.

3.4.2 Environmental safety regulations

Legal and administrative controls can play a significant part in reducing environmental health risks during some emergencies. For example, regulations specifying the conditions under which hazardous materials must be transported and stored can include some provisions governing protection from disasters. This can sometimes reduce the risk of uncontrolled discharges during a sudden large-scale emergency. Environmental quality and industrial safety rules are very important in this regard. However, without adequate inspection and vigorous enforcement, their effectiveness will be reduced.

The international transportation of toxic wastes and the relocation of polluting industries from industrial to developing countries may present great hazards, and some countries can ill afford to pay for industrial and environmental health inspection.

Zoning and land-use planning are another area where rules and regulations can dramatically reduce risks. However, these are difficult to enforce where poor people have no choice about where to live or how to earn a living. Related, but more specialized regulations govern the location and/or design of essential facilities, such as schools and hospitals.

Building codes, such as wind-loading codes or earthquake-resistant standards for new buildings, have been very effective in reducing the loss of life and property in extreme events. For example, in Darwin, Australia, the 1974 tropical cyclone destroyed only 3% of buildings engineered to wind-resistant codes, as opposed to 50–60% of non-code constructions (Smith, 1992).

3.4.3 Reducing the vulnerability of environmental health infrastructure

Vulnerability may be reduced through the location, design and maintenance of environmental health infrastructures. Hazard mapping may reveal quite straightforward risks, e.g. a water-treatment plant sited in a flood plain, on an earthquake fault, or next to a chemical facility, and may be used to identify priority locations for hazard-mitigation measures, such as flood-control dykes and avalanche-deflection walls. However, the decision concerning the appropriate action to take in such cases may not be equally straightforward. Decision criteria may include the cost of relocating or protecting the facility and the risk that damage to sewage-treatment plants will pose a threat to health.

For further information on the protection of health facilities, see Pan American Health Organization (1993).

3.4.4 Protecting other facilities

Laboratories should be protected from disasters so that they are immediately available during relief and recovery activities for testing water, soil and other materials for contamination, and for the analysis of biological samples as part of epidemiological surveillance. Although priorities for protection should include water-supply systems, waste-treatment plants and laboratories, other installations are by no means unimportant.

Adequate storm drains can contribute to flood mitigation. If they are blocked by landslides or other disasters, they should be repaired so that flooding does not occur as a secondary hazard. Sanitary landfills and facilities for waste storage, collection and disposal can produce significant secondary hazards if they are flooded or burned during a disaster, or if they are so unstable and improperly sited that they contribute to a mass debris flow. The water supplies and sanitary facilities of hospitals and health centres should be examined for possible weaknesses in emergencies. Cost-effective ways of strengthening them may exist. Part of the general hospital or health-centre plan, to which environmental health managers should contribute, should be the provision of alternative arrangements for water, power and heat if centrally supplied services are interrupted.

One example of international support for such a review of infrastructure for vulnerability reduction is UNESCO's Educational Buildings Programme. This has helped to develop prototypes for, among others, schools resistant to earthquakes (in Armenia and Nepal), schools resistant to severe tropical storms (in Costa Rica and Viet Nam) and schools on stilts to avoid flooding (in Bangladesh and Sri Lanka).

3.5 Preparedness and planning

3.5.1 The national emergency planning process

This section is concerned with planning to respond to disasters, rather than planning to mitigate or prevent them.

The overall context of environmental health planning is the national health policy on emergencies. See Section 3.2 on policy development. Annex 1 provides an overview of a national emergency planning process. Plans developed at each level should relate to plans at other levels, to produce a hierarchy of coordinated plans from national to local levels. This is illustrated in Figure 3.2.

In addition to participating in overall health, water supply, and sanitation sector planning for emergencies, those in charge of water-supply and waste-disposal systems should also be responsible for the planning process within their own facilities. Each water-supply and waste-disposal institution in a country (or district) should carry out a review of its resources (both human and material), and of the vulnerability of the components of its system to various hazards, and prepare plans for temporary repairs.

In the case of emergency shelters and temporary settlements, alternative planning options at the national/regional level will be based on scenarios for a variety of situations and involving different numbers of shelters and settlements, their locations, the numbers of people accommodated, and the resources available and required. There should also be a well-understood and agreed method of assessing people's immediate environmental health needs and for satisfying them with whatever resources are available. For more information on assessments, see Chapter 4.

All agencies dealing with environmental health should know before an emergency occurs how the following tasks are to be carried out:

— liaison with other health departments/organizations and with the appropriate emergency coordinating body;

Figure 3.2 **The hierarchy of disaster-management plans**

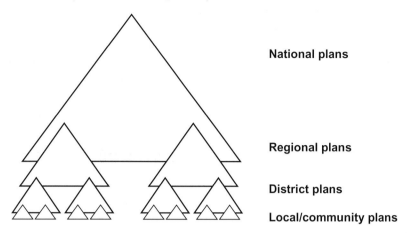

National plans

Regional plans

District plans

Local/community plans

— the evaluation of immediate public health conditions and risks;

— the evaluation of damage to public sanitary installations and the provision of advice on remedial measures;

— the evaluation of shelter and food needs;

— the mobilization of personnel and equipment;

— emergency action to control or eliminate environmental health hazards (often secondary to the immediate hazard);

— the emergency restoration of water-supply and waste-disposal systems, etc.;

— reporting on conditions and on the measures taken.

With the aid of a plan that provides guidance on these points, environmental health staff in an area should be able to provide information on the following:

— the location and magnitude of known damage;

— any structural or functional damage to water-supply and waste-disposal systems, etc.;

— the size and location of populations with inadequate water, shelter, and sanitary facilities;

— the repair resources available;

— estimates of repair times;

— estimates of special needs for environmental health at hospitals and other institutions;

— local capacity for disaster response.

3.5.2 A general model for disaster-preparedness planning

National, regional, district, and local emergency plans share many general characteristics so that the sequence of planning steps shown below will apply to all of them.

1. *Identify the hazards and estimate their effects*
   This is the process of vulnerability assessment, as described in Section 3.3.1.

2. *Assess the likely needs*
   This involves making a preliminary list of everything that will have to be done before, during and after the emergency. It may be helpful to assess needs in terms of percentages, e.g. $X\%$ of the people affected will need assistance with shelter, $Z\%$ will have to be provided with food, etc. This assessment should be done by considering local capacity and the extent to which additional external resources will be required to respond to unmet needs. Where several types of emergency

are expected, estimates should be tabulated to compare probable needs. The different types of needs should then be quantified, according to likely numbers of people affected. The main types of need to consider are early warning, clothing, health care, evacuation, food, sanitation, shelter and water.

3. *Discuss the needs*

   This step involves including as many people as possible in the planning process. They are likely to think of things which may have been overlooked (e.g. specific cultural factors) and make constructive suggestions for improvements.

4. *Determine the operational procedures and review existing priorities* (see step 9)

   This step provides the framework for emergency operations. When planning for a range of emergencies, hazards should be prioritized, so that initial planning is concentrated on the most serious potential emergencies. The fundamental policies on which the plan is based should be set out, e.g. minimizing the effects of the emergency; public participation in the planning process; self-reliance; adequate treatment of all victims; phasing out; planning principles which should be highlighted; and the overall framework of the plan. Goals should be set and approved by the highest appropriate authority; this will help to provide a stable management environment when an emergency occurs. Responsibility should be delegated wherever possible, to give maximum scope for individual initiative. A plan that seeks to control everybody and everything from one central point is a poor one and will almost certainly fail.

5. *Assign the responsibilities*

   The pattern of responsibilities will have started to emerge during the previous steps. This is the time to clarify them so that everybody is clear about who is responsible for what. They can then prepare their own plans to meet their respective responsibilities. To facilitate coordination, all individuals should be encouraged to work out how to do their jobs, drawing on their own initiative and special expertise, and to discuss their intentions beforehand.

   A useful tool for defining roles and responsibilities for planning and action is stakeholder analysis. This is a participatory process that aims to:
   — identify and define the characteristics of key stakeholders;
   — assess the manner in which they might affect or be affected by the programme/project outcome;
   — understand the relations between stakeholders, including an assessment of the real or potential conflicts of interest and expectation between stakeholders;
   — assess the capacity of different stakeholders to participate.

   For further information on stakeholder analysis, see DfID (1995).

Box 3.2 Responsibility for environmental health in disasters and emergencies

There is seldom a single environmental health manager responsible for emergency planning. In most countries, particularly in urban areas, numerous local government bodies and private enterprises are responsible for environmental health infrastructure and services, with little coordination between them.

It is not only professional sanitary engineers and public health workers who must be involved in emergency planning. All community health, humanitarian and development workers should be part of the planning process, together with community representatives. Focal points for emergency planning should be clearly defined, but should not necessarily be the local authorities.

6. *Make an inventory of local capacity and available resources*

Few jobs will be completely self-contained and resources will have to be shared. All common resources needed for an emergency response, including human resources, materials, transport, special equipment (e.g. earth-moving, water-purification) and money should be listed in the inventory. Local capacity should be included in this inventory.

7. *Review steps 2–5*

This is the time to compare needs with resources and to create reserves. It is usually helpful to tabulate. Shifts and rest periods should be taken into account in human resources planning.

8. *Identify critical areas*

These are the areas where potential responses will be subjected to the greatest strain and which need strengthening beforehand. They are also the areas which need monitoring most closely when the plan is implemented.

9. *Confirm priorities*

The priorities identified in Step 4 and discussed in subsequent steps need to be confirmed in the light of an understanding of both needs and resources. Priorities can change with time.

10. *Finalize the plan*

A rigid format is not essential. What matters most is that the plan should be easy to read, though where more than one plan is required it will obviously be helpful if there is a standard layout. A suggested simple format is:

- *Situation.* A brief description of the hazard, its likely effects, the needs arising from it and the planning assumptions.
- *Aim.* A clear and concise statement of the aim of the plan.
- *Concept of operations.* A brief description of the overall policies, framework and goals of the plan.
- *Allocation of responsibilities.* A clarification and assignment of roles and tasks (as determined in Step 4).
- *Coordination.* Reporting procedures, channels of communication and arrangements for establishing and effecting appropriate coordination.
- *Annexes.* The main part of the plan should be as simple as possible. Details can be given in annexes, including diagrams showing coordination procedures and supporting plans prepared by individual departments to meet their respective responsibilities.

It may be helpful to write parts of the plan in the form of:

- *Standing operating procedures.* These are routine procedures to be followed in certain circumstances, such as for the handling of warnings, or the procedures to be used in emergency operations centres during an operation.
- *Standing orders* containing long-term organizational and administrative details.
- *Checklists and emergency operating procedures.* These may make the total plan more bulky, but it will not be necessary for everybody to read the whole plan; what they need to know is how they fit into the overall concept and the details of those parts of the plan which are directly applicable to them. Supporting plans should stand on their own. All paragraphs should be numbered for easy reference.

11. *Practise the plan*

The planning process is in itself a very valuable learning experience. As time passes, however, familiarity with the problem and the plan will fade. Plans should therefore be reviewed, updated and practised regularly so that the people who will be responsible for implementing them are brought up to date. Simulations can help to identify weaknesses in plans, which can then be remedied before the event. It is probably better to republish a whole plan than attempt to issue amendments.

12. *Evaluate the plan*

If an emergency occurs and the plan is implemented, the effectiveness of its implementation should be evaluated so that lessons can be learnt and applied.

The planning process is a valuable learning experience that should be used to develop the skills of individuals and organizations (see Chapter 16 for further information on human resources development).

For further information on planning methods, see Pan American Health Organization (1982, 1983); Carter (1991); Natural Disasters Organization (1992); and World Health Organization (1999a).

3.5.3 Strategic plans and operational plans

Strategic plans are essential to ensure that disaster prevention and emergency preparedness take place within the overall framework of the disaster-management cycle. They also enable monitoring of governmental and private-sector policies and activities to encourage them to take long-term vulnerability into account.

Operational plans are specific plans prepared for dealing with future events that may be uncertain in timing, magnitude, location and effects. In such plans, therefore, the emphasis is on preparedness for response. They may include measures such as establishing communications and management information systems; stockpiling or identifying materials and equipment; identifying routes and sites for evacuation; or identifying and notifying personnel so that the emergency response may be rapid and effective. It is essential that operational plans are practised and revised, to ensure they remain appropriate to the hazards identified. Practising operational plans is a useful training exercise (see Chapter 16).

3.5.4 Participatory methods in planning

Participatory planning must involve people from the start of the planning process. It is not enough simply to ask them for their opinion of a plan that has already been drawn up. This means listening to people in the communities concerned with disaster management plans. This is not always easy because planners and people in the community often have different priorities and perceptions. For example, an environmental planner may think that improving drainage in an informal urban settlement is most important, while the residents of this poor neighbourhood may view the prevention of crime or malnutrition as more urgent. Drainage, or at least the health problems and possible flood risk produced by poor drainage, is probably one of the priorities of residents as well, but not the first priority. A flexible and community-responsive planning process will sooner or later have to consider drainage, but will reach that point in a roundabout way. The

---

Box 3.3 Community risk assessment: a powerful training tool

Representatives of a small town, urban neighbourhood or rural community are invited to join planners in the visual inspection of the area that they inhabit. Existing hazards and vulnerabilities are discussed. A highly localized risk analysis is produced in this way, and local participants also discuss the appropriate response to those risks. Past disasters are recalled. Lessons of other people's experience are discussed. In this way, the locality studies itself. A core group of knowledgeable and motivated volunteers is developed, who can help to train others in the community, possibly on a paid basis.

best starting point for locally-based strategic emergency planning in this case might be a neighbourhood proposal for street lighting (as a means of reducing crime) or for a community garden to be created in vacant land (as a means of reducing malnutrition). Once the residents' priorities are recognized and they feel more in control of their environment, there will probably be greater public support for improving drainage.

Beginning with the priorities and perceptions of the community, good will and the credibility of the planning process can be established. The neighbourhood group developed around these initial projects can then turn its attention to other issues including hazard reduction and emergency preparedness. Once a neighbourhood or community group has been established, it can play an active part in both disaster prevention/mitigation and emergency preparedness.

The same group of participatory techniques used for vulnerability assessment can be used for community-based planning for emergencies. See Section 3.3.5.

3.6 Institutional learning and memory

One of the keys to improving emergency preparedness is the ability of organizations and individuals to learn from previous disasters and to incorporate that learning into practice. However, many of the lessons are *not* learned, mainly for two reasons.

First, staff turnover in government at all levels is such that some staff may never experience certain types of disasters. Elections and other changes in government reinforce the effect of retirement and transfer and disrupt the continuity of administrative experience. Second, there is often a desire to re-establish the "normal" state of affairs as soon as possible after an emergency. Even when institutional changes that would prevent future disasters are clearly needed, these can be overlooked in the rush to re-establish "normality". Nevertheless, there are things that can be done to ensure that lessons are learned.

3.6.1 Evaluation of emergencies and disasters

It may be possible to make the periodic review of emergencies and disasters a governmental responsibility, to ensure that experience is shared with the various ministries concerned and to keep politicians and legislators up to date with current hazards and preparedness measures. It must be emphasized that whatever the institutional form that this body takes, it must have support at the highest level or the institutional memory of disasters can still be lost in the "noise" of competing bodies (such as those concerned with economic growth, national security, etc.).

One way to ensure that the evaluation lessons become included in practice is to integrate national experience into professional training curricula.

3.6.2 Vulnerability analysis of major projects

A related, but broader, challenge is to institutionalize the thorough appraisal of past and present investment policies as they affect vulnerability to hazards. Sometimes, where a major project requires large-scale population resettlement, there is some public assessment of the effects of such resettlement on health and livelihood. Often these effects are not mentioned in the public record or have been defined as "external" to the financial calculation justifying the investment. Some major projects have effects on vulnerability that are of long duration, and those employed in them should be considered more vulnerable to hazards and included in the high-vulnerability category, at least until investigations prove the contrary. The records kept should include a detailed account of how such large-scale changes in the landscape came to be made, what the expected benefits were, and what the present consequences are.

3.6.3 Using rules and regulations concerning environmental health and hazards

The institutional memory of disasters can also take the form of the body of rules and regulations that have grown up in response to known hazards. Environmental health activities normally take place within a comprehensive framework of rules and regulations. Usually, this framework has grown out of years of experience and analysis, and contributes substantially to public safety.

The activities of environmental health staff will often be defined by regulations that indicate the types of monitoring they must perform, the levels of service expected, and the actions to be carried out when specific problems are identified.

The health and safety of environmental health staff themselves is also being given increasing emphasis in many countries, as well as the safety of the public when environmental health activities are being carried out. For example, the safe storage and use of chemicals employed in vector control are governed in most countries by legal provisions or administrative regulations.

3.7 Warning indicators

3.7.1 Early warnings

An extremely important component of preparedness, prevention and mitigation is the capacity to obtain and use early warnings of impending hazards or threats. There are limitations and obstacles to the timely forecast of extreme events, however, and a number of factors can also limit the effectiveness of warnings in influencing public behaviour (see Box 3.4). Both sets of constraints must be borne in mind by environmental health managers.

Warning systems vary greatly, as does the amount of forewarning that they give. Warnings must give sufficient time to enable environmental health preparedness and prevention activities to be carried out.

3.7.2 Slow-onset hazards

In the case of slow-onset hazards, such as drought and certain outbreaks of plant, animal and human disease, there is often a long warning time. Meteorological services are increasingly capable of reliable forecasts of climate patterns several months to one year in advance. The 1997–1998 El Niño event, which affected climatic conditions worldwide from June 1997 until April 1998, was predicted in early 1997. However, lacking specific thresholds or marker events, authorities often wait until the process is far advanced before action is taken.

Box 3.4 **Risk perception**

The perception of risk is not universally the same. It can vary from culture to culture, by socioeconomic class and even by individual. For example, many farmers live on the slopes of active volcanoes or in the flood plains of rivers because they perceive the balance of benefits to risks as favourable. However, some risks are not consciously chosen, but simply thrust upon people because information is not made available and there is no public discussion. In other cases, people may be aware of risks, but believe that they have no alternatives to their present behaviour. For example, the urban poor may live on steep slopes prone to landslides during heavy rain or in ravines prone to collapse during earthquakes, but may believe that they have nowhere else to live. It is especially important in complex societies containing many cultures and socioeconomic interests to ensure that a thorough discussion of risks by representatives of all groups is an integral part of the counter-disaster planning process.

Environmental health indicators, in combination with routine activities carried out by veterinarians, nutritionists and epidemiologists, can be used to provide early warnings of some of these slow-onset hazards. Some African countries have systems for early warning of famine, which are linked to nutrition surveillance. In Botswana, for example, monthly returns from weighing and measuring children in well-baby clinics are automatically screened for anomalies. These data, together with crop and livestock data, are used to trigger a variety of timely drought-response measures, including supplementary feeding, public works as a form of income supplement and the exemption of affected families from paying taxes (Walker, 1989).

3.7.3 Hazards with moderate warning time

A number of hazards have an intermediate range of warning times. Those responsible for environmental health should be among the first to be informed by the authority issuing the alert or provisional warning, in advance of any public announcement. An effective communication system should be established and the readiness of supplies, equipment, transport, communications and personnel should be confirmed.

There may also be specific actions that managers can take to increase the level of protection of vital facilities or to prepare for possible evacuation. For instance, a volcanic eruption can usually be foreseen by a few days, if not as long as a few weeks or even months in advance, and the affected population can be evacuated in good time. Ash fall from volcanoes can contaminate and clog water-storage facilities and treatment plants and, with sufficient warning, steps can be taken to protect water supplies from this hazard.

Heavy snowfalls can be forecast with moderate accuracy a few days in advance. If access to isolated areas is likely to be difficult, managers can confirm that the local environmental health services are well supplied with spare parts, chemicals, etc.

Slope stability studies can signal an acute risk of avalanches or mudslides as a result of predicted heavy rain. Fairly straightforward models can then provide at least several days' warning. Such hazards can destroy or harm vital facilities that have not yet been moved to safer sites following a review of location. Steps may have to be taken to evacuate these facilities and confirm the readiness of back-up facilities.

Many meteorological hazards have warning times measured in hours or days. Flash floods in semi-arid and arid watersheds are perhaps the most sudden form of meteorology-related hazard. Other river flooding takes place more slowly; where there is a dense hydrographic network of stream gauges connected by telemetry, models allow quite reliable flood warnings to be given many hours in advance. Following a flood warning, standing orders for low-lying facilities, such as water- and sewage-treatment plants, should be implemented (e.g. removal of vital records to upper stories, protection of electrical equipment, sand-bagging of entrances, etc.). A careful review of the area most likely to be affected by the flood may reveal the existence of a population in danger of being cut off. If so, efforts should be made to pre-position water tankers on higher ground in the area concerned.

Cyclones can be detected by weather satellites in the form of small cells several days in advance of landfall. However, the communication of this information has been problematic. First, cyclones can change their course unpredictably. In 1977, the landfall of the storm that devastated the Indian state of Andhra Pradesh was not in the area expected, even though the storm itself had been tracked for days. Second, a warning system may not be understood or believed by the people at risk. See Section 4.2.1.

3.7.4 Warning of industrial accidents

Advance warnings of large-scale accidents in industry, transportation, etc., are limited by the nature of the events concerned. For example, in Bhopal, India, there was no advance warning of the cloud of methyl cyanide that descended on the residents. In the case of the explosions in the sewer system of Mexico's second largest city, Guadalajara, in 1992, citizens had been complaining for several days to the authorities about the smell of petrol.

Frequent inspections of high-risk factories and, for example, bridges and dams can reveal structural weaknesses. There is often reluctance to shut down key facilities, however, because of the costs involved and, in some cases, a misplaced reliance on a tendency to overdesign. Environmental health workers often have a role to play in the inspection of potentially hazardous industrial plants and in liasing between the factory management and the public.

3.7.5 Warning of refugee movements

Civil unrest or war in one country should alert the relevant authorities of neighbouring countries that an influx of refugees is possible. Several weeks' or even months' warning may be provided. Arrangements can then be made to receive and accommodate refugees, especially where there has been a prior history of cross-border movements and where food, medical supplies, blankets and tents or tarpaulins have been stockpiled (United Nations High Commissioner for Refugees, 1999).

If any generalization is possible about the full range of warning systems, it would be that social and political receptivity to warnings lags behind the technology that provides them. Often the warning messages are passed from one government agency to another without ever being transmitted to the population who need them. It is also fair to say that community participation in warning systems has not been adequately fostered. In addition, existing national warning systems often involve the provision of information by a variety of government departments or even by nongovernmental agencies, other countries (in the case of international river systems and refugee movements), or international agencies (especially regarding weather forecasting and famine early warnings). Integration of this information in a timely and concise way is vital if the decision to issue a warning is to be effective.

3.8 Further information

For further-information on:

- health assessment of projects and investments, see: Lee (1985), Birley (1991, 1992, 1995);
- urban development and health, see: World Health Organization (1987a), Hardoy & Satterthwaite (1989), Tabibzadeh, Rossi-Espagnet & Maxwell (1989), World Health Organization (1991a), Bradley et al. (1992), World Health Organization (1992b), International Institute for Environment and Development (1993), Satterthwaite et al. (1996), United Nations Commission on Human Settlements (1996);
- rapid appraisal in health planning, see: White (1981), Werner & Bower (1982), Annett & Rifkin (1989), Organisation Mondiale de la Santé (1989), Scrimshaw & Hurtado (1989), Manderson, Valencia & Thomas (1992), von Kotze & Holloway (1996);
- rapid appraisal in environmental management, see: Hope & Timmek (1987), Raintree (1987), Chambers, Pacey & Thrupp (1989), Cullis & Pacey (1992), Hiemstra, Reijntjes & van der Werf (1992), and Kumar (1993);

— hazard mapping, see: Foster (1980), United Nations Office of the Disaster Relief Co-ordinator (1991), Smith (1992), Collins (1993), de Lepper, Scholten & Stern (1995), Waugh (1995);
— community emergency preparedness, see: World Health Organization (1999a);
— warning systems, see: United Nations Office of the Disaster Relief Co-ordinator (1984), Drabek (1986), United Nations Office of the Disaster Relief Co-ordinator (1986), Walker (1989), Dymon & Winter (1993).

4. Emergency response

Emergency response is the phase of the disaster-management cycle that often attracts the most attention and resources. During this phase, environmental health services may have a great impact on the health and well-being of affected communities. However, the impact achieved in the early days of the response is largely a test of previously-planned local and national preparedness and mitigation measures. Moreover, the way the emergency response has been planned and the way the emergency is managed will have a significant influence on post-disaster recovery and future development possibilities. The emergency response phase should therefore be seen as a critical part of the disaster-management cycle.

Emergency response is sometimes a cyclical process, involving repeated assessment, planning, action and review, to respond appropriately to needs and capacities as they evolve. It starts with an initial assessment and may be triggered spontaneously by the disaster event, or officials may authorize the mobilization of people and resources. Rapid and effective mobilization is facilitated by proper disaster preparedness.

4.1 Assessments

Following a disaster, rapid and effective action is needed to save lives, protect health and stabilize the situation, to avoid making the emergency worse. But even in an acute emergency, an assessment, however brief, is needed to ensure that any action undertaken is effective. This section deals primarily with two types of assessment: rapid initial assessments to establish the nature and scale of the emergency and the likely need for external assistance; and detailed sector assessments to plan, implement and coordinate a response. Other types of assessment are required at various stages of the response, such as continual assessment (i.e. monitoring or surveillance) and assessments for postemergency rehabilitation.

In acute emergencies, initial assessments should be rapid and produce the information required to start an appropriate response. In less acute emergencies, or once an acute situation has stabilized somewhat, a more detailed assessment is needed to design longer-term measures with adequate provision for monitoring and management. More thorough assessments are needed for recovery and resettlement programmes. Whatever form the assessment takes, it is essential that information is collected and rapidly transmitted in a way that makes it clear what actions should be taken and why.

4.1.1 Purpose of emergency assessments

Emergency assessments should allow the following (Adams, 1999):

— an initial decision to be made on whether assistance is needed;
— a decision to be made on whether local capacity is adequate or external resources are required;
— priorities for intervention to be established and an intervention strategy identified;

— necessary resources to be identified;
— base-line data to be collected, to facilitate monitoring;
— information to be collected for fund-raising and advocacy work.

4.1.2 Process of assessments

It is important to use standardized processes and standard report formats for assessments, to ensure objectivity and to enable the humanitarian response to be made in proportion to the needs identified. Assessment questions should be considered before field work, and information recorded in a way that can be understood by decision-makers who may not visit the disaster area. When several teams assess different geographic areas their findings can be compared and resources directed to where they are most needed. Training on assessment techniques is an important element of emergency preparedness for environmental health services.

Checklists can be a useful way to ensure that assessments are thorough and that no important issues are missed. Checklists may be found in a number of publications, including: International Federation of Red Cross and Red Crescent Societies (1997a); Sphere Project (2000); United Nations High Commissioner for Refugees (1999); and United States Agency for International Development (1988). Checklists should be used with common sense and good judgement to ensure that each emergency is assessed according to its specific characteristics.

Assessments often begin with a brief review of information about the area and the population affected, the type of disaster and the environmental health infrastructure that may have been affected. Accurate information on disasters such as floods may be rapidly available from satellite images of the affected area. When combined with preliminary information from the disaster area, this can provide a rapid overview of the situation and an indication of likely damage and needs. In some cases, it may be possible to start organizing an initial response on the basis of this second-hand information.

Field-based assessments allow preliminary information to be confirmed and the details necessary for organizing specific relief to be gathered. The process may start with an aerial view of the disaster area, or an overview from a high point on a hill or tall building. For assessment staff from outside the affected area, discussions with local colleagues may provide a similar overall picture of the situation, which allows field assessment work to concentrate on areas of most pressing need. Information available might include health data; approximate figures on the number of people affected, displaced, killed and injured; the number of houses and other buildings destroyed; and the major impact of the disaster on water supplies and sanitation.

It is most important to work with local partners and government agencies to ensure that assessments seek to find information that is not already available and that information gathered is shared with interested parties. Assessments should be coordinated, and new staff arriving in a disaster-affected area should contact whatever body has been established to coordinate the emergency response before carrying out field assessments.

4.1.3 Field assessment techniques

First-hand information may be gathered in the field using a variety of techniques, including the following:

— on-site visual assessment, with both structured and nonstructured observation techniques (e.g. a health observation walk);
— expert measurement and testing (e.g. water quality testing, or diagnosis of mechanical failure of a pump);
— surveys, to provide statistically valid information from a sample of the population;

— interviews with key informants, community leaders, groups of disaster-affected people, focus groups or household members;

— participatory techniques, such as ranking or diagramming, to gain a rapid understanding of the way the disaster has affected different parts of the population and what peoples' own assessment of the situation and options for response might be.

Whichever assessment techniques are used, they should be adapted to the urgency of the situation and the degree of detail and accuracy needed to mount an appropriate response.

There is growing acceptance that disaster survivors themselves should be partners in the relief process. Relief is far better done *with* people, rather than for them. For the most part, a disaster-affected population will take action itself. Professional health staff need to take into account existing coping mechanisms used by groups of survivors and be willing to reinforce any spontaneous activity that appears to be appropriate. It is vital also to explore the survivors' own perceptions of their needs, which may differ from the views of those providing help. This is an important complement to more formal systems of "needs assessment" (Campbell & Chung, 1986; Pan American Health Organization, 1987). Effective intervention is almost always characterized by consultation and by efforts to empower those for whom help is intended.

4.1.4 Organizing an emergency assessment

A field assessment, particularly following a large-scale disaster, requires organization, resources and management in the same way as any other professional activity. Where teams of people are required, they need to be mobilized, briefed and often trained before starting the assessment. Environmental health staff may often carry out assessments in teams with specialists in related professions, such as engineering, health and social welfare, from other government departments or organizations. In such cases, close coordination is needed between different institutions and a clear management and reporting structure should be established. Assessment teams need to be given clear terms of reference and be aware of the type of information and recommendations that are expected from their work.

Staff carrying out assessments may also carry out initial relief activities simultaneously. For instance, a team visiting an isolated water treatment works may carry with them spare parts, fuel or treatment chemicals. However, a sensible balance must be found between the need to act quickly and the need to gather sufficient information to ensure that action is effective and appropriate. It is usually more effective to concentrate on assessment activities that enable an appropriate and substantial response to be launched than to spend time on initial relief activities, even when this sometimes means not responding to obvious needs during assessment work.

The provision of material and other support to assessment teams is discussed in section 4.5. Further details on technical assessments are provided in the relevant chapters in Part II.

4.2 Evacuation

Evacuation can be an important component of prevention, preparedness and response. It involves the temporary transfer of a population (and to a limited extent, property) from areas at risk of disaster to a safer location. Environmental health staff are involved in ensuring that evacuations do not create health hazards.

4.2.1 Disaster warnings and emergency instructions

The following points should be borne in mind when designing and implementing disaster warnings and instructions for public evacuations or other emergency measures (adapted from Walker, 1989):

— language used should be simple and non-technical;
— if different warning systems are used, they should not give conflicting messages, or people will tend to ignore them;
— messages should state clearly the exact nature of the impending threat and its implications for the target population;
— the potential victims of a disaster should be clearly identified.

Even if the warning creates awareness of an impending disaster, people may fail to react, and it is likely that environmental health workers will be part of a broad effort to persuade the population that the warning must be taken seriously.

Radio broadcasting is likely to be restored relatively quickly and should be used to the fullest extent. Reliable information will enable the survivors to understand the situation, how the problems are being addressed, and what steps they should take to ensure their safety and the success of the relief operation.

4.2.2 Organized evacuation

Organized, pre-impact evacuation is commonly carried out on a massive scale in some countries in response to warnings of tropical storms (e.g. in India and the USA). Various forms of evacuation may be organized as a precautionary measure in response to the threat of air attack or other military action.

Organized post-impact evacuation may also occur in response to industrial accidents and after earthquakes (e.g. in the severe winter conditions following the Armenian earthquake of December 1988). Officially supported and comprehensively organized population relocation has also occurred extensively after volcanic eruptions.

4.2.3 Spontaneous evacuation

Spontaneous pre-impact evacuation commonly occurs in response to a perceived threat, such as tropical storms, volcanic eruptions, droughts, floods and chemical or nuclear accidents. Military operations can also set off massive migrations. Communities facing severe food shortages may move *en masse* in search of food or income to avoid starvation.

Post-impact spontaneous evacuation occurs in response to the loss of shelter or essential services in an area. In tropical storms and flooding, there is a tendency to move to the periphery of an affected area, especially where some existing services remain, or to higher ground or raised roads, such as happened in Bangladesh and Mozambique. In many emergencies, those relocating will move quickly to stay with friends and relatives, in preference to staying in public facilities (public buildings, schools, stadiums, military camps, etc.).

4.2.4 Environmental health services on evacuation routes

Travel time in evacuations should be kept as short as possible, but where longer journeys are necessary, the support of environmental health personnel is required. People travelling long distances on foot require considerable support to reduce risks to their health.

Clean drinking-water should be provided, preferably at periodic rest stations along the way, at the rate of three litres per person per day in temperate climates, rising to at least six litres per day in hot desert areas. Safe water should also be provided for personal hygiene. Ideally, water should be disinfected with chlorine or another appropriate chemical. If possible, evacuees should be shown how to choose safe water sources. Non-perishable food should also be provided.

At rest stops, excreta and solid wastes should be buried in holes or trenches. These should be at least 60 centimetres deep and, when the contents reach 30 cm from the ground level, should be backfilled with excavated earth and trampled down. Where the evacuation is likely to take several days, the use of temporary toilets should be considered.

Where appropriate, existing facilities such as hotels, schools and offices may be temporarily taken over as evacuation rest stops, and their water supplies and toilets used.

When evacuation is on foot, as is often the case, rest-stops should be provided every two hours' walk, if possible, and evacuees should be given information about road conditions and access to water, food, shelter and medical assistance on the next section of the route.

Special precautions may be needed to protect people living along evacuation routes from possible health risks due to the passage of the evacuees, particularly from defecation on the roadside, which may require clean-up activities.

4.2.5 Environmental health problems associated with evacuations

Any large-scale population movements into an area are of primary concern for environmental health. Such movements involve settlement in marginal conditions, usually away from services. In particular, people are often moved into areas where there are no piped water supplies.

Relocation can result in high population densities, associated with wholly inadequate water supplies and sanitation. There is almost always an increased risk of faecal–oral transmission of diseases related to poor hygiene.

Other risks include contact with pathogens not found in the home area (e.g. the malarial parasite), including those transmitted by vectors unfamiliar to the evacuated population. Generally, the evacuated population will be more susceptible to these diseases than the local population, as occurs in areas endemic for malaria.

The relocation of a population into high-density emergency settlement will usually greatly increase the risk of outbreaks of common childhood diseases. Measles is a particular risk when the population has low immunization coverage. Health conditions and nutritional status before displacement are also important.

Evacuation can also place people in the vicinity of unfamiliar environmental hazards (e.g. dispersal into damaged industrial areas where a range of toxic substances are stored).

4.2.6 Influencing settlement in evacuations

Patterns of settlement can sometimes be closely controlled in organized evacuations. To this end, it is necessary to:

— avoid creating points of high density at any stage of the movement, including at organized transit centres and final destinations;
— deal with potential conflicts in priorities during the planning stage. For example, staff security, logistics and distribution are sometimes facilitated by high-density settlements, but this may be to the detriment of public health;
— ensure that the capacity of the services can meet the demand at all times, particularly at times of peak—not average—predicted flows.

Influencing the patterns of settlement in self-evacuation is much more difficult. The authorities will have to take a number of major decisions:

— when to encourage such movements and when to discourage them;

— whether to risk the concentration of people or to encourage dispersion;

— the choice of site;

— the choice of organizations to provide services.

Attention to managing population flows is crucial, to avoid creating health and security problems. The most serious environmental health problems can occur where population movements are blocked or channelled in such a way that local requirements vastly exceed supplies. A common misconception among decision-makers is that health risks can be controlled by concentrating displaced people. The reverse is true. The health risks of evacuation will generally be exacerbated, rather than controlled, by concentrating people at centres. Dispersal is generally a more effective strategy.

The provision of services of any type tends to attract settlement and is one means of encouraging a population to move into designated areas. Preplanning, in terms of prior identification of temporary settlement points and arrangements for immediate staffing in an emergency, may help staff encourage patterns of settlement that match available water supplies and logistics capacity, and maintain an acceptable balance between settlement size and accessibility.

Where possible, displaced people should be warned of specific risks. For example, in damaged urban areas, a displaced population may be tempted to drink run-off water from a waste site or from a damaged industrial plant.

In some settings, poor relations between host and displaced populations can exacerbate tension and create local security problems. Relations with the host population needs to be carefully considered and local people be involved as much as possible in the choice of potential sites.

4.2.7 Strengthening services in host communities

Whether the evacuation is officially organized or spontaneous, there will be a need to strengthen the environmental health services in the area of influx. Priority may need to be given to locations with:

— very large, dense, underserved settlements;

— settlements with poor public-health indicators and/or with a risk of epidemics;

— settlements without adequate supplies;

— large numbers of people sheltering in large buildings, such as schools, office blocks and warehouses;

— poorly functioning hospitals, clinics and feeding centres;

— substantial numbers of people with special needs, unaccompanied children, the elderly and disabled;

— understaffed and poorly equipped laboratory services.

Good relations with both the host community and the evacuees is essential in gaining cooperation. In addition, lay people with useful skills among both the evacuees and the host population should be encouraged to volunteer their services.

4.2.8 Problems with temporary emergency settlements

The coverage provided by environmental health services in reception areas is likely to be patchy and in some locations it may be difficult for evacuees and staff to cope.

Some of the more difficult problems include:

■ Inappropriate choices of settlement sites. These sites are usually forced settlement sites and the problems include: no reliable water supplies; a high water-table (which complicates sanitation); the risk of flooding; and the presence of disease vectors (particularly malaria mosquitoes). For more details on site selection and planning, see Chapter 6.

■ Random defecation. This is hard to control when populations have no experience of, or access to, latrines.

■ A population that is too frightened, too hostile, or too socially fragmented to collaborate effectively.

■ Extreme difficulties in case-detection and epidemic investigation. This situation can occur because of continual movement of the population, often combined with insecurity. It is particularly difficult to estimate the size of populations when there is extensive movement between centres.

An adequate number of staff accompanying groups of displaced people can be effective in reducing environmental health risks. A balance may have to be struck between using rescue resources to bring essential supplies to large populations *in situ*, and removing relatively small numbers of people from areas at risk elsewhere. Policies for dealing with such situations must be established during the planning stage.

4.3 Environmental health measures in the emergency phase

4.3.1 General objective and activities

The general objective of environmental health measures in the emergency phase may be described in terms of health indicators, particularly the crude mortality rate (see section 2.2.5), and the incidence or prevalence of key environmental health-related diseases. It may also be described using indicators of service provision, e.g. the amount of water available per person per day, or the number of people per functioning toilet. It is important to establish a broadly agreed objective and indicators for immediate actions. This will help to avoid the risk of a grossly uneven or disproportionate response that leaves part or all of the affected population vulnerable for an unnecessarily long time, and to focus efforts where they will produce the greatest and most rapid health benefits.

Overall public health priorities in the emergency phase include ensuring access to food, shelter, health care, water supplies and sanitation facilities, control of communicable disease, and public health surveillance.

Specific environmental health measures in the emergency phase aim to reduce loss of life and protect health by changing the adverse conditions of the physical environment affecting or endangering health. These measures can include the provision of shelter, water supplies, sanitation, vector control and the burial of the dead, as well as measures to protect food, control epidemics and communicable disease, and to limit chemical and radiation hazards.

Priorities in the acute emergency phase include:

— providing facilities for people to excrete safely and hygienically;
— protecting water supplies from contamination;
— providing a minimum amount of water for drinking, cooking and personal and domestic hygiene;
— ensuring that people have enough water containers to collect and store water cleanly;
— ensuring that people have sufficient cooking utensils, equipment and fuel to cook and store food safely;
— ensuring that people have the knowledge and understanding they need to avoid disease;
— ensuring that people have soap for hand washing;

— containing or removing sources of chemical or radiological contamination, or evacuating people, to ensure they are no longer exposed to these hazards.

4.3.2 Priorities for emergency response

It is not possible to define a universally applicable order of priorities for emergency environmental health measures, as each situation demands a specific response. The priorities following a population displacement in southern Africa, where a cholera epidemic is imminent, are likely to be different from the priorities following a tornado in the United States. To make rational decisions about priorities, and to revise those priorities as the situation changes, means that an adequate assessment must be combined with basic environmental health and epidemiological principles.

In practice, several priorities usually need addressing simultaneously, as they are closely related, both epidemiologically and operationally. For instance, containing and disposing of human excreta is an important aspect of protecting water supplies from contamination; providing water collection and storage vessels and increasing water production are both needed to ensure the adequate collection and consumption of water for personal hygiene.

Although the most effective environmental health measure in most emergencies, in terms of public health impact, is ensuring that basic water supplies and facilities for safe excreta disposal are provided to the affected population, serving hospitals and feeding centres may be more urgent in some situations (e.g. when a large number of people have been injured, or a significant proportion of the population depends on mass feeding centres).

Refuse collection and disposal, drainage and vector control are usually lower priorities than water supply and excreta disposal. However, malaria may rapidly become the most important health risk after a disaster, and an environmental and health surveillance system should be established rapidly, to enable a rapid response to a malaria epidemic. Again, priorities differ from situation to situation and change for each emergency as it evolves, so establishing and using epidemiological and environmental surveillance systems is also a high priority.

Support for laboratories, stores and offices used for the emergency response should be provided rapidly, to ensure that assessment, response and monitoring are effective.

Services should be established, or re-established, as rapidly as possible, either through setting up temporary systems, or through the repair and/or temporary modification of existing systems. For more information on this, see the relevant chapters of Section II. The complete repair and reconstruction of services after a major disaster can take years. This book is concerned mainly with the early stages of the emergency repair and recovery of essential facilities for maintaining environmental health.

4.3.3 Hospitals and relief centres

In an emergency, existing centres providing specialized care will probably have already become the focus of organized relief activity. Small numbers of supervisory environmental health staff can often improve conditions greatly by:

— supervising any emergency modifications to water and sewerage systems, including improvising the repair of damage;
— providing emergency facilities for the disposal of wastewater and solid wastes;
— ensuring the destruction or safe disposal of medical wastes (e.g. dressings, syringes, etc.);
— supervising the hygiene of food services;

— supervising arrangements for washing, cleaning and disinfecting facilities, equipment and materials;

— monitoring the water distribution arrangements to ensure equity of access to water.

Where first-aid posts and temporary health facilities are required, the following environmental health considerations should influence their location and organization:

■ First-aid stations should be located in open spaces, but sheltered from intense heat, cold or rain.

■ They should be far enough from potential secondary hazards (fire, explosion, flood, landslide) or the effects of earthquake aftershocks to be safe, but reasonably close to sites where the injured are concentrated, so as to minimize the need for transportation.

■ A safe and adequate water supply, drainage for wastewater, latrines and hand-washing facilities for first-aid workers should be provided.

■ The proper disposal of medical wastes should be organized as soon as possible.

In some places, mobile emergency hospitals along the lines of military field hospitals will be available. The environmental health considerations applicable to these facilities are the same as those listed above.

4.3.4 Environmental health in search and rescue operations

The most effective search and rescue action is usually taken by people in the affected community before national and international teams are mobilized. Training and support can help local people involved in search and rescue work more effectively and safely.

Environmental health staff may find themselves directly involved in local search and rescue activities, and may be required to provide leadership or technical assistance. In addition, environmental health workers are likely to be involved in providing:

— services for hospitals and medical facilities;
— services for emergency operation centres;
— potable water supplies for organized rescue teams;
— assistance in assessing the risks from hazardous materials during rescue activity and information on the location of hazards. In the case of volcanic eruptions, this can include information on ash toxicity and any other effects;
— information about high-occupancy buildings to help in allocating rescue resources;
— advice on emergency water and sanitation for large, isolated and trapped populations;
— advice on handling human and animal corpses;
— direct assistance with the retrieval, transportation and temporary storage of human bodies.

In addition, environmental health services may be able to provide the following support:

— communications equipment to link newly organized rescue teams;
— fuel supplies for generators, and compressed gases for cutting equipment;
— transportation for specialist teams;
— specific equipment, such as power saws, drills, cutting devices, jacks, air bags;
— portable generators for lighting and water supply;
— support facilities for large volunteer teams.

There needs to be a clear policy on the use of limited specialist resources during the relatively disorganized early stage of an emergency. For example, generators, water storage equipment, transportation and tools can quickly become dispersed and lost in an unco-ordinated rescue effort. A record should be kept of where each major item of equipment is taken or used, and who is responsible for it.

4.4 Organization of environmental health activities during emergencies

Organizational arrangements will be specified as part of the planning process described in Chapter 3, with the aim of providing the framework for a common understanding of the roles and responsibilities of all parties, and ensuring a timely flow of information. An example of an organization chart for emergency environmental health activities is shown in Figure 4.1 Table 4.1 shows typical numbers of environmental health personnel needed in an emergency.

4.4.1 The place of environmental health in the organization of emergency activities

It was emphasized in Chapter 3 that environmental health planning for emergencies and disasters takes place in the context of an interlinked set of coordinated planning processes. This is also true of organizational structure. Thus, environmental health activities have their place in the broader health sector organization for emergencies and disasters, while the health sector, in turn, is part of the national sectoral organization for emergency activities. Figure 4.2 provides an illustration of this.

Figure 4.1 **Specimen organization chart for emergency environmental health activities[1]**

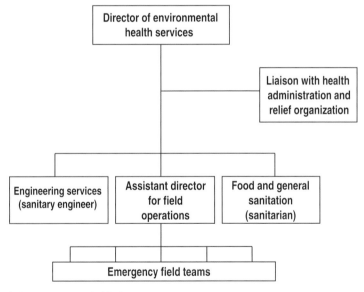

[1] Source: Assar (1971).

Table 4.1 **Numbers of environmental health personnel needed in an emergency[1]**

Population affected	Number of personnel		
	Sanitary engineers	Sanitarians	Auxiliaries
Less than 1000	—	1	1–2
1000–10 000	—	1	2–5
10 000–50 000	1	2	5–10
50 000–100 000	1–2	2–3	10–15
For each additional 100 000	1	2	10

[1] Source: Assar (1971).

Figure 4.2 **Health organization for emergencies and disasters**[1]

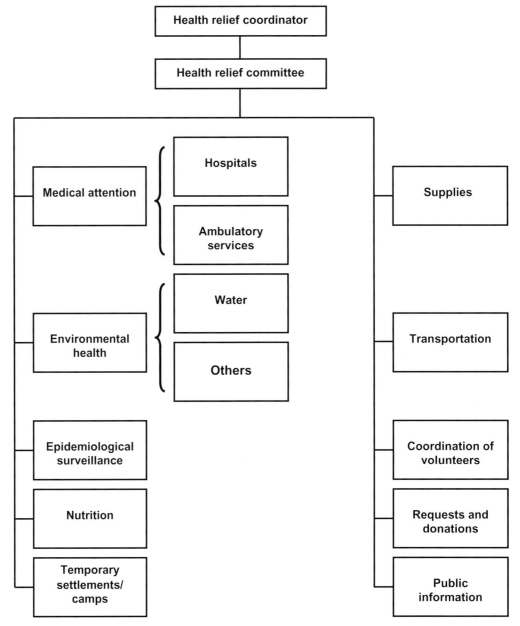

[1] Source: Pan American Health Organization (1981).

Environmental health personnel will liaise and cooperate in many ways with other health workers, Red Cross/Red Crescent society staff and other community workers. For example, environmental health staff are likely to be stationed in large shelters, reception stations, short-term camps, and longer-term settlements for displaced people and refugees. In addition, they are also likely to be required in hospitals and health centres to repair or manage any water and sanitation installations on site, and advise on measures to maintain environmental health quality when facilities are used by very large numbers of people. This is all the more important because of the tendency for health-care centres to become gathering points for survivors.

4.4.2 Emergency field teams for assessment and initial response

Following a rapid initial assessment that may have identified general environmental health problems, small, mobile emergency teams should be created, coordinated by a field supervisor. These teams should be responsible for assessing environmental health needs; liaising with local health workers; identifying needs for priority water supplies; sanitation; vector control; and surveillance in specific operational areas. Each team should have its own transportation, communications, and supplies for subsistence and professional activities in the disaster-affected area. These resources should be prepared and checked as part of emergency preparedness.

Teams should be in frequent radio or telephone contact with their supervisor for reporting, receiving information and requesting support.

Teams of five to seven people are often most effective, ensuring a sufficient number of people with complementary skills and levels of experience, but small enough to be mobile, reactive, and easy to manage and support. They should be prepared and equipped to deal with all expected environmental health needs.

The teams will need assistance if a major health threat arises for which they are unprepared (e.g. a larger than anticipated number of refugees or evacuees, unexpectedly severe industrial contamination requiring specialized chemical treatment, or a serious outbreak of vector-borne disease). A key function of the field teams is to request additional assistance, based on their assessment of local needs and capacities. Personnel and equipment, as well as transportation, should be held in reserve in preparedness for such requests.

Ideally, specialists in engineering and food hygiene should accompany field teams in areas where there are large city water-supply and sanitation systems to be dealt with, or where mass feeding will be required.

4.4.3 Other specialized emergency environmental health functions

"Food and general sanitation" in Figure 4.1 refers to environmental health measures in mass feeding centres, the management of mortuary services, and the monitoring of the general environmental health situation (in collaboration with epidemiological surveillance). A functional link with veterinary services may be required if there are many animal carcasses or large numbers of stray animals.

Staff in a central office should be responsible for collating information on the status of water facilities and environmental health needs as it comes in from field teams and engineering staff. This information can be used to prioritize the allocation of resources and to formulate messages to the public. Specialized equipment for this purpose should be stockpiled and its location identified before it is needed. The means used to identify and record locations can be as rudimentary as file cards, graph paper, base maps, hand calculators and coloured pencils, or as elaborate as GIS (see Section 3.3.5).

4.4.4 Coordination of emergency response activities

Arrangements must be made at every level for collating and sharing essential information, and for taking decisions on resource use. Such arrangements can range from a simple committee meeting of community leaders or local administrators, to a complex, preplanned, purpose-built emergency operations centre. The basic aims are:

— to share and interpret data on existing threats and urgent needs;
— to identify priorities for collective action;
— to identify useful resources that are actually available;
— to allocate resources as effectively as possible in relation to the priorities identified;

— to seek and identify ways of filling resource gaps;
— to prevent duplication of programmes and overlapping roles;
— to minimize gaps in services.

Coordinating groups should include a senior environmental health specialist. He or she must be able to evaluate the public-health implications of data provided by other organizations. The specialist should also be able to collate and present the implications of events in the public-health sector in the wider context of the relief operation, and to explain the reasons for specific strategies.

Coordination may be led by government departments, interdepartmental bodies, provincial or district authorities, or international organizations (such as UNHCR in refugee emergencies). Whatever coordination arrangements are made, they should be understood and respected by all involved, to ensure a rapid and appropriate response to the emergency.

Effective communications are essential in an organized relief response. Staff should always be aware of the possibility that someone else might be able to use a particular item of information; a willingness to share information across organizational boundaries may be as important as specific technical issues.

Coordinating the activities of international organizations may present particular challenges. For more information on this, see Section 4.11.

4.5 Personnel management in emergencies

Personnel managers in emergencies and disasters face unusual problems, and special arrangements often need to be made to ensure an effective and rapid emergency response. The staff will generally be working for long hours under difficult and possibly dangerous conditions. Many staff may be absent as a result of death or injury, transportation difficulties, or concern for family needs and survival. Emergency procedures should be designed that can function adequately with reduced staff numbers. Replacement management staff need to be identified and legally empowered in advance to take over in the absence of those originally designated. A flexible approach is needed to allow staff to use their full range of skills, even if that means changing accepted roles and responsibilities.

4.5.1 Professional functions

Well-trained people are needed at policy-making levels, for technical services, surveys, and overall planning and supervision. They may include managers, engineers, medical doctors, epidemiologists, or environmental scientists, depending on the availability of personnel and the specific responsibilities concerned. The most important requirement, apart from experience and managerial skills, is the ability to communicate.

Workers from a number of related fields are needed to assist professional environmental health staff in making surveys, and to control water quality, food sanitation and waste disposal. They will also assist in vermin control and with the work of auxiliary personnel. These workers may come from a wide variety of backgrounds, but appropriate training courses and experience should prepare them for their roles in emergencies. They may include medical assistants, nurses, pharmacists, and humanitarian and welfare workers who have been trained in emergency environmental health work.

Auxiliary personnel are needed to monitor the functioning of all sanitary installations; to supervise food hygiene, vermin control, disinfection and volunteers; and to provide health education. The auxiliaries should have received formal education or training in the main aspects of environmental health, since they will have to carry out the bulk of the field work.

4.5.2 Flexibility in the use of human resources

In emergencies, environmental health measures may be carried out by a variety of people. As well as professional environmental health staff, such people may include primary health-care workers, social welfare workers, teachers and other development workers. They may be the only people available to take charge of meeting the immediate needs for water, shelter and sanitation, especially in isolated localities. This should be borne in mind when designing training programmes and when organizing mobile field teams of trained environmental health specialists, to ensure that these other workers are adequately supported and that their capacities are used to best effect.

4.5.3 Cooperation with the private sector

If too few public sector environmental health workers are available, they may be supplemented by private sector workers, including:

— industry-based and consulting civil and sanitary engineers;
— private laboratory personnel;
— dairy workers;
— industrial cleaning staff;
— railway and airline sanitation workers;
— commercial pest-control operators;
— teaching staff at universities and institutes with expertise in environmental health and sanitary engineering.

Water company employees may also be available to supplement environmental health personnel, although in some situations these companies may also be facing the problems of increased work and absenteeism, and might even require assistance from the environmental health agencies.

4.5.4 Working with volunteers

Volunteers will usually come forward in an emergency, often from existing community-based organizations, youth groups and sports clubs, etc. They may be able to provide skilled and unskilled help, and provide a communications channel with the affected community. They may be vital actors in the recovery process.

All volunteers will need to be supervised by qualified environmental health personnel to ensure that they work effectively and that they take no unnecessary risks (particularly with chemical or radiological hazards, such as when using chemicals for vector control).

4.5.5 Facilities for emergency personnel

The facilities required by emergency personnel will vary substantially according to the customary level of basic support, the task involved and the local conditions generated by the emergency. Broadly, however, all facilities will have common requirements, including:

— basic personal needs;
— family support;
— safety and security;
— emotional support and counselling;
— office facilities;
— facilities for maintaining transportation and communications.

4.5.6 Support for specialist activities

In addition, some emergencies will require specialist facilities and support, including specific safety services; storage for special equipment and supplies; repair facilities for equipment; computer equipment; and specialized laboratory services. These requirements will, in most places, be fairly limited and concerned mainly with carrying out assessments, investigating disease outbreaks, vector control and monitoring a limited number of chemical and radiological hazards.

Personnel who carry out assessments and investigate outbreaks of disease should have good access to communications and be given priority for transportation. Special arrangements should be made for samples to be sent back to laboratories.

Environmental health agencies in a disaster-affected region will generally bring in specialist staff from elsewhere in the country. In large operations, personnel from various other departments and organizations may also be attached to the operation, possibly in addition to international staff. If volunteers are recruited in large numbers, basic local facilities for registration, introduction and briefing will be needed.

4.5.7 Subsistence needs of personnel

Emergency personnel will need to be supported while they give support to others. Work may involve long hours in isolated situations without power supplies, safe drinking-water and waste disposal. Workers also run a relatively high risk of exposure to unfamiliar diseases. A relief worker who falls sick becomes part of the problem, rather than part of the solution.

To maintain morale and efficiency, emergency workers will need access to clean water and food, and facilities for sleeping, washing and cooking. Cash for personal and official expenses is also required.

Tents, stoves, cooking utensils, lamps, water containers, blankets, sleeping bags, chairs and tables, packaged rations, and other camping equipment may be needed, and should therefore be included in the supplies stored for emergencies. Environmental health services must provide for their own personnel. To depend on relief agencies for food and shelter is unwise and unfair; these agencies will already have more than enough to do to provide for victims.

4.5.8 Security and safety needs of personnel

In many areas, security is likely to be a major problem, particularly for female emergency workers and those in charge of valuable equipment. In all post-disaster situations, and particularly during times of conflict, agencies should provide all necessary security arrangements for their staff. These include an assessment of the security situation; appropriate guidelines for staff, depending on the level of insecurity and the nature of the risks; appropriate transportation and communications equipment; safe places to sleep; secure places to store equipment and vehicles; permits and photo-identification; up-to-date security briefings and information on current risks; and evacuation arrangements and procedures for staff in case of need. For further information on security, see: International Federation of Red Cross and Red Crescent Societies (1997a); United Nations (1998); United Nations High Commissioner for Refugees (1999); and van Brabant (2000).

In post-disaster situations there are many other threats to the health and safety of staff. The working environment tends to be unsafe, as a result of damage to buildings and roads, infectious diseases, or lack of appropriate equipment for reconstruction. In addition, the need to act fast, the great risks faced by the affected population, and the lack of close monitoring all discourage staff from applying health and safety procedures strictly. Managers need to encourage staff to apply correct health and safety procedures, and ensure that they have the means to do so. Adequate selection, briefing and supervision of volunteers are necessary to ensure their health and safety during relief activities.

Buildings used by staff must be safe and should be inspected by a qualified structural engineer after any emergency that causes structural damage. Where toxic substances, such as insecticides, are used, safe and lockable storage must be provided in buildings, together with arrangements for washing and showering. Even under the best conditions, simple but strict safety precautions should be observed.

Provision should also be made for the general health care of emergency workers. They may be injured or fall ill, especially under the stress of long hours and working under difficult conditions. A suitable medical centre should be identified early on, and arrangements should be made for medical evacuation, if necessary.

4.5.9 Psychological needs of personnel

Some environmental health personnel may need welfare support and counselling when dealing with death and disruption on a large scale, following the death or injury of family members or friends, or because of loss of housing and personal effects. Support can be provided by other team members and friends but, wherever possible, professional help should also be available.

To remain effective, emergency workers need to know that their families are alive and are provided with basic security and personal support. It is particularly important to provide all available information about the fate of family members and close friends. Staff will need to be reassured that support is being provided to any injured family member and to young children or other dependants in the family. When extended families or neighbours are unable to help, providing official support may be the best way to ensure that essential staff are able to concentrate on their jobs.

To reduce stress during long and intensive operations, particularly those in insecure situations, recreational and rest periods need to be planned, preferably away from the operational area.

4.5.10 Administrative support for personnel

Basic administrative support will be needed. The organization responsible for environmental health will need to update and safely store details of staff addresses and present places of deployment. There should also be a system for recording the number of hours worked in the field, any injuries sustained on the job, and any emergency payments made.

Relief and monitoring operations generate substantial amounts of information, and details of projects and proposals for repair and reconstruction have to be submitted to the appropriate authority. Basic emergency sets of office equipment, including storage for files, card indexes and computers/printers will be required, especially where additional field offices have to be set up.

Portable office units or containers make it easier to set up lockable and relatively weatherproof storage in remote or damaged areas. A support team, including an individual fully responsible for finding accommodation and making the necessary arrangements, should also be considered. Requirements for communications equipment, photocopying and file storage usually increase in an emergency. Lockable storage will be needed for more expensive equipment.

Newly-assigned staff and teams from outside the region will need information on the extent of any damage, the location of damaged facilities, the organization of the emergency operation, and a security and safety briefing. Newly-assigned staff should also be briefed on any traditional, religious, or cultural customs of the affected community that they should be aware of.

4.6 Equipment and supplies

4.6.1 Types of equipment needed

Lists of equipment and supplies for environmental health will generally need to be drawn up locally, taking account of local practices and conditions, and can be at almost any level of sophistication. The needs to be met may range from those of the rural village to those of a major urban conurbation. This book is primarily concerned with the more basic requirements. Even basic needs, however, may include specific requirements for more complex items, such as computers and communications equipment.

Standardized equipment, including forms for reporting and for requesting supplies, that is developed and held as a preparedness measure, makes operations faster and more consistent, and makes response training easier and more effective.

The categories of equipment to be considered include:

— equipment for personnel;
— equipment for emergency water supplies;
— equipment for emergency sanitation;
— materials, tools and consumables needed to repair and operate damaged urban water and sanitation networks;
— equipment for vector control;
— items used in monitoring and surveillance;
— laboratory equipment and materials;
— maps, reports and other materials that provide information on the area and the disaster, and allow information to be updated and communicated;
— administrative and office items.

A selection of items needed is given in Annex 2.

4.6.2 Procurement

There is no need for environmental health agencies to stock all the items that they need, as long as they can be purchased locally, or brought into the area rapidly when needed.

In many countries, the procedures for requisitioning supplies are complicated and lengthy, and some supplies may need to be brought in from another country. To avoid delaying the response, emergency personnel should not delay the requisitioning and purchasing of urgently needed equipment in a disaster.

Heavy equipment is usually very expensive and need not be stored by environmental health services. It is usually available from the army or from the highway or public works departments. Certain supplies, such as kitchen utensils, temporary shelters, etc., may be the concern of relief agencies. The environmental health requirements for these supplies can be discussed with other agencies involved in relief work.

Lists of essential chemical supplies, pipes, fittings and jointing materials, tools for a mobile repair unit, spare pumps and power units, trucks, tanks, etc. can be prepared, in collaboration with the officials in charge of water- and sewage-treatment works. Follow-up is necessary to ensure that the equipment and supplies for the emergency operation of water and sewage systems are purchased and then stocked in such a way as to facilitate their speedy delivery and use.

4.6.3 Specifications

It is important that the equipment and supplies stored for emergency use conform to standard specifications, so that they are robust, appropriate to emergency conditions and reliable. The United Nations system, the IFRC and several international NGOs, such as Oxfam and Médecins Sans Frontières, have developed detailed specifications for relief items, based on many years of research and field-testing.

Field staff should use standard equipment lists, or give detailed specifications when ordering equipment and supplies, to avoid procurement and logistics staff supplying the wrong items, or items that cannot be used efficiently. Ministries of works or ministries of water supply will often be able to provide standard specifications for approved water supply and sanitation equipment.

4.6.4 Storage and distribution

There are various storage options. Planners should designate sites for storage in advance, if possible. Suitable sites may include commercial warehouses, or water supply and sanitation service depots, where suitable buildings and stores management procedures already exist. If necessary, items can be transported in lockable containers that can be left on or near the site of operations. The supplies required for most environmental health activities in emergencies are generally simple to store and handle. However, secure storage and handling arrangements and staff training may be needed for water-treatment and vector-control chemicals, and large storage spaces and mechanical handling equipment may be needed for heavy or bulky pipes, pumps, valves, etc.

Inventories should be regularly reviewed by environmental health staff and updated. Periodic tests must be carried out to ensure that the equipment is always in working condition. The same equipment should be used for training purposes, but should always be repacked carefully after each training exercise, and any lost or damaged items noted on the inventory.

Some equipment may be used in routine environmental sanitation operations and will not need to be stockpiled specifically for emergencies, but there should always be an adequate reserve. Supply of these items should be planned within the overall local emergency planning framework. There may be competing demands for this kind of equipment, in which case priorities for its use, and mechanisms for coordinating its use, need to be established.

To ensure that essential items are always available, supplies in, supplies out and stock levels should be closely monitored and coordinated with field staff. It is important to record the end destination for items in the stock records, to monitor that they are being used appropriately and to provide reliable reports.

4.7 Transportation and logistics

Transportation is needed for a range of environmental health operations during emergencies, including:

— moving assessment and operational teams;
— road clearance;
— moving people affected by disaster;
— moving equipment and supplies;
— trucking water;
— moving human bodies;
— moving solid waste;
— moving animal corpses (especially after floods and cyclones);
— repair and reconstruction.

The organization of transportation should be planned in advance. Vehicles and their supporting services are expensive and it is difficult to assemble reliable fleets at short notice. An organization should estimate what and how much it will need to move, and arrange for its existing resources to be increased during an emergency, if necessary. Any organization responsible for environmental health may eventually find itself using a wide variety of different vehicles, all of which will need maintenance and spare parts at some stage.

4.7.1 Types of vehicle required

It is essential to select the right vehicles for the specific tasks envisaged. For example, in damaged urban areas, a major problem may be debris that can damage tyres and suspension systems. In such cases, tractors with clearance equipment, and personnel vehicles with robust tyres and suspension systems, would be appropriate vehicles. High ground-clearance light trucks with diesel engines will be useful in all regions affected by tropical storms where there is extensive flooding of roads. In earthquakes and some floods and storms, roads may be severely damaged or blocked by landslides, so that trucks and four-wheel drive vehicles for personnel may initially be required.

Environmental health agencies may need:

— ordinary cars to use for office administration;
— four-wheel drive personnel vehicles;
— minibuses to collect and transport staff;
— trucks;
— rubbish collectors and vacuum (sewage) trucks;
— fuel and water tankers;
— bulldozers and other road-clearance equipment;
— graders;
— compacters;
— cranes;
— cargo-handling equipment (e.g. forklift trucks);
— boats.

4.7.2 Sources and numbers of vehicles required

Although possible sources of vehicles can be designated at the planning stage, information may be needed quickly in an emergency on what vehicles are actually available and from what sources. It may be possible obtain vehicles from:

— the environmental health organization;
— government agencies, including public works departments and the armed forces;
— contractors;
— vehicle hire companies;
— other partners, e.g. nongovernmental organizations.

The numbers of vehicles required will depend on local conditions and on the size of the population and area concerned.

Each team should have its own vehicle. Transportation requirements increase substantially when dealing with visitors, including international aid staff and the press. The use of vehicles for administrative tasks is often substantial and usually underestimated. Vehicles may spend long periods waiting at liaison meetings and banks, queuing to collect goods held at customs, etc., or moving between shops and factories in a search for local supplies.

Disruption of public transportation may make it necessary to set up a temporary shuttle service to bring staff to and from work. Vehicle allocation should also allow for liaison with volunteer groups and local self-help groups.

4.7.3 Repairs and maintenance

In some countries, up to 40% of public vehicles may be out of action because of breakdowns, and shortages of fuel or spare parts. There may not be much time for repairs in emergencies. Extra vehicles should be made available to replace those that have broken down or have been damaged in accidents.

When operating a vehicle fleet, even on a short-term emergency basis, it is essential to consider the availability of fuel, tyres, spare parts and trained mechanics; how to provide support for drivers; and how to supervise vehicle movements and security. Trained drivers and competent vehicle mechanics can substantially increase the efficiency of a vehicle fleet by keeping more vehicles on the road for longer periods.

Other requirements include:

— safe storage of fuel, equipment and supplies;
— stocks of tyres (widespread debris generally increases wear and tear);
— transportation planning and control staff to establish policies and supervise operations;
— ensuring that all vehicles, including hired vehicles, have the proper documentation;
— arrangements for cash payments for fuel, drivers' salaries and living allowances, or hire of vehicles.

4.7.4 Road operations: transportation logistics in field operations

It is important to plan for transportation operations beforehand, since there will rarely be time to do so at the height of an emergency. For road operations, efforts should be made early on to determine road conditions and operating constraints. Information should be coordinated and shared among organizations involved in the emergency response.

Information may be needed on:

— breaks in road networks;
— road capacity (including bridge loading limits, and any restrictions on height and width);
— the potential effects of any adverse weather conditions;
— the availability of fuel;
— security conditions;
— round-trip times;
— the possibility of staying in radio or telephone contact.

4.7.5 Air operations

When air transportation is to be used, specialist advice should be sought on airport capacity and aircraft landing requirements. Account should also be taken of equipment (including lifts and lighting) and labour requirements for unloading, and arrangements for safe refuelling and for restarting engines. Staff should liaise closely with the personnel of national airlines and private air transportation companies. Access to some routes and airfields may be controlled, and staff may need clearance and permits, even in emergencies. For further information on air operations, see United States Agency for International Development (1988).

4.7.6 Other modes of transportation

Depending on local geography, the state of the infrastructure, and other factors, alternative modes of transportation may be used to supplement air and road transportation. In emergencies, railway systems (which are often state-owned) can be mobilized to transport supplies and people quickly at relatively low cost. In countries with navigable rivers, it may be possible to transport less-urgently needed fuel, building materials and water by boat. Early in the relief operation, managers and logistics staff should plan to deliver high-volume supplies by cheaper, often slower routes. This will mean estimating consumption and creating the necessary stocks to allow for a longer delivery time.

4.7.7 Pooling of transportation services

Organizations sometimes collaborate by providing transportation services to each other. For example, an additional pool of heavy vehicles may be available from government sources and can be used to augment existing departmental transportation resources. There may also be large public or private workshops that can provide services to the operation as a whole. However, policies on allocation and scheduling will need to be agreed.

The public works department or the armed forces may be able to provide transportation for environmental health personnel to travel to isolated areas to gather health data, or to move heavy equipment needed to repair water supplies.

In countries where there is an existing refugee or food-relief operation, a large, specialized, relief transportation organization may have been developed over several months or years. Such an organization can be of considerable value in any disaster, provided that a reliable system for the receipt, clearance, transportation and storage of valuable shipments has been established. If necessary, environmental health planners should establish working relationships with any such organizations before an emergency occurs.

For large-scale operations, or those involving the handling of valuable items, it is important to designate an internal or shared transportation/logistics support group, with staff responsible for:

— port and airport clearance;
— commodity tracking and scheduling;
— vehicle allocation, management and maintenance;
— driver support and payment;
— storage.

4.7.8 Vehicle priorities

It is necessary to prioritize vehicle allocation, and essential tasks should be given the highest priority. In particular, some vehicles should be reserved for prompt survey and investigation, and for relocating personnel in emergencies.

Emergency operations centres may be responsible for vehicle allocation and may establish a joint scheduling unit. In practice, however effective the coordination arrangements may be, it is important for field teams to be relatively self-sufficient in fuel, replacement tyres, spare parts and other essential requirements during the emergency period.

4.7.9 Field logistics systems

Whatever the mode of transportation chosen, a system for tracking and receiving valuable items is required. Staff should be assigned to clearly identified tasks for receiving such goods. It is important to establish as quickly as possible written procedures for handing over valuable items. This will involve establishing a commodity-control chain, with documentary controls such as supplies request forms, waybills, bin cards and stock reports. Signatures and identification should be required for all receipts.

Vehicles and their cargo are highly valuable. Staff should be briefed on the importance of providing lockable storage for tools and equipment, and on arranging for overnight security when parking vehicles containing valuable goods and equipment.

4.8 Telecommunications

Telecommunications are the foundation of an effective emergency response on any scale. If installed from the start, they will ensure that the information on the situation is adequately transmitted, facilitating rapid reaction and personnel security.

Use of standardized equipment allows an efficient telecommunications service to be provided with good user support and at a lower cost in the long run. The system used must be based on experience and field feedback. Training, advice and maintenance must be arranged, and in a large-scale emergency response, one or more telecommunications technicians may be required to carry out these tasks. Nonstandard telecommunications systems should be used *only* after consultation with the local authorities responsible for telecommunications and/or with relief agencies operating in the area.

It is essential that personnel are trained in the use of telecommunications equipment, basic communications procedures and radio discipline, to avoid miscommunications and blocked communications channels.

4.8.1 Types of telecommunications equipment

The most basic communications equipment available worldwide include the following:

- *Telephone.* Traditional telephone communications tend to be seriously disrupted in sudden emergencies, as a result of damage to switching equipment, network disruption, or loss of electrical power. If telephone lines of different quality are available, the possibility of obtaining better lines should be investigated. Certain companies or United Nations agencies can sometimes provide good satellite lines. The standard satellite communications system used by IFRC is the Inmarsat system. Satellite communications systems are becoming cheaper to purchase and run. Associated equipment for voice, fax, email, telex and data is available. Mobile telephones are increasingly affordable and more widely used in emergency situations.
- *Fax.* A fax machine should be purchased locally if the supplier can install and maintain it. A dedicated, good-quality telephone line is highly recommended. The fax and telephone should not normally share the same line.
- *Email* and other internet services. These may be accessed through fixed telephone connections, mobile telephones, satellite links, or high-frequency (HF) radio. Email communication is increasingly replacing telephone and fax communications in emergencies.
- *Telex.* This is used less and less, but where it is available, it still provides a reliable and cheap method of communicating text.

Radio technology is widely used in emergency operations. Its two great advantages for emergency situations are that it is independent of damage caused to fixed communications systems, and that it has the capacity to transmit to a number of different users at the same time. This is very important for rapidly transmitting security information and instructions. All staff who are to use radios should be trained in their use. A number of different systems are available, including the following (International Federation of Red Cross and Red Crescent Societies (1997a):

■ *HF radio.* HF and short-wave radios (operating at 3–30 MHz) are suitable for short-, medium- or long-range contacts (up to several hundred kilometres), depending on the frequency chosen. HF radio can be used for voice (single side band, SSB) or written messages (PACket TOR or PACTOR technology; see below). The quality of the HF radio link depends on wave propagation; this may vary, depending on many parameters such as the time of the day, the distance to be covered, solar activity, etc. HF radios need a heavy battery or mains power supply, and radio sets are usually fitted in vehicles and buildings.

■ *TOR system.* Telex Over Radio (TOR) is used for transmitting text over HF. However, this system is rapidly being replaced by PACTOR technology (see below), that offers error-free links, as well as full ASCII data transmission.

■ *PACTOR system.* This system provides text and data transmission on HF radio. A PACTOR modem is connected to the radio and to a personal computer running a specific software application called GLPLUS. It can also be used for text transmission contact with normal TOR stations.

■ *Very high-frequency (VHF) radio.* This is generally used for local voice communications, e.g. in a city or a camp. The quality of the communication is generally good, as FM (frequency modulation) is used. Small portable radio sets are available, but these have a short range. A good VHF network needs a fixed base, plus mobile and even repeater stations. Typical VHF radio ranges are (Davis & Lambert 2002):

— handheld to handheld: about 5 km, depending on terrain;
— vehicle to vehicle: about 20 km, depending on terrain;
— vehicle to base: about 30 km, depending on terrain;
— base to base: about 30 km, depending on terrain.

■ *Repeater set.* A repeater set receives and then retransmits VHF radio signals on another frequency at a higher power. Placed high, a repeater set will give far better range than point-to-point radio communications systems. However, the breakdown of a repeater may disable the entire radio network. Installation of a repeater is recommended only if a telecommunications professional is permanently available in the area.

4.8.2 Sources of radio communications

Alternatives may include:

— pre-established emergency radio networks;
— groups of amateur radio operators;
— armed forces or police radio;
— couriers (to supplement radio, or for when radio is not available).

Where radio equipment is widely used, it is essential to ensure that frequency allocations match the traffic likely to be carried.

Local regulations for the use of radio and telephone communications should, if possible, include provision for emergency use by accredited international teams that bring their own equipment with them.

4.8.3 Developments in telecommunications

This is a complex and fast changing area, and continues to be a subject of discussion by national governments, telecommunications coordinating groups, and international relief agencies, but a consensus on basic communications frameworks for international humanitarian relief is emerging. Details of current international conventions, and the options available for telecommunications support and coordination within a United

Nations framework during emergencies, are available from the United Nations Office for the Coordination of Humanitarian Affairs (OCHA) in New York.

Low-cost, satellite-linked mobile telephones are becoming more widely available and will revolutionize field communications in remote areas.

4.9 Financial procedures

Contingency planning must cover access to sufficient cash for essential local purchases and for emergency spending on repairs and other urgent work. Rapid procedures for approving contracted services (or standing arrangements) are also necessary.

Transparent and simple methods should also be established for accounting for these financial decisions. In general, more elaborate rules for the purchase of materials and contracting of services may have to be suspended in disasters to give environmental health personnel the flexibility to overcome deficiencies and replenish any stocks that have run low, are damaged or are inaccessible. Streamlined and precise procedures for granting authority for such transactions, and authorization limits for different staff levels therefore need to be established in advance.

Well-designed budgets that accurately reflect the activities to be carried out are an essential tool for financial management, allowing transparency in financial decision-making and a realistic basis for financial planning and management. In emergency situations, budgets may need to be revised from time to time as the situation changes, or as new information on needs and resources becomes available. It is important for managers to stay in close contact with funders, to facilitate the process of renegotiation.

Provision for audits and for exchange of financial information between field staff and programme administrators is necessary to ensure that systems for financial control are established and operated correctly. It is usual for very large amounts of money to be spent rapidly in emergencies and extra care is needed to ensure that money is not wasted or diverted.

Field staff may be given the responsibility for managing the budgets for the work they carry out. In such cases, it is essential that up-to-date and reliable financial information is provided to them so that they can monitor and control spending.

Senior staff need to carry out financial forecasting to ensure that current and future needs for funds are met. Cash planning is necessary to avoid field staff running out of cash for urgent local expenditures. If large amounts of cash are used for local purchases and paying casual labourers, then special cash-handling procedures may be needed, to enable field staff and office staff to work safely and avoid losses.

Field staff should be aware of the need to provide information for writing financial reports. Their job is made much easier if they are provided with standard financial reporting forms. The increasing use of portable computers for field work means that financial information can be recorded electronically by field staff, reducing the number of calculation errors and the need for data entry in a central office.

4.10 Rules, standards and guidelines in disaster response

There is an inevitable tendency in areas affected by disasters to relax the application of day-to-day administrative procedures and to reduce the scope of, or abandon, many regular monitoring tasks. Staff will be under intense pressure as they assist in re-establishing a basic framework of public health. However, basic rules for the application of professional standards are needed to ensure an effective emergency response and accountability for the considerable resources mobilized.

International guidelines, such as the *World Health Organization Guidelines for Drinking Water Quality, Volumes I and II*, and national guidelines concerning environmental health provide a framework within which field staff should make local judgments about appropriate emergency actions. Where existing international and national guidelines and standards are not considered to be applicable, then the reasons for this need to be explained at some stage.

In addition to existing public-health and safety rules in a given country or locality, and regulations governing the work of environmental health workers, the other agencies involved in relief operations will have their own rules and standards; see for example, International Federation of Red Cross and Red Crescent Societies (1997a); United Nations High Commissioner for Refugees (1999), and Section 4.10.5.

4.10.1 Importance of rules and guidelines in emergencies

The very conditions in which rules and regulations are widely perceived to be least appropriate may in fact be those in which clear standards and guidelines are most needed. An essential element of environmental health management is the identification and reduction or mitigation of risks. In disasters, and during post-disaster recovery, every kind of improvisation may be attempted, often by people unaware of the direct risks involved or the wider effects. Examples include:

— the patching and reconnection of parts of water-supply systems using improvised and leaky joints;
— connecting to unsafe drinking-water sources, and improvising plumbing in mass-care centres, resulting in back-siphonage;
— indiscriminate use of toxic agricultural insecticides in attempts to control insect vectors;
— mass feeding operations in which critical aspects of food hygiene are neglected;
— inappropriate clean-up after industrial accidents that may give rise to new risks, such as the introduction of hazardous chemicals into watercourses.

Rules and guidelines, when applied in an appropriate way, ensure that rapid and innovative action can be taken in emergencies, without creating new risks and damage to infrastructure.

4.10.2 Basic principles for creating rules for emergencies

First, it is essential to ensure that rules and regulations for emergencies are as straightforward as possible, are appropriate for situations where there is a clear risk to large numbers of people, and make minimal demands on staff time and resources. A balance must be struck between attempting to avoid catastrophic breakdowns in public safety, and encouraging initiative and creative contributions to recovery. Responsibilities for specific tasks should be assigned to designated individuals in an organization; replacements should be nominated to take over if these individuals become casualties or are unable to make contact.

Second, written authorizations or permits to carry out specific measures and to take specific decisions should be provided, and this fact should be made known as widely as possible both before and after an emergency. Certain relief and recovery tasks, such as the recommissioning of parts of water-supply systems, vector-control activities and the emergency disposal of hazardous wastes, should be "signed off" by a responsible individual.

Finally, the risk of inappropriate and dangerous decisions and actions should be reduced by controlling access to the most important resources and facilities, and by screening and briefing any new staff or volunteers. When possible, essential safety measures should be summarized, using pictures as well as words, if necessary, in a single, robust and easily carried document (e.g. a coloured, laminated card, or simply a clearly duplicated sheet of paper, that can be stockpiled alongside operational supplies).

4.10.3 Special rules in areas of high potential public-health risk

The following major risk areas must be subject to detailed control and regulation, even under extreme emergency conditions:

— the continued operation or recommissioning of large water-supply systems that have been damaged;
— the selection of sources for emergency water supply;
— the emergency disposal of toxic materials, especially soluble industrial waste;
— large-scale feeding.

Specific guidelines on the selection and application of pesticides for disease vector and nuisance pest control will also need to be widely publicized. In some circumstances, special rules will be necessary for handling the dead. See Chapter 14 for further details.

4.10.4 Rules concerning foreign relief workers

In disasters with an international dimension, where relief workers from many countries may be involved, certain legal and administrative difficulties are almost inevitable in some form or other.

Foreign professional staff, including medical personnel, engineers and other technicians, will generally not be licensed to practice in the affected country, and special regulations may be needed to allow them to do so. Increasingly, arrangements for employing international specialists are becoming formalized by agreements between governments and with international agencies and nongovernmental organizations. Examples include UNHCR's arrangements with specialist agencies and technical consultants, and IFRC's Emergency Response Units and Field Assessment and Coordination Teams. Associations of specialists have been formed, with specific operating rules and requirements for the prior screening and accreditation of personnel. Under these conditions, problems of licensing are very much easier.

4.10.5 International standards and codes of conduct for humanitarian response

For many years, international nongovernmental humanitarian agencies have been developing and using guidelines and professional approaches to humanitarian work. Examples include technical manuals, training courses, financial procedures and equipment kits. Since the early 1990s, there has been considerable collaborative work to create and apply codes of conduct and standards, to improve their performance and accountability. Some of the more important initiatives are described below.

The Code of Conduct for the International Red Cross and Red Crescent Movement and NGOs in Disaster Relief. This code of conduct, published in 1994, sets out ten principles that govern the work of subscribing agencies, and makes important recommendations to the governments of disaster-affected countries, donor governments and intergovernmental organizations to facilitate application of the code of conduct.

The Sphere Project Humanitarian Charter and Minimum Standards in Disaster Response. This builds on the humanitarian principles described in the Red Cross/NGO Code of Conduct, and provisions of international human rights law, international humanitarian law, and refugee law to describe the core principles that govern humanitarian action and asserts the right of populations to protection and assistance. Minimum standards are set out for humanitarian action in the fields of water supply and sanitation, nutrition, food aid, shelter and site planning, and health services. These standards are based, as far as possible, on existing guidelines and standards, and are accompanied by key indicators and guidance notes to help staff translate the standards into practical actions in the field. Sphere Project minimum standards are referred to in the technical chapters in Part II, where relevant.

The Humanitarian Accountability Project. This project aims to establish the means for people affected by disaster to comment on the performance of international and local systems of humanitarian assistance, so that performance and accountability in humanitarian action can be improved at all levels. To this end, a staff member should be "in-post", whose role is to listen to people involved in disasters and emergencies, such as agency staff, affected communities, donors and others, and to help make an assessment of the humanitarian response, and encourage improvements where necessary.

Staff who are likely to be involved in an emergency response should be aware of these and other initiatives governing the work of international agencies, as part of preparedness planning.

4.11 International assistance

Primary responsibility for disaster relief almost always rests with the government of the affected country. Prior planning is needed both for requesting international health assistance and for handling such assistance. As far as possible, requests should be based on the field assessment of conditions. It may be appropriate to discuss major requests with local WHO offices and with the staff of major international relief agencies in the country, many of whom may have extensive previous experience.

4.11.1 In-country coordination

All requests for assistance should be made by a single government body and all offers of assistance should be received by this body for onward transmission to those concerned. This will usually be the responsibility of the national disaster council or ministry of internal affairs. Health staff linked to the council should be the final authority; they should be informed of all proposed medical and environmental health inputs, and should be able to regulate and control any shipments.

United Nations organizations and specialized agencies such as WHO, UNICEF, UNHCR, and the World Food Programme (WFP) are responsible for providing advice and assistance to the government, in accordance with their mandates, and are often represented in the national disaster council. They will also provide technical assistance and material support. IFRC is normally represented in-country by the National Red Cross or Red Crescent Society.

Under certain conditions, joint coordinating arrangements for specialist support may be appropriate. In some emergency operations, medical advisers (pharmacists, laboratory specialists) may already be attached to the national health ministry. If a major additional requirement for supplies suddenly develops, coordination can often be improved by appointing representatives of the department of medical supplies, and advisers on medical supplies and pharmaceutical matters, as joint coordinating secretaries for international relief supplies.

Within the health sector, a senior health official coordinating the environmental health response should act as a liaison and contact point for international agencies and organizations. He or she should be able to communicate with the staff responsible for coordination at the regional and district levels, and should thus be in a position to provide information on needs and resources in the affected area.

The multitude of inputs from international, multilateral and bilateral sources of assistance following a major emergency or disaster have frequently overwhelmed capacities for coordination in recipient countries. In the last few years, OCHA has been responsible for the coordination of humanitarian assistance in complex emergencies.

4.11.2 Forms and functions of international assistance

In the environmental health sector, the international assistance that can be provided may include:

— expertise and assistance with planning and implementing activities;
— components for emergency repairs to damaged water-supply systems;
— tanks, pumps, piping components and tools for emergency water supplies for large concentrations of people;
— resources (funding for vehicles, fuel and spare parts) to support the emergency delivery of water by road tanker;
— laboratory and water-testing equipment.

4.11.3 Integrating international staff and local specialists

Well-qualified international staff can make a substantial contribution to relief work. In particular:

■ They show people that, despite the overwhelming problems, there are ways of imposing order on the situation.
■ They recognize that what people can do in a short time is limited and help local officials focus on what they can actually cope with. They encourage local staff to seek out those problems where intervention is likely to be both feasible and effective.
■ They encourage staff to use information as a management tool, and to use appropriate methods to ensure that the information that they use is accurate and representative.

Experience suggests the importance of integrating international staff and local specialists. The latter are more likely to be aware, for instance, of local practices in the use of water sources and other local resources, and be better able to assess the feasibility of adaptations for emergency use. They will also be more aware of seasonal variations and local organizational constraints, and be better able to communicate directly with survivors.

4.11.4 Guidelines on employment of international assistance teams

Ideally, countries should establish guidelines on the employment of international assistance teams. The guidelines should cover the following areas:

— ability to meet internationally recognized standards for qualifications and proficiency;
— self-sufficiency in personal needs and equipment;
— commitment to remain in country for a certain length of time, or until certain activities have been completed;
— ability to react sufficiently quickly and with sufficient staff and other resources;
— knowledge of the country, or experience in the technical area concerned;
— recognition by, and support from, the United Nations agency concerned (e.g. UNHCR in refugee emergencies);
— capacity and commitment to enable members of the local population to participate in their operations.

It is important to avoid situations in which teams arrive with high-technology equipment, remain for only short periods of time, and then withdraw without stabilizing the situation in the longer term.

Sophisticated equipment for water-supply systems or vector control is useless in the longer term if supplies of spare parts are not continued, qualified repair and maintenance staff are not available locally, and local people are not properly trained to operate the equipment. Similar problems have occurred in refugee operations, where international specialists have built sophisticated, electronically operated water-treatment and pumping systems and then departed, leaving no blueprints and making no arrangements for the supply of spare parts or planned maintenance. Such arrangements are expensive and often fail more catastrophically than those they replace.

4.12 Further information

For further information on:

— assessment techniques, see: Scrimshaw & Gleason (1992), Beaglehole, Bonita & Kjellström (1993), Good (1996a), International Federation of Red Cross and Red Crescent Societies (1997b), Médecins sans Frontières (1997a), Baker et al. (1999), World Health Organization (1999b), Davis & Lambert (2002);

— public health in disasters and emergencies, see: Goma Epidemiology Group (1995), Perrin (1996), Médecins sans Frontières (1997a), International Federation of Red Cross and Red Crescent Societies (2000), International Federation of Red Cross and Red Crescent Societies, Johns Hopkins University (2000);

— human resources, see: International Committee of the Red Cross (2001), People in Aid (1997);

— equipment, transportation and logistics, see: de Ville de Goyet (1993), United Nations Development Programme, Inter-Agency Procurement Services Office (1995), Adams (1999), United Nations High Commissioner for Refugees (1999), Davis & Lambert (2002);

— telecommunications, see: International Federation of Red Cross and Red Crescent Societies (1997a), United Nations High Commissioner for Refugees (1999), Davis & Lambert (2002);

— international humanitarian codes of conduct and standards, see: International Federation of Red Cross and Red Crescent Societies, International Committee of the Red Cross (1994), Sphere Project (2000);

— coordination, see: Dufresne & Thompson (1996).

5. Recovery and sustainable development

5.1 From disasters to development

5.1.1 The transition from relief to recovery

A distinction is usually made between immediate measures taken to support life and sustain morale, and the later activities dedicated to re-establishing the economic, social and cultural life of the people concerned and rebuilding damaged areas. In this book, the first group of activities is called *relief*, while the second is collectively referred to as *recovery*.

There is no clear-cut boundary between the relief and the recovery periods. It is important to emphasize that the disaster-management cycle is an unbroken chain of human actions whose phases overlap (see Chapter 1). Since the disasters change social, political, economic and even demographic realities irreversibly, there can be no return to the predisaster situation. In addition, people begin almost immediately to rehouse themselves and to re-establish their social and economic networks after a disaster (Bates, 1982; Aysan & Oliver, 1987; Oliver-Smith, 1986a, 1991). Certainly, by the time the relief phase is changing into recovery, most people have very clear ideas about what they want to do to rebuild their lives. It is essential to take their views into account when planning for recovery.

An account of recovery and development in Mexico City after the earthquake of 1985 is given in Box 5.1.

5.1.2 Sustainable development

The World Commission on Environment and Development (also known as the "Brundt-land Commission") has defined "sustainable development" in terms of livelihood security. A system is sustainable if it provides all people with secure livelihoods, in ways that do not compromise the ability of future generations to achieve secure livelihoods (World Commission on Environment and Development, 1987a).

Livelihood is defined as access to adequate food and cash to meet basic needs. *Security* refers to secure ownership of, or access to, resources and income-earning activities, including reserves and assets to offset risk, ease shocks and meet contingencies. *Sustainable* refers to the maintenance or enhancement of resource productivity on a long-term basis (World Commission on Environment and Development, 1987b).

Throughout this book, three key concepts are continually emphasized:

— organization that is responsive to local needs;
— improvisation;
— incremental improvement.

These three principles can and should be carried over into the period of full repair of infrastructure, economic rehabilitation and physical reconstruction of neighbourhoods and communities, and become a permanent feature of sustainable development.

> **Box 5.1 Recovery and development in Mexico City[1]**
>
> Following the earthquake in Mexico City in 1985, an innovative housing reconstruction pro-
> gramme provided almost 50 000 housing units in a way that directly involved neighbourhood
> associations, tenement groups and church organizations in decision-making. This strengthened
> the social capacity for mitigating, coping with and recovering from any future disaster.
>
> Furthermore, the programme, called "Renovación Habitacional Popular" (RHP) created 115
> 000 new jobs in the construction industry that were filled almost exclusively by locally recruited
> workers. This strengthened the community's economic base and helped local people to rebuild
> their livelihoods. The reconstruction plans included space for workshops, commercial spaces
> and houses, and laid the foundation for sustainable livelihoods.
>
> RHP also strengthened the alliance between the public and private sectors. The RHP task
> force included experts seconded from private sector organizations, as well as experts from
> the public sector. The public sector provided institutional support, a timely flow of information
> and funds, and shortcuts in bureaucratic procedures. The private sector contributed practical
> experience in finance, design, construction and management.
>
> When construction was complete, RHP was dissolved, preventing the institutionalization and
> bureaucratization of the recovery process.
>
> [1] Source: Pantelic (1991).

5.1.3 Increasing individual and institutional capacity

Increasing the capacity of people to offset risk, absorb shocks and meet contingencies
is central to the goal of sustainable recovery. Reconstruction of a damaged area is not
limited to the erection of new buildings. An integrated development process is required
that should embrace the full redevelopment of the affected area according to the needs
of its population.

Long-term recovery from a major disaster is inevitably a slow and difficult process.
No society is ever the same after a disaster, nor should it be. Disasters reveal weaknesses
and deficiencies in society's ability to protect itself, especially its more vulnerable
members. Those concerned with environmental health should learn the lessons that disasters teach about the health of the population, and the resilience and responsiveness
of health facilities, including water supplies and sanitation systems. They can help to
draw out the more general lessons that will result in prevention, mitigation and increased
preparedness.

Emergencies and disasters often provide an opportunity for new voices to be heard
in society: emergent community-based organizations express the needs of disaster-
affected people (Anderson & Woodrow, 1989; Berke et al., 1993) and can become a permanent force for change and sustainable development once the emergency is over.

After major disasters, countries have often introduced new legislation and established
new institutions and programmes. They have also adopted building codes; regulated
land use; controlled dangerous industrial processes and the transportation of toxic
chemicals; provided insurance and credit for vulnerability reduction; improved early
warning systems; increased preparedness; and improved the coordination of emergency
response. All of these initiatives and changes offer environmental health planners and
administrators opportunities to promote health and safety, and all are part of the overall
recovery process.

5.2 Assessment for recovery

Continuing relief efforts, such as the provision of emergency shelter, water, sanitation,
etc., will not produce recovery alone. By the very nature of the emergency response,

such activities are often not well integrated into long-term development processes. More importantly, during the relief phase, populations are often supported by outside resources that are not sustainable in the long run. At a certain stage, people in camps must either return home, become integrated with the host population, or settle in a third location. Similarly, the self-sheltering population will need to support itself either in its old neighbourhoods or communities, or elsewhere.

The reconstruction of housing and of water-supply and sanitation systems are priority areas. The information required for long-term planning and policy-making are outlined in the following sections.

5.2.1 Reconstruction of housing

Before long-term plans for the reconstruction of housing and other forms of shelter can be drawn up, the following information is required:

- The *number of people concerned*, their geographical distribution, age groups, etc.
- The *number of houses damaged and destroyed* and the standard and pattern of housing before the disaster.
- The *number of families already engaged in repair* or rebuilding; the way in which they are organized; the incorporation of risk-reducing features in rebuilding; the assistance they may require and the possibility of encouraging low-cost risk-reducing techniques.
- The *available resources* (land, labour power, skills, materials, equipment, access to transportation, and financial resources to support self-help).
- *Remaining hazards* that may be faced by people settling on certain sites.
- *Economic data* (previous rent levels, land prices, costs of materials, and the source and amount of funds available for investment in housing).

Housing policy should take this information into account and a thorough consultation process should be carried out, with special efforts made to hear the opinions of people who may not normally be heard in the community. The goal is to find answers to the following questions:

- What agencies should provide assistance to self-help rebuilding or engage directly in housing construction, and what partnerships with community organizations and the private sector are possible?
- Should new housing be built on the previous site or elsewhere, bearing in mind that residents may have pre-empted this decision by beginning to rebuild or by occupying vacant land with the intention of building there?
- Should particular groups or families be given special consideration in rehousing?
- Are there ways of encouraging those engaged in self-help rebuilding to incorporate new safety features against earthquakes, wind, flooding, etc., as appropriate?
- Is it necessary to lower building standards that do not affect health or safety in order to build quickly and affordably (Davis, 1978; Hardoy & Satterthwaite, 1981; Aysan & Oliver, 1987; Oliver-Smith, 1991)?
- Is it necessary to introduce new industries and techniques, and start training building workers, etc., especially in low-cost safety improvements? Some nongovernmental organizations have considerable experience of such training (Cuny, 1983; Maskrey, 1989).
- Should changes be made in the laws governing landlord–tenant relations?
- Is it necessary to modify the laws governing land ownership, or access to vacant land for building, as well as zoning regulations? Is compulsory public purchase of hazardous terrain necessary and possible?
- Does legal ownership need to be established to provide security of tenure?

■ To what extent are the people involved able and willing to contribute financially and otherwise to reconstruction?

■ Are laws needed during the recovery period to regulate speculation in urban land prices and the prices of building materials (McAuslan, 1985)?

■ Are new arrangements needed to provide financial support for house repair and new housing (Alexander, 1993)? The question is particularly relevant to the use of special credit lines, low-interest loans, revolving loan funds, and loan guarantees to encourage the adoption of new safety features or health improvements, e.g. the credit facilities supporting Lesotho's urban and rural sanitation campaign for building ventilated improved pit (VIP) latrines (Blackett, 1990).

■ How can the "informal" construction industry that exists in many countries be stimulated to work with residents attempting their own repairs? Hardoy & Satterthwaite (1981) describe how use was made of a large number of artisans and traditional builders rather than giving all the work to established formal-sector contractors. Support could also be given to women's groups attempting to break into the construction industry (see Carr, 1984).

For examples of self-help reconstruction, see Box 5.2. For examples of incorporating safety features during reconstruction, see Box 5.3.

Box 5.2 **Self-help reconstruction in Guatemala**[1]

The 1976 earthquake in Guatemala left thousands of people living in substandard housing in many neighbourhoods of Guatemala City.

Leaders of several working-class neighbourhoods on the outskirts of the city joined local church workers and students from San Carlos University in a land invasion that provided more than 1000 families with new, more stable terrain for rebuilding their homes. Faced with such large-scale, popular action, the National Housing Bank (BANVI) agreed to buy the land and the Emergency Committee of the Calvary Church (CEMEC) agreed to build 1500 houses ($26 m^2$ each), a health station, a 10-room primary school, a market, a church, a park, a slaughterhouse and a first-aid station. BANVI also agreed to lay out and gravel streets, and help provide electricity, potable water and drainage.

The participating families agreed to engage in decision-making, commit three weeks of labour to house construction, and pay a mortgage of $US 8–10 per month.

The title to a house was transferred after a year of proper care and use as the owner's family residence.

[1] Source: Oliver-Smith (1991).

Box 5.3 **Incorporation of safety features during reconstruction**

During the recovery period, those engaged in self-help rehousing should be encouraged to incorporate new safety features against earthquakes, wind, flooding, etc.

One example of this is the successful promotion of lightweight aluminium sheeting as a roofing material, instead of the traditional heavy ceramic tiles that proved lethal in the 1976 earthquake in Guatemala (Bates, Farrell & Glittenberg, 1979).

Another, is the use of metal straps to tie down roof rafters against strong winds, a low-cost innovation introduced in many places following cyclone/hurricane disasters in recent years (Davis, 1986).

Other work includes research on strengthening existing adobe (mud brick) construction.

5.2.2 Reconstruction of water-supply and sanitation systems

Once damaged systems have been repaired, and services to the disaster-affected population are adequate for protecting life and health, longer term reconstruction should be planned. The following information is required:

- The number of people affected, their geographical distribution, age groups, etc.
- People's access to protected water supplies and sanitation systems and the pattern of water-related diseases before the disaster.
- The data (meteorological, hydrogeological, hydrological, and other relevant data) needed for planning improvements in water supply and sanitation in these areas.
- The results of an evaluation of emergency response and urgent repairs and measures (i.e. whether and how emergency measures have actually improved access to protected water and sanitation, and decreased the amount of water- and sanitation-related disease).
- The activities carried out by the people themselves to improve water supplies and sanitation in the disaster-relief phase (including the predisaster activities of community-based and nongovernmental organizations), and whether these activities incorporate low-cost improvements and health safeguards.
- The availability of labour, skills, materials, equipment and financial resources for assisting the community to continue the improvements, or for extending water-supply and sanitation systems, and the feasibility of collecting basic relevant data if none has been collected.

Questions of water supply and sanitation policy will arise that are similar to those raised by self-help housing, as follows:

- What agencies should provide assistance to those engaged in improving water-supply and sanitation systems?
- Should particular groups be given special consideration?
- To what standards should new and improved water-supply and sanitation systems be constructed? (This is especially relevant in drought-prone areas during the period of recovery, which can be quite prolonged). Should lower standards be accepted temporarily, or should reconstruction be used as an opportunity to provide better water supplies than before the disaster?
- If new industries and techniques are introduced, is it necessary to train water-supply construction workers, such as highly skilled well-digging teams?
- Are any changes required in the laws governing the ownership or control of water resources?
- Are new banking and credit arrangements needed to stimulate community-based improvement of water supplies and sanitation?
- Should a price be set for the water or sanitation services provided by utilities and, if so, how should it be done?

5.2.3 Secondary damage assessment

Whereas primary damage assessment involves the rapid appraisal of deaths, injuries and disease, and identification of damage to infrastructure, material resources and services, secondary damage assessment is concerned with the impact of the primary damage on the economic, social and cultural life of survivors. Since sustainable livelihood security is the goal of both recovery and sustainable development, the assessment of such damage should be concerned with the following three kinds of loss or disruption.

Loss of livelihood, including:

— loss of capacity through physical disability or emotional disturbance due to the disaster;

— loss of employment if the place of employment fails to reopen, or reopens only after a long delay;

— loss of tools, raw materials, family labour (through death or injury), or other workers, or markets for the self-employed artisan;

— loss of arable land (due to landslides, salt spray, flooding, a river shifting its course, desertification, etc.), livestock, seed or farming equipment;

— loss of boats, nets, other equipment, fishing grounds (due to silting, beach erosion, etc.), or markets for fish;

— loss of access to common resources such as pastures, forests, wetlands used for gathering fuel or fodder, or for obtaining craft materials, etc.;

— loss of access to public resources such as tenancy on an irrigation scheme, a government contract, etc., as a result of physical damage to public installations, bureaucratic disruption, or emergency reallocation of government funds to disaster relief;

— indebtedness as a result of coping with a disaster, attempts to replace any one of the livelihood items mentioned, or attempts to rebuild a house; likelihood that indebtedness will cause a further loss of resources (through distress sale of land or animals, mortgaging of crops, etc.).

Loss of social cohesion, owing to:

— multiple deaths in a family;

— separation of family members;

— being a refugee or a displaced person;

— loss of status in the neighbourhood, community, or family as a result of relying on support from outsiders;

— the weakening or destruction of a community-based organization, such as a cooperative, trade union, women's group, or mutual aid group;

— loss of political influence at the municipal, state/regional, or national level because of deaths of party leaders, damage to party property, etc.

Loss of cultural identity, owing to:

— the destruction of significant cultural sites, places of worship, or religious objects;

— the death of an important cultural/religious leader in the disaster;

— the disruption of important cultural rites because of the disaster and its aftermath (e.g. the site of celebration has become inaccessible, or it is impossible to gather the necessary number of people to perform the rite);

— the minority status of the culture among refugees or displaced persons;

— the need to violate food taboos or other cultural norms to survive in the aftermath of a disaster;

— dependence on the government or outside donors for long periods of time, with the consequent erosion of self-confidence and initiative.

For information on the rehabilitation of livelihoods in Somalia and on the importance of cultural values in successful resettlement, see Boxes 5.4 and 5.5, respectively.

5.2.4 Secondary vulnerability assessment

The various kinds of losses discussed above under the headings of livelihood, social cohesion and cultural identity can create new vulnerability to future disasters or make exist-

Box 5.4 **Rehabilitation of livelihood in Somalia**[1]

During 1993 there was sufficient stability in Somalia to allow a dramatic improvement in support for sustainable livelihoods. The settled agropastoral people in the interriverine zone in the south of the country were provided with seed and implements to begin farming again. Marketing infrastructure was also re-established. A major veterinary campaign was launched to immunize livestock, and water points were rehabilitated. These economic measures were complemented by the reconstruction of basic health care and education infrastructure and the re-establishment of local government.

[1] Source: Wisner (1993).

Box 5.5 **Importance of cultural values in successful resettlement**

Oliver-Smith (1991) reviewed a series of post-earthquake resettlement attempts in Guatemala, the Islamic Republic of Iran, Peru and Turkey. He found that site, layout, housing type and popular input were significant variables in explaining success or failure of the scheme. Besides the physical properties of the site, cultural values that differed from group to group were important in defining acceptable layout, housing and the mode of community participation.

Resettlement can dramatically change a way of life. For example, Skopje, Yugoslavia, was a closely-knit city with a strong mediaeval Ottoman heritage before the 1963 earthquake. Reconstruction converted it into a low-density, linear city, 24 km long, changing the lifestyle of its citizens for ever (Davis, 1975). In other cases, efforts have been made to preserve the identity of settlements during post-disaster reconstruction (Alexander, 1993).

ing vulnerability worse. Failure to recover, or partial recovery, makes it more likely that people will be more vulnerable to the next stressful situation. Recovery planning must therefore identify such people (or groups) and meet their needs for rehabilitation and reconstruction.

5.3 Recovery planning

The answers to the questions raised in the previous section do not constitute a restoration "plan" by themselves. They relate to only a few of a very large number of subsectors of critical importance for restoration and sustainable development. Even complete answers to all possible policy questions would not constitute a plan, although that is precisely what many published restoration "plans" actually look like.

A thorough evaluation of the relief response up to the point at which recovery planning begins may reveal that secondary damage to livelihoods, social cohesion, or cultural integrity have been left unaddressed or even unintentionally made worse. In addition, a survey of peoples' responses to such secondary damage may reveal coping mechanisms that can be reinforced or encouraged during recovery.

In many countries, a specific governmental body is created for the purposes of coordinating and directing rehabilitation and reconstruction. Elsewhere, an ad hoc task force consisting of officials from a number of ministries takes this responsibility. In yet others, it is the national counter-disaster agency that also coordinates recovery. Whatever the organizational form adopted, it is essential to ensure close liaison between the body responsible for recovery and that concerned with disaster management (hazard assessment, preparedness, warning, relief, etc.). Decisions taken in the course of recovery (e.g. the decision to resettle a large number of people in a new site) could themselves create serious hazards. As noted above, observed patterns of community self-help during the relief phase are highly relevant to the design of recovery programmes.

It is also necessary to guarantee that the body responsible for recovery is represented and has a strong voice in all routine economic planning and can review all major economic decisions and comment on their possible effects on hazard vulnerability. For example, it makes little sense for the recovery agency to provide loans to farmers to produce grain for the national market if, with no prior consultation, a different planning commission decides to import a large quantity of grain.

Finally, post-disaster recovery requires true community involvement in planning and implementation, based on close consultation between planners, policy-makers and the communities concerned. For example, the affected population must be strongly represented on the body that directs recovery. People will have begun their own individual family and community "programmes" for recovery long before the officially designated body meets for the first time. Such local initiatives are healthy signs of adjustment and coping with the post-disaster situation. They should be incorporated, coordinated, and extended as part of the recovery planning process. As a minimum, these self-help activities should be the starting point for a dialogue between planners and the people concerned. However, it should not be assumed that such activities, carried out under severe resource constraints, represent all that people could do to satisfy their desires or commitments for the future. The people affected by recovery plans must be equals in the planning process. The process of participatory planning was discussed in Section 3.5.

5.4 Recovery in different contexts

Recovery commonly takes place in two very different situations. The first is that of self-sheltering populations (i.e. those that have sought short-term public shelter, but have remained in or near their original homes and sites of livelihood activity no matter how severely damaged these may be). The second is that of populations living in longer-term camps for displaced persons or refugees.

5.4.1 Self-sheltering or short-term evacuees

In this situation, livelihood options may be severely affected, but social cohesion and cultural identity are probably less so. Short-term evacuees will quite probably be far advanced in self-help activities, and there are also likely to be a variety of pre-existing community-based organizations and emerging self-help organizations active among them. Close consultation with representatives of the affected people is vital; they will often take the lead, making requests—sometimes quite detailed and professional— through their community organizations.

Financial credit and technical assistance are probably the most important things that an official recovery agency can provide. Means of ensuring financial accountability on the part of such organizations are a legitimate concern of the government, and they must be taken seriously and dealt with in good faith. Some legal assistance may be needed to control speculation and hoarding at a time when high land prices or monopoly pricing of building materials, replacement livestock, well-digging equipment, etc., could be a serious obstacle to self-help efforts. Likewise, assistance with questions of land tenure may be an appropriate role for the recovery agency.

5.4.2 Resettlement

Under many circumstances the worst possible plan is to resettle (i.e. permanently relocate) the people affected by a disaster. First, they are likely to resist such attempts; this has happened repeatedly in a variety of countries (see Box 5.6). Second, such resettle-

---

Box 5.6 People's resistance to resettlement

Resistance to resettlement is often mentioned in the literature. Cases come from many countries: Guatemala, Indonesia, Turkey, the United Republic of Tanzania and Yugoslavia. When people reluctantly move to a new site, they often drift back to the old one over a period of years (Oliver-Smith,1991; Pantelic, 1991). The town of Yungay, Peru, was totally destroyed in 1970 by a mudslide triggered by an earthquake. Some 4500 people died. However, there was a potent sense of solidarity among the 500 survivors, who demonstrated a strong will to rebuild their town despite government efforts to get them to settle elsewhere (Oliver-Smith, 1986b).

Box 5.7 Meeting the challenges of Mount Pinatubo: successful resettlement in the Philippines[1]

In 1991, Mount Pinatubo erupted, killing more than 900 people, destroying or damaging more than 100 000 houses, and displacing some 1.2 million people. A typhoon occurred during the eruption and torrential rains turned the *lahar* sand spewed from the volcano into massive mud flows.

The Philippine National Red Cross (PNRC) engaged in a huge relief effort, beginning with evacuations a few months before the major eruption.

During the recovery period, PNRC also undertook the resettlement of some of the displaced families in permanent new villages, placing the emphasis on sustainable livelihoods, assisted self-help housing, and infrastructure.

Livelihood opportunities included fish, pig, goat and poultry farming; vegetable, mushroom and orchid production; and garment making. Housing is being improved gradually by residents with basic building material provided by PNRC. For instance, in New Maligaya Red Cross Village, forest officials allowed settlers to cut trees killed by heavy ash fall from the volcano. These became the frames for their new houses. Infrastructure in the new villages included protected water supplies, health centres and schools. A variety of non-profit general stores, multipurpose cooperative societies and other economic institutions were also created.

These resettlement efforts were carried out in cooperation with various Philippine government ministries, local government, and private industry. One private company, the Zambales Electric Company, cooperated in extending electricity supplies to New Maligaya Village at the request of the local mayor and PNRC.

[1] Source: Belen (1992).

---

ment programmes are complex and costly. Their complexity means that a long time is needed to study and prepare them, after which the people are even less inclined to move. If people are moved without adequate planning and preparation, a great deal of economic hardship, disease and even loss of life can occur.

Resettlement has sometimes been strikingly successful, as in the Philippines in 1991, when people forced from homes on the slopes of Mount Pinatubo were helped to establish new livelihoods in a new location (see Box 5.7). However, failures generally outnumber the successes and there are always dangers and high costs. The population concerned may sometimes remain in place, but require income support and vocational training because the disaster has destroyed the livelihoods that previously supported them. Affected populations are sometimes able to use their political power to persuade governments to invest quite large sums in restoration or resettlement schemes.

5.4.3 Rehabilitation and reconstruction for long-term camp residents

Permanent options for residents of a camp are: to become economically independent and integrated with the host population; to return home; or to leave for some other destination (possibly a third country in the case of refugees).

UNHCR has often successfully provided refugees with land, tools, seeds, livestock, etc., and enabled them to establish local livelihoods. However, this is very difficult to achieve. Success depends on local culture, economic feasibility and political commitment. Recovery planners can probably be of most assistance in the economic sphere.

Refugees with essential skills may find well-paid employment locally, but many have little to offer but their labour power. Some become caught in a vicious circle of landlessness and low income. This can erode their already limited capacity for coping with future emergencies and increase their vulnerability.

Where there is much vacant land, arrangements can be made locally for its use by camp residents. If, throughout its history, the camp has shared facilities with the host population, such as a school, a health centre, or a water supply, it is more likely that such arrangements can be made.

The repatriation and resettlement of refugees at home is the second possibility. This requires assurances of security. Returnees may find that their property has been confiscated, or their claims to land and property disputed. They will certainly need considerable support to finance farms or small businesses. Even when international movements are the result of large-scale disasters, such as drought and desertification, return may still be sought by some refugees. A large investment in land restoration may then be required and recovery planning must be coordinated with overall economic plans in the country concerned (Scott, 1987).

Rehabilitation and reconstruction can also be applied to camp sites following the return of residents to their home communities. The water supplies, drainage and electrical distribution systems may sometimes be of value to nearby communities, and long-term sustainable development of the camp sites for agricultural, industrial, recreational, or educational purposes may be possible.

In Macedonia, following the return of Kosovar refugees to Kosovo in mid-1999, UNHCR was responsible for cleaning up and rehabilitating eight camp sites that had at one time held over 100 000 refugees. Most of the sites were either within or near villages and small towns. Following the return of the refugees, UNHCR held a series of meetings with local municipalities, national communities and international donors to encourage further development of the sites, using the infrastructure that remained. By the end of 1999, good progress had been made and development plans and funding commitments were available for at least one-half of the sites.

For further information on economic development by refugees, see: Christensen (1985); Kibreab (1985, 1987); and Harrell-Bond (1986).

Information on the linkage between resettlement and development in Mozambique is given in Box 5.8.

5.4.4 Chronic conflict situations

In situations of chronic disruption to livelihoods and to environmental health services because of conflict, there is no possibility of recovery and long-term sustainable development. In these situations, the affected communities remain vulnerable to the direct and indirect impacts of violence, including destruction of water-supply and sanitation infrastructure, or repeated displacement, both of which may make installation of permanent infrastructure inappropriate. The challenges facing environmental health agencies in these situations are great, but they may learn useful lessons from the affected communities themselves about strategies for operations that do not rely heavily on fixed

> **Box 5.8 Linking relief and development in Mozambique[1]**
>
> Following the 1992 peace accord, the focus of most aid programmes in Mozambique shifted from emergency relief to rehabilitation. Approximately 3 million internally displaced persons and 1.5 million refugees were assisted in returning to their home areas. Although many households rapidly restarted crop production, they remained vulnerable because basic services had not been rebuilt. Distributing cash was more appropriate in some cases than distributing a standard bundle of food, seeds, tools and selected household items. Cash allowances gave the returnees the ability to choose what they needed most and helped to revitalize the local economy.
>
> [1] Source: Whiteside, 1996.

material resources for their success. For instance, hygiene promotion activities; or community health-worker training that enables communities to make informed choices about selecting temporary water sources; or practicing simple diarrhoea management all maintain their value even when people are displaced or their settlements are damaged. However, sustainable improvements in environmental health can only be achieved in situations of peace and relative stability.

5.5 Post-disaster environmental health activities and sustainable development

5.5.1 Vulnerability reduction

A sustainable livelihoods approach to recovery focuses on encouraging the development of people's capacity through their access to food, cash and other basic resources and a corresponding reduction in their vulnerability to disasters. Sustainable livelihood security provides the resources that people will eventually use to improve their standards of housing, water supply, sanitation, food safety, dietary security and personal hygiene. Exposure to disease vectors and pests will also be expected to decline correspondingly. Improved nutrition will increase resistance to disease.

People with livelihood security will be less likely to live on a grossly hazardous site (steep, unconsolidated slope; frequently flooded area; low-lying, unprotected coastal areas prone to frequent storms, etc.). They will also have time to attend meetings and to become involved in community-based organizations that will represent their interests politically.

5.5.2 Specific implications of sustainable development in environmental health planning

This section is based on two premises about sustainable development. The first is that sustainable development is linked with economic growth (although the two are certainly not identical). If this is true, then where sustainable development occurs, average household disposable income should rise, allowing spending on improvements in water supply, sanitation and food safety. The pricing of such items and services is crucial. They cannot usually be fully subsidized, since the cost is difficult for governments to bear for a large population, but a sliding scale of subsidies may be considered, so that the lowest income earners are also able to make improvements. There may be substantial local or national economic activity generated by households' spending on sanitary improvements.

The second premise is that sustainable development stabilizes or even improves the ecological basis of livelihoods. If this is true, environmental health planners should be able to count on a number of direct and indirect positive effects of low-cost, "green" design and redesign of technology in rural and urban areas. For example, they will be able to count on more accessible water sources because the afforestation and protection of watersheds will raise groundwater levels and reduce sediment streams. Soil conservation should have a similar effect. The same activities reduce the risk of landslides, floods and strong winds (Pryor, 1982). Use of highly toxic agricultural pesticides and other agrochemicals should decline as farmers turn to integrated pest management and nitrogen fixation, composting and mixed farming for nutrient cycling. Thus, pesticide resistance in disease vectors would be expected to decline, as well as poisoning from the misuse of pesticides. These effects would be additional to the environmental improvement provided by design and engineering approaches to vector control.

The development of local renewable energy sources (solar, wind power, small-scale hydroelectric power plants) should make water pumping possible and have other indirect environmental health benefits, such as reduction of in-house air pollution. The production of methane (bio-gas) from animal manure as an energy source can have secondary sanitation benefits, in addition to providing cleaner and healthier cooking facilities.

Affordable and accessible rural energy supplies can also make possible a variety of food processing and preserving industries that can increase income, food security, and food safety. Rural energy supplies also make possible the lighting of houses at night, thus increasing the numbers attending continuing education, including adult literacy and health-education classes.

The combined effect of rising income and ecological improvement can jointly stimulate improvements in environmental health. Such improvement, in turn, could reinforce improvement in other sectors. The sum of all these improvements can be a residential and livelihood environment in which the frequency and impact of disasters decrease.

5.6 Further information

For further information on:

— the links between relief, recovery, and development, see: Fernandez (1979), Rubin & Barbee (1985), Anderson & Woodrow (1989), Quarantelli (1989), Pantelic (1991), Oliver-Smith (1992), Berke, Kartez & Wenger (1993), Voluntary Health Association of India (1993), International Federation of Red Cross and Red Crescent Societies (2001);

— the psychosocial aspects of disaster management, see: Quarantelli (1980), Lima (1986), Dynes, DeMarchi & Pelanda (1987), Butcher et al. (1988), Lystad (1988), World Health Organization (1989a), Austin (1992), Ignacio & Perlas (1994), World Health Organization (1996a), International Federation of Red Cross and Red Crescent Societies (1998);

— self-help reconstruction, see: Haas, Kates & Bowden (1977), Davis (1978), Kreimer (1979), Hardoy & Satterthwaite (1981), Turner (1982), United Nations Office of the Disaster Relief Co-ordinator (1982a), Cuny (1983), Skinner & Rodell (1983), Maskrey (1989), de M. Monzon (1990);

— the dangers of resettlement, see: Hansen & Oliver-Smith (1982), Harrell-Bond (1986), Cernea (1988), Clay et al. (1988).

PART II

Technical aspects

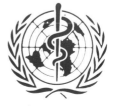

6. Shelter and emergency settlements

6.1 Introduction

The environmental health conditions faced by people are largely affected by the location and organization of the site where they are obliged to live in the days, weeks or months after a disaster. Security, the presence of a suitable water supply and the conditions necessary for adequate sanitation are probably the three most essential factors to consider when choosing and equipping, or improving a site for disaster-affected people. The quality of shelter available has a great impact on health and well-being. Environmental health managers and sector specialists such as water engineers should therefore be directly involved in decisions about selecting, equipping or upgrading emergency settlements and, in some cases, they may have to lobby hard to ensure that suitable sites are chosen. Once decisions have been taken and people settle, it becomes very difficult to move them to a better site.

When locating or planning emergency settlements, their long-term economic, social and environmental impacts on the surrounding area should be carefully considered.

Shelter needs may vary, depending on the nature of the disaster and the emergency situation created. This chapter considers the examples of: people who seek and organize their own temporary shelter; those who are obliged to take shelter in public buildings, offices etc; and those who are displaced to an unbuilt site where all shelter, water supply and sanitation facilities need to be provided.

6.2 Assistance to self-sheltering populations

After sudden disasters within limited areas, or where relatively few people are displaced by conflict, people generally house themselves. They find accommodation with neighbours or family members, or make temporary shelters within the ruins of their former homes. They will usually have found accommodation long before relief teams have begun to provide tents or other help. People are generally very reluctant to move away from their neighbourhoods following such a disaster. However, in extreme situations (e.g. very cold weather; the threat of explosion or toxic gas; possible secondary flooding or mass movement of debris) survivors should be evacuated.

In general, it is probably best to support the efforts of survivors to house themselves, through the following actions:

- Advising people attempting to house themselves in the ruins of their previous home on the structural integrity of what remains.
- Discouraging people from staying in homes that are definitely unsafe (e.g. in danger of collapse due to earthquake aftershocks); they should be informed of the danger and encouraged to move to a safer location.
- Providing as much assistance as possible when the ruins can be strengthened by reinforcement and temporary repairs. Timber, jacks, nails, tools and plastic sheeting and tarpaulins for temporary roofs or walls should be made available.
- Informing people who prefer not to evacuate a devastated neighbourhood about the nearest safe water supply or the measures that they can take to ensure the

safety of drinking-water (filtering, boiling, disinfecting, storing in closed contain-ers, etc.). Also, instructing them in the safe disposal of waste, including where and where not to defecate, and in the importance of oral rehydration therapy for chil-dren with diarrhoea, even if the available water is moderately contaminated.

- Informing people that water supplies may be contaminated. Surface water may be contaminated by sewage and debris in the wake of floods. Water from roof catch-ments may be contaminated by ash and dust that will have to be filtered out. Infor-mation about simple household methods of filtration, sedimentation, storage and disinfection should be provided (see Chapter 7).
- Distributing a stock solution of bleach or water chlorination tablets (e.g. sodium hypochlorite) at central pick-up points in each neighbourhood for home water disinfection. Careful instruction is required on the proper use of chlorine solu-tions and tablets, and this may be possible only where communities are well orga-nized and there is a history of good relations with the health authorities. Water purification tablets are an expensive option.
- Providing buckets for collecting water from a safe supply and containers with lids for storing it.
- Providing blankets and kerosene lanterns for illumination at night.
- Advising people on the status of sanitation systems, and providing temporary alter-native sanitation facilities if existing systems can no longer be used.

6.3 Short-term shelter in existing buildings

In many situations, such as in northern Iraq and several countries of Eastern Europe and the former Soviet Union during the 1990s, people may independently seek shelter in buildings such as schools, community centers, offices, sports facilities, and even railway carriages and wagons. Such buildings are often also used for organized short-term evac-uation centers.

The evacuation centre should be as close as possible to the neighbourhood or rural community concerned, but far enough from the disaster site to avoid secondary hazards. This avoids the additional stress and health dangers of a long journey, and enables survivors to have access to their former dwellings, which is psychologically important.

Buildings used as short-term reception areas should be thoroughly inspected by a suitably qualified person, to ensure that they are not structurally damaged, or sited near potential secondary hazards.

Such buildings will probably have at least some running water and toilets, and some may even have kitchens. For large numbers of people, however, these will have to be sup-plemented. Military barracks or youth camps are usually better equipped for large numbers of people, but have the disadvantage of often being sited further away from population centres.

Whatever the buildings used as temporary accommodation, it is very important that they are only used for a short period, and that they are cleaned and maintained inten-sively, to avoid a rapid deterioration in environmental health conditions.

The following points should be taken into consideration in relation to buildings used for temporary shelter (Assar, 1971; United Nations High Commissioner for Refugees, 1999; Sphere Project, 2000):

- People sleeping on beds or mats should have a minimum of 3.5 m² of floor area or 10 m³ of air space. In rooms with high ceilings, double bunk beds may be used.
- Beds or mats should be separated by a minimum distance of 0.75 metres.
- Adequate ventilation is required. The amount of fresh air needed is approximately 20–30 m³ per person per hour. It may be necessary to provide mechanical venti-

lation. Whenever possible, smoking and the use of cooking fires in the shelter should be strongly discouraged.

■ An ambient temperature of 15–19 °C is desirable, but lower temperatures can be tolerated with warm clothing. In cold climates, buildings may need extensive repairs and modifications for winter conditions, particularly in conflict situations where windows and insulation material may have been removed or destroyed.

■ To avoid very high temperatures in hot climates, buildings can be modified to increase shade, ventilation and thermal capacity.

■ Buildings should have emergency exits and fire escapes; the flues of stoves used for space heating should extend outside the building; overloading of electrical circuits should be avoided; lanterns and lamps should be placed or suspended so as to avoid dangers; and liquid fuels should be stored outside the building. Clear instructions on fire hazards and safety practices should be displayed in conspicuous places and drawn to the attention of residents; fire-fighting equipment should be available and properly maintained. A group of volunteers from among the survivors should be taught about the possible fire hazards and trained in the use of fire-fighting equipment.

■ Access to sufficient water for drinking, cooking, and personal and domestic hygiene should be provided.

■ One wash basin should be provided for every 10 people, or 4–5 metres of wash-bench for every 100 people; there should be separate benches for men and women, and waste receptacles at each bench. One shower head is needed for every 50 people in temperate climates and one for every 30 people in hot climates. Floors must be disinfected daily.

■ Arrangements must be made for human waste disposal. Water-flushed toilets may be available in existing buildings if the water supply has not been interrupted. Outside latrines should be located within 50 metres of the building, but at least 20 metres away from the kitchen, dining hall and water supply.

■ One refuse bin of capacity 50–100 litres should be provided for every 12–15 people. The bins should have tightly fitting lids. Special arrangements for the collection of refuse may be needed if the normal collection service is interrupted.

6.4 Site selection and arrangement of emergency settlements

When existing buildings are not available, one possibility is to use tents or makeshift shelters made of plastic sheets, tarpaulins, or local materials, such as palm thatch, in a secure location where water, sanitation and food can be provided. Emergency settlements for refugees and displaced people need to be established rapidly. However, they may be in service for months or even years, and it is usually impossible to know at the outset of an emergency how long the emergency settlement will exist. Therefore, the measures listed below are designed to provide healthy living conditions for disaster-affected people in both the short term and the long term. Specific long-term issues are discussed in Section 6.5.

The requirements that ensure that temporary camps are healthy environments are considered below (Assar, 1971; United Nations High Commissioner for Refugees, 1999; Sphere Project, 2000).

■ The site should be free of major water-related hazards such as malaria, onchocerciasis (river blindness), schistosomiasis (bilharzia) and trypanosomiasis (sleeping sickness). If these diseases are endemic, care should be taken to avoid or control vector habitats and provide personal protection against mosquitoes, blackflies, tsetse flies, etc.

■ The topography of the land should permit easy drainage and the site should be located above flood level. Rocky, impermeable soil should be avoided. Land covered with grass will prevent dust, but bushes and excessive vegetation can harbour insects, rodents, reptiles, etc., and should be avoided or cleared. Wherever possible, steep slopes, narrow valleys, and ravines should be avoided. Ideally, the site should have a slope of 2–4% for good drainage, and not more than 10% to avoid erosion and the need for expensive earth-moving for roads and building construction.

■ Whenever possible, the area should be naturally protected from adverse weather conditions.

■ Areas adjacent to commercial and industrial zones, exposed to noise, odours, air pollution and other nuisances should be avoided.

■ Areas sufficiently close to blocks or rows of shelters should be identified for sanitation and waste management. The residential area of the camp should face the prevailing wind to avoid odours from latrines.

■ There should be ample space for the people to be sheltered and for all the necessary public facilities such as roads, firebreaks (areas without buildings and with little or no flammable vegetation) and service areas (30 m² per person, or 45 m² per person allowing for small gardens, but not for full-scale agricultural activities). Areas for public spaces, markets, etc. should be defined from the beginning.

■ Food distribution areas should be organized so as to create safe conditions for people collecting food, as well as for those distributing it.

■ To facilitate the management and control of communicable diseases, camps should hold no more than 10 000–12 000 people, or should be subdivided into independent units of no more than 1000 people.

■ Drainage ditches should be dug around the tents or other shelters and along the sides of roads, especially if there is a danger of flooding. Care should be taken to lead water away from shelters, latrines, health centres, and stores. Persistent areas of stagnant water that are difficult to drain can be backfilled, or covered with polystyrene balls or a thin layer of oil, to control insects. Water points should also have adequate drainage to avoid mud.

■ The site should be provided with at least two access roads for reasons of security and to reduce the risk of the site being cut off due to floods or other problems with roads.

■ The surface of roads can be sprinkled with water to keep dust down. Sullage wastewater can sometimes be used to keep down dust on dirt or gravel roads. Restricting traffic and imposing speed limits can also help to reduce dust.

■ Shelters should be arranged in rows or in clusters of 10–12 on both sides of a road at least 10 metres wide to permit easy traffic flow and access by ambulances or firefighting vehicles. In tented areas, there should be at least 2 metres between the edge of the road and the tent pegs.

■ Built-up areas should be divided by 30 metres wide firebreaks approximately every 300 metres. Firebreaks can be used for locating roads and recreation areas.

■ Shelters should be spaced 8 metres apart so that people can pass freely between them without being obstructed by pegs and ropes. This spacing also helps to prevent the spread of fire. If this is not possible owing to a lack of space, the distance between shelters should preferably be at least twice the overall height of each shelter, and should never be less than 2 metres. A separation greater than 8 metres may lead to open defecation and should be avoided.

■ There should be a minimum of 3.5 m² per person inside the shelter in warm climates where cooking is done outside, and 4.5–5.5 m² per person in cold climates where cooking is done inside the shelter.

■ Shelters may be tents or prefabricated units, or may be built out of plastic sheeting together with timber, stone and thatch. Where plastic sheeting is used, it is common to provide one piece, 4 metres by 6–7 metres, per household.

- Small shelters with few occupants are preferable to large shelters with many occupants.
- In cold weather, kerosene stoves or other heating appliances should be provided and people should be instructed in their use; every precaution must be taken to prevent fires and explosions.
- In the absence of electric lighting, wind-proof kerosene or oil lamps, or battery-operated lanterns, should be provided for lighting shelters, toilets and roads.
- Natural ventilation should normally be adequate for temporary shelters such as tents.
- The site chosen should be within reasonable distance of an ample source of good water and, ideally, near some high ground from which water can be distributed by gravity; water sources should gradually be improved and protected once basic needs are satisfied. No one should have to walk more than 500 metres to a water point, and there should be at least one water point for every 250 people.
- Where there is no piped water, water tanks should be installed on both sides of the road (see also Chapter 7).
- Refuse bins should be provided (see also section 8.5).
- Latrines or other facilities for excreta disposal should be provided (at least one toilet per 20 people), and gradually improved as time and resources allow. The dangers of indiscriminate defecation should be emphasized in health education. See Chapter 8 for information on emergency excreta disposal. Maintenance of toilets must be given priority in health education and camp organization (see also section 8.3).
- Bathing, laundry and disinfection facilities should be provided, and health education should emphasize the importance of frequent hand-washing. One double-sided ablution bench (3 metres long) should be provided for every 50 people (see Chapter 7).
- The camp site should be cleaned regularly according to a prearranged schedule. Participation by camp residents in the cleaning of the camp should be encouraged. Young residents can be organized into teams responsible for cleaning and reporting possible health and environment problems.
- Separate accommodation is necessary for unaccompanied children, with provision for adults (welfare staff and/or community volunteers) to stay with them; there should be at least one adult per shelter or room. These children may be very disoriented and frightened, and may also have special nutritional needs (United Nations Children's Fund, 1986). The shelters should be situated near the nutritional rehabilitation centre and field hospital, and as far from sources of secondary hazards, noise and contamination as possible.
- In conflict- and famine-related disasters, many people may be suffering from malnutrition and debilitation when they arrive, so specialized services such as intensive or therapeutic feeding may be needed. Intensive feeding or nutrition rehabilitation units should be provided with up to 15–30 litres of potable water per bed per day. Also, special care needs to be given to latrines and other waste-disposal facilities used by parents, children and staff. Means for hand-washing by all staff and parents concerned with child feeding are also important. For the design and management of therapeutic feeding units, see World Health Organization (2000a).

6.5 Longer-term issues for emergency settlements

When emergency settlements exist for more than a few weeks, a number of social, environmental and health issues need to be considered to ensure that the health and well-being of the settlement population are sustained and that long-term costs of maintaining the settlement infrastructure and services are kept under control. Some of the short-term risks to health may be managed during the emergency phase, but when communities are obliged to remain in emergency settlements for a long time, a number of psychosocial and other health problems associated with alienation, overcrowding, and loss of control and purpose, demand special attention.

Longer-term settlements need more sustainable and durable water-supply and waste-disposal systems, laundries and wastewater facilities. As far as possible, these facilities should be designed and constructed so that local authorities and local residents can maintain them with a minimum of external resources. Regular monitoring and repair schedules need to be established and managed.

The need for recreational facilities may become greater. The safety of areas where children play must be ensured. If a stream or lake offers the opportunity for swimming or water sports, community volunteers should act as lifeguards.

Children should be prevented from entering dangerous parts of the camp or its environment, and encouraged to use recreational areas with swings, seesaws and other amenities that can be easily made from locally available materials. Fences should exclude all camp residents from dangerous areas, e.g. those where fuel and pesticides are stored.

In longer-term camps, schools, places of worship, workshops, bakeries, etc., may be planned or grow up spontaneously. Care should be taken to provide them with appropriate and adequate water-supply, sanitation and drainage systems.

Where camp inhabitants spontaneously set up workshops or carry out commercial activities—a sign of social and emotional health and much to be encouraged—care should be taken to ensure that there are no health hazards, such as smoke or fire from a bakery or pottery, liquid effluent, and flies from an abattoir or butchery. It may be best to zone the camp so that such activities are confined to an industrial quarter.

6.6 Community participation in environmental health management

Community participation is the key to success in camp management and in preparedness planning and health education. Enabling people to participate in the decision-making process and implementation of environmental health measures is an important part of empowerment and building resilience.

Committees, including representatives of camp inhabitants and camp authorities, should be set up to involve residents in issues such as camp management, land use, health, water supply and sanitation. In this way, the needs and views of those living in the camp can be voiced in an organized forum. Difficulties in such matters as the distribution of water, or the taste of treated water, can quickly be brought to the attention of the health authorities, and the committee can suggest solutions. This participatory approach is much more likely to be effective in finding solutions than a centralized, top-down approach.

Participation also empowers the inhabitants, who are in danger of becoming passive, dependent and depressed in a camp environment. The camp will, in effect, become their home for some time. Participation in decisions about the layout of the camp and the gradual improvement of the facilities can increase residents' sense of being at home.

It is very important to ensure that the women in the camp are adequately represented on the camp health committee. Special arrangements may have to be made to involve women in decision-making, even where they are not normally seen in public or involved in public affairs.

Basic sanitation regulations (e.g. those concerning the disposal of wastes, the times and places for various uses of streams or other water sources, etc.) should be discussed with the health and land-use committee. In this way, it is more likely that people will cooperate and that conflict will be minimized.

6.7 Further information

For further information on:

— site selection and layout, see: United Nations Children's Fund (1986), Delmas & Courvallet (1994), Shook & Englande (1992), Good (1996b), Jensen (1996), Chalinder (1998), Adams (1999), United Nations High Commissioner for Refugees (1999), Sphere Project (2000), Davis & Lambert (2002);

— shelter, see: Davis (1981), Howard & Spice (1981), United Nations Office of the Disaster Relief Co-ordinator (1982b), Médecins Sans Frontières (1997b), United Nations High Commissioner for Refugees (1999), Sphere Project (2000), Davis & Lambert (2002).

7. Water supply

7.1 Water-supply preparedness and protection

Water-supply problems arise in all phases of the disaster-management cycle. As with all other elements of emergency management, water supplies can be designed and maintained in ways that help to reduce the health impacts of disasters.

It is useful to distinguish between large-scale, formal water-supply systems (e.g. urban water-supply systems) and small-scale, scattered supplies. The distinction is not so much between urban and rural areas, as one based on the level of technology and the institutional arrangements for management, maintenance, and protection. Whether the affected systems are rural or urban, sanitation surveys may be necessary to identify the main health hazards (World Health Organization, 1997a).

Water sources are exposed to a variety of hazards that may damage or contaminate them, but they can be protected against disasters to some extent. This section is concerned mainly with ways in which improvements to existing water supplies can make them more resistant to damage.

7.1.1 Establishing and protecting small-scale decentralized supplies

Kinds of damage to small-scale water supplies

Roof catchment systems are often damaged by wind in tropical storms. People who depend on canals are vulnerable to chronic and acute pesticide poisoning or, where the canal drains an industrial zone, poisoning from the release of toxic chemicals. Unlined canals may also be easily washed away or broken during floods, so cutting water supplies. Shallow wells in areas with a high water-table are more prone to contamination from flooding than are deep boreholes. They may also dry up sooner in a drought. Hillside springs may be destroyed in a landslide. Wells near rivers can be contaminated and filled with sand during unusual flash flooding. All piped systems are subject to breaks and disruption during earthquakes, landslides or civil strife. Dug wells and boreholes are particularly vulnerable during wars, since bodies or toxic materials can be dumped in wells, and borehole pumps sabotaged.

Routine forms of protection

In all activities to provide or improve water supplies during "normal" times, it is important that those responsible are aware of the specific hazards to which water sources might be subject. This hazard mapping should be as much a part of the planning of water-supply systems as other factors, such as water quality and taste, distance to users, and capital and recurrent costs.

Simple modifications in design can sometimes help to protect the water source from an extreme natural event or industrial accident. For instance, flexible plastic pipe is more resistant than rigid pipe to earth tremors.

Some basic improvements, such as raising the head wall of a dug well, and providing a cover and outward-sloping concrete apron around it, simultaneously provide additional protection from contamination due to floods and run-off into the open hole, and short-circuit seepage from nearby puddles; they also prevent contamination by debris and animals falling into the well.

If the surface or groundwater could be affected by toxic hazards, it is probably better to avoid the water source. Providing an alternative water source should then be a high priority.

Need for consultation with water users

Many people use multiple sources of water. Some will prefer certain sources for drinking-water and others for laundry, bathing, watering animals and irrigation.

Wherever a hazard, or the potential for disruption of the water supply, exists, the primary health-care workers or other development personnel should discuss alternative drinking-water sources with the people concerned. These discussions should take place before an emergency arises. A delegation from the local health committee or safety committee should visit the alternative sources regularly to check on their status. Where recent improvements in water supply have resulted in former sources being abandoned, the committee may want to discuss the desirability of providing some minimal maintenance at the old site to preserve it for use in an emergency.

There should also be local contingency plans for rapidly ensuring the safety of such reserve sources of drinking-water. These will usually involve stockpiling a limited amount of chemicals to disinfect the source (taking into consideration the shelf-life of these chemicals), plus fencing to exclude animals. Depending on the economic base of the community or neighbourhood concerned, the discussion may go on to consider the provision of alternative or reserve water for livestock, small-scale industry, or irrigation; however, the first priority should always be water for drinking, cooking and personal hygiene.

7.1.2 Establishing and protecting large-scale, centralized supplies

Types of hazard

The location of sources and the design of water-supply systems are critical in emergency and disaster preparedness. Hazards to catchments (e.g. forest fires or chemical contamination), reservoirs (drought, earthquake, contamination, landslides), pumping and treatment plants (flood, earthquake, fire, explosion, chlorine gas leaks), as well as to the distribution system (earthquake, flooding), need to be taken into account in siting, design and contingency planning. Sabotage may pose a hazard to all stages of a water-supply system.

Strengthening existing systems

Weak points in distribution systems, such as river crossings, open canals, landslide scars, etc., or places where pipes cross earthquake faults, should be strengthened (see Figure 7.1). Low-lying, flood-prone facilities can be raised or protected with levees or bunds. Reserve electrical generators can be provided if necessary, as well as a stock of pre-positioned replacement pumps and pipes for emergency repairs. Standardization of pumps, pipes and fittings, etc. is important, so that spares and equipment can be sent as temporary replacements from an unaffected town.

Systems based on rapid sand filtration can be made less vulnerable to disasters by appropriate staff training and by including emergency provisions at the planning stage that will help cope with prolonged high turbidity, power failures and shortages of chemicals. Emergency provisions include extra stocks of chemicals, stand-by power generators and emergency prefiltration storage/sedimentation capacity.

Figure 7.1 **Reinforcement of water pipes crossing streams or gullies[1]**

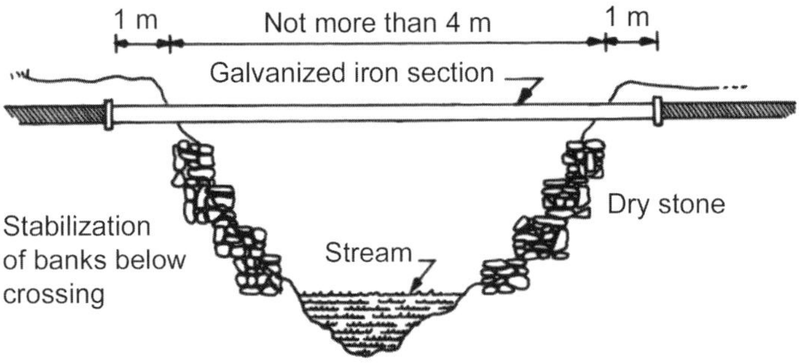

[1] Sources: American Water Works Association (1984), Jordan (1984).

Staff should be rigorously trained in the action to be taken in an emergency to assess the state of the water-supply system and to restore and ensure its integrity from the standpoint of health and the environment.

Long-term investment decisions

Long-term design and investment decisions should also take into account the possibility of disaster. For instance, slow sand filters, which can be adequate even for large cities (e.g. London and Amsterdam), are less vulnerable than other treatment systems to hazards, such as interruption of chemical supplies and power supplies (Pickford, 1977). Decisions on routing water-transmission mains and distribution networks should also take into account the possibility of damage due to natural causes, such as earthquakes and landslides, and to sabotage.

7.1.3 Preparation for displacement emergencies

When a risk of population displacement is identified in the vulnerability assessment (see Section 3.3), steps should be taken to prepare for such an event, taking into account the likelihood of displacement, the likely numbers of displaced people, displacement routes, and likely destinations. Preparedness measures may include: identifying water sources along displacement routes and at potential temporary settlements; pre-positioning stocks of lightweight water equipment (pumps, flexible reservoirs, pipes and taps) and supplies (fuel and water treatment chemicals); identifying and training staff; and holding discussions with local communities along displacement routes about access to water sources. During a large population movement, it may be very difficult to move staff and equipment along the congested roads, so it is important to establish a local response capacity.

7.2 Emergency water-supply strategy

7.2.1 Situations demanding an emergency water-supply response

Short-term water-supply needs and emergency measures may differ in the following types of situations:

— short-term emergencies affecting rural or unserved periurban communities;
— short-term emergencies in urban situations where a central water service is available;
— short-term emergencies involving population displacement and temporary shelters;

— long-term displacement emergencies that result in semipermanent emergency settlements.

These situations are considered in turn in sections 7.2.3–7.2.7.

7.2.2 Emergency response strategy

Priorities

The first priority is to provide an adequate quantity of water, even if its quality is poor, and to protect water sources from contamination. A minimum of 15 litres per person per day should be provided as soon as possible (Sphere Project, 2000), though in the immediate post-impact period, it may be necessary to limit treated water to a minimum of 7 litres per day per person (United Nations High Commissioner for Refugees, 1992a). If this is the case, then people may use an untreated water source for laundry, bathing, etc. Water-quality improvements can be made over succeeding days or weeks.

The main public health priority is usually to provide a basic water supply to the affected population. It is often better to organize separate human and material resources for providing water supplies for hospitals, nutrition centers, etc., so that work on the general water supply is not delayed. Hospitals will soon be swamped with cases of water-related disease if the general water supply is not sufficient. However, priorities should be defined for each situation, on the basis of an assessment (see Section 7.3).

Gradual improvement of water supplies

In all situations, a successful emergency response in the water-supply sector depends on improvisation and gradual improvement of water supplies, progressing from basic services during the emergency and recovery phases, to more sustainable services in the long term, when installations should be more robust and less vulnerable to disasters. These improvements should be incremental, wherever possible. In other words, emergency measures should be designed and implemented in such a way that they can be built upon later. However, this may not be possible, and temporary measures that require complete replacement after weeks or months may be required, such as the use of lightweight petrol pumps and flexible tanks.

Assessment, monitoring and review

The most effective emergency water supply measures are ensured through a process of assessment, monitoring and review. Assessment is required to identify needs, damage and resources, so as to be able to respond appropriately and with maximum impact; monitoring of activities and the context is essential to ensure that the water supply activities are carried out as planned, with timely indications of problems and unmet needs; and periodic reviews of the situation and the response are essential to ensure that the response remains relevant to the needs and resources of the communities affected by the disaster. Assessment of damage, resources and needs in the water-supply sector is discussed in Section 7.3.

Hygiene promotion and participation

The emergency water-supply response should be carried out with, or as part of, a hygiene promotion programme that works with the affected population to respond to disasters to reduce risk, increase resilience and mitigate the impact of disasters on health. This should ensure the design and maintenance of water systems that meet the needs of all the groups involved, including women, the elderly, children and the disabled. Opportunities for participation should be sought in assessment, monitoring and review, as well as in programme design and implementation. See Chapter 15 for more information on hygiene promotion and participation.

7.2.3 Rural emergencies

Rural communities are usually less vulnerable than urban communities to disruption of water supplies in disasters, as their supplies are generally decentralized and based on simple technology, and there are frequently alternative sources available. However, certain hazards, such as floods and droughts, may have a greater impact in rural areas than urban areas. This section is concerned principally with floods and droughts, although other hazards, such as earthquakes, landslides and conflict, may produce the same type of damage.

Floods

If the usual water source is not damaged or contaminated and is still safely accessible to the population, it is necessary only to monitor the source and react quickly to increased numbers of cases of diarrhoea. However, if the accustomed source is contaminated, commonly the case after floods, an alternative source should be sought or water should be chlorinated before consumption until the source can be disinfected and protected (see Section 7.4.3). In any case, preventive disinfection will help reduce the health risks associated with contaminated water.

Emergency repairs to damaged supplies may include repair or replacement of pumps; repair of spring catchments; repair of gravity supply pipes and distribution systems; and providing steel or plastic tanks to replace broken concrete reservoirs. It is common to find in rural areas that a significant proportion of water supply installations are out of order, owing to long-term problems with maintenance and repair. These installations may be brought back into service as part of the emergency response.

Droughts

Even if populations do not migrate in search of food during a prolonged drought, they will seek new or alternative sources of water. Diseases caused by water shortages, such as trachoma and scabies, increase during droughts. The incidence of diarrhoea and water-borne diseases such as cholera may also increase because of lack of water for washing, and intensive use of a small number of water supplies vulnerable to contamination. Drought itself can therefore constitute an emergency, even if reserves of cash, food and livestock are sufficient to avoid food shortages.

In droughts, water quantity is an absolute priority and health staff should cooperate with the government public works or water-supply departments, and with nongovernmental organizations and others involved, to ensure that attempts are made to increase the yield of existing water sources or to find additional ones.

During droughts, there is also often a problem of water quality, because of increased pressure on water sources that remain, many of which may be unprotected. Measures for protecting sources used for multiple purposes are described in Section 7.4.1.

Water trucking may be needed following disasters that affect rural water supplies, though this is more expensive and difficult to organize than in urban situations. See Section 7.4.4.

7.2.4 Emergency water-supply measures in urban areas

Damage likely

When urban water-supply systems are damaged, it is useful to distinguish between damage to water-distribution networks, damage to the source, and damage to the treatment and pumping facilities. Different components are susceptible to different hazards. In most earthquakes, for example, the following components of urban water-supply systems are usually damaged:

— house service connections;
— power supplies;
— control systems;
— trunk mains;
— service reservoirs;
— pumps and treatment plants.

Priority should be given to identifying areas of the city in which water supplies have been disrupted or contaminated, but which do not have alternative local sources, as well as periurban populations that are not normally served by central distribution, but are nevertheless in need of water because of the disaster. Special measures may need to be taken to ensure continued water supply to prisons and hospitals.

Damage to chlorine gas storage facilities may pose an extreme danger and require the evacuation of the surrounding area. Well-trained staff with specialist equipment are needed to deal with this.

Meeting immediate needs

Such areas and populations will need emergency supplies trucked to distribution points or piped in from unaffected areas. An alternative to trucking water into these areas or to providing emergency piped connections is to use mobile purification units connected to the nearest untreated source (see Section 7.4.4).

Alternative temporary water sources and treatment plants may sometimes be available from dairies, soft-drink bottling plants, breweries, or even large swimming pools (see Box 7.1).

In urban areas, it may be necessary to ration or restrict water use while repairs are being made, to ensure that the available water is being used according to agreed priorities. These priorities should be decided on the basis of an assessment, and should be discussed and agreed with agencies working in related sectors, such as health, water supply, sanitation and public works. Where water rationing is required, it is essential that water users are informed of the reasons for this, and the way in which the rationing system is to work.

Where sanitation relies on water-borne systems, relatively large quantities of water may need to be provided quickly, to ensure that those systems function, otherwise a sanitation crisis is likely.

Rapid repairs to urban water systems

If the water-treatment plant or pumping stations are flooded, the flood water should be pumped out and equipment cleaned and disinfected. Damaged mains and feeders should be repaired as quickly as possible. The quick coupling and plastic patching of pipes, and the use of accelerators in concrete and cement can speed repairs, but technicians in the water company need to have practised these techniques (hence the necessity of training exercises). It is also sometimes possible to bypass damaged sections. Good records, maps of the system, and a good stock of spare parts and tools are also essential.

> Box 7.1 **Water emergency in Puerto Limón, Costa Rica**
>
> In 1991, an earthquake affected the Atlantic coast and hinterland of Costa Rica. Water mains were broken in the coastal town of Puerto Limón, and landslides increased the sediment and turbidity of the Banano river which supplied water to the town's water-treatment plant. Within 8 hours of the earthquake a team of water engineers from the national water company (AYA) decided on twin approaches to the urgent problem of providing the town of 40 000 people with water. Contact was made with a major soft-drinks bottling company in San José, the capital. The management agreed to convert its entire plant to filling 2-litre bottles with clean water. Within 18 hours of the earthquake, the first planeload of bottled water arrived, and the local plant requested additional plastic bottles from Miami. In all, some 130 000 litres were provided during the first three days.
>
> Simultaneously, work began damming a small creek, about 3 km from the water company's pumping station. This source was not affected by landslides and sediment. Although there was no road, access was gained by four-wheel drive vehicles up the stream bed. Temporary pipe was laid above ground to bring this new water supply to the pumping station. From there, water could be pumped to the treatment plant which had not been seriously damaged by the earthquake. Treated water was then distributed by tanker truck to the town until water mains were excavated and repaired. People reused the bottles that had been provided. During the critical first few weeks, 20% of water requirements came from springs that had been unaffected and 80% from the Banano River.
>
> Within 60 days, additional water was added from wells drilled along the course of the main pipe from the treatment plant to the town and fed directly into the system; 120 breaks in the main pipelines had been repaired; and service was available for 6 hours a day. Within 90 days, another 200 breaks in the distribution network had been repaired, and deeper wells had been dug to supplement supplies from the new diversion works on the Banano River.

After repairs, the new sections of pipe should be disinfected by filling them with a strong chlorine solution (100 mg/l) for one hour, or a weaker solution for a longer period (e.g. 50 mg/l for 24 hours), and then flushed through with treated water before being put back into service.

The review of water-system status should include catchments and reservoirs. Where a dam or reservoir wall has been badly damaged and is dangerous, the reservoir should be partly or completely drained.

Following floods and damage to sewerage systems, it is wise to ensure a continuous water supply with adequate pressure and to increase the free residual chlorine level to as high as 1 mg/l to prevent contamination through the entry of polluted water into the distribution system. This high level of free residual chlorine should be a short-term measure that is discontinued as soon as flood-waters have receded and the risk is reduced.

In general, emergency repairs should aim to restore conditions as nearly as possible to those that existed before the disaster, rather than attempt any substantial upgrading of the service. However, the real risks of a cessation of funding after the initial repairs have been made should also be taken into account. In addition, any opportunity should be taken to incorporate into the system some basic protection against similar disasters and other local hazards.

7.2.5 Supplies for affected periurban areas

There may also be a large demand for water in areas of a town or city that have not previously been served by the water company. The short-term methods adopted to meet these needs may be similar to those described above for rural areas (i.e. existing sources should be repaired and disinfected; and water should be trucked in if nothing else can be done, etc.). However, the emergency can be an opportunity to develop new water sources for an unserved urban population. This is an incremental improvement that contributes to longer-term vulnerability reduction. See Section 7.4.1 for a description of water sources.

Failing all other means of providing safe water, residents should be advised on how to treat water in the home when this is realistic, using one of the methods described in Section 7.4.3.

7.2.6 Short-term displacement and temporary shelters

Providing emergency water supplies to people during their displacement and while they are in temporary shelters, such as transit camps, is made easier if prior preparedness measures have been taken (see Section 7.1.3). However, it is often impossible to prepare for displacements, and staff are obliged to respond without prior preparation. Where possible, existing and known water sources should be used to supply people on the move and in transit shelters. Temporary solutions, involving water trucking and lightweight, mobile equipment, are more appropriate than solutions designed for gradual improvement. The situation should be reviewed frequently to estimate likely numbers of people to be catered for, their health status, and the length of time they are likely to be in need of emergency water supplies.

7.2.7 Long-term emergency settlements

Long-term emergency settlements, such as refugee camps that may exist for several years, present specific challenges and opportunities. The potential for epidemics of enteric disease is higher in a weakened population living in crowded conditions for a considerable time, particularly in settlements that form spontaneously, without adequate site selection and planning (see Chapter 6). On the other hand, more time is available for gradual improvements in the water supply, as well as for intensive health promotion and training of water-supply staff and other health and environmental workers.

Early in the life of emergency settlements, when displaced people continue to arrive, often in large numbers and in a poor state of health, water supplies may be totally inadequate, and emergency systems need to be set up rapidly to reduce the risk of epidemics. As in other situations, priority should be given to providing the minimum quantity of water needed for drinking, cooking, and personal and domestic hygiene. In large settlements, while the distribution system is being constructed, people may need to travel to the water-treatment installation to collect water. As the distribution system is extended, water is brought gradually closer to peoples' shelters, so encouraging increased water consumption. Priorities for developing the system should be set according to unmet needs and the pattern of water-related disease in the settlement.

The techniques and equipment used for water-supply systems in emergency settlements are described in section 7.4. The emergency water equipment developed by a number of agencies, described in section 7.4.5, is particularly suitable for population displacements and emergency settlements.

7.3 Assessment

Following a disaster, an assessment of damage, available water resources and unmet needs enables staff to direct resources where they are most needed.

7.3.1 Assessment of damage and available water resources

In urban areas, a thorough assessment of the post-impact status of the entire water-supply system should be undertaken, while taking steps to meet the immediate, emergency water needs of the population. This assessment should consider the following types of damage:

— contamination of the water source and damage of the raw-water intake;
— damage to the water-treatment works, including structural damage, mechanical damage, loss of power supply and contamination due to flooding;
— damage to pumping stations;
— pressure failure in all or part of a water distribution network, allowing backflow;
— damage to both sewerage and water mains in the same locality, with local seepage into water pipes where the pressure is reduced;
— badly repaired plumbing in domestic or public buildings, resulting in back-siphonage;
— failure to disinfect a contaminated source correctly, or to maintain an adequate chlorine residual throughout the system.

In rural areas, the damage and resources assessment should be simpler, as installations are less complex. The following information on water resources is required:

— the current availability of supplies from all sources, the causes of supply problems (e.g. dry streams and wells, pipe breaks, dams empty, tanks damaged or silted up, roof catchments destroyed, etc.), and alternative sources and their status;
— the causes or indicators of contamination (e.g. human or animal bodies in the water, discoloration of the water, high turbidity, unusual smell, saltiness, diarrhoea or other possible water-related illnesses in the population).

Although simpler than urban assessments, rural damage and resources assessments usually take longer to carry out because of the distances involved. Information may be gathered by local health and community workers, using standardized procedures and reporting formats, to enable priorities to be set.

7.3.2 Needs assessment

An assessment of unmet needs is usually carried out at the same time as the assessment of damage and water resources, and by the same people. However, in urban situations, engineering staff may focus on assessing damage to infrastructure, while environmental health staff assess the degree of unmet need. In such cases, it is important that the two areas of assessment are well coordinated so that the information they provide can be usefully combined.

The unmet-needs assessment should identify the population affected by insufficient or contaminated water supplies; the quantity of water needed for various purposes (e.g. for drinking, other household uses, agriculture, livestock, industrial uses); how often it will be needed; and any additional treatment, storage and distribution facilities needed.

Figure 7.2 shows a needs and resources assessment that covers all the general issues in planning an emergency water-supply system. The particular assessment in Figure 7.2 was developed for refugee emergencies, but something similar can be adapted for use in each country or region, and can provide a helpful guide for environmental health field teams.

Figure 7.2 **Needs and resources assessment: general considerations for planning an emergency water-supply system**

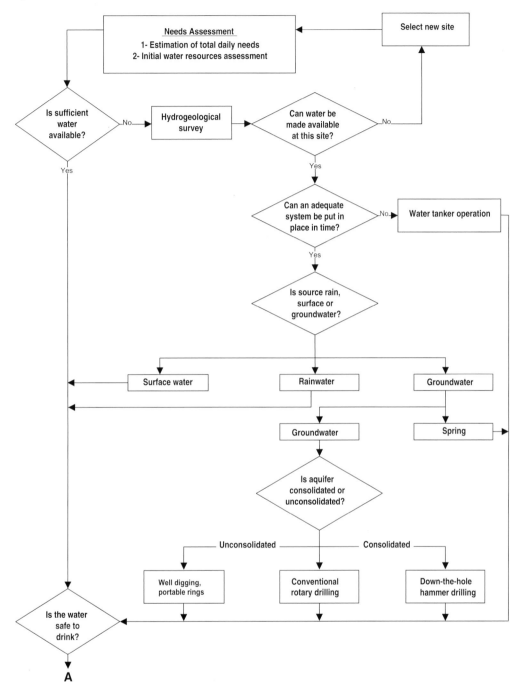

7.3.3 Needs and standards

When designing an emergency response, it is important to set objectives that are based on both general and specific agreements about needs. A number of agencies have been using standards for general guidance in setting targets for emergency water-supply interventions for many years.

For example, the minimum personal allowance of water for drinking, cooking and hygiene is set by the United Nations High Commissioner for Refugees (1992a) at 7 litres per day per person over a short emergency period. In most situations, however, water needs are much higher, as follows:

Figure 7.2 **(Continued)**

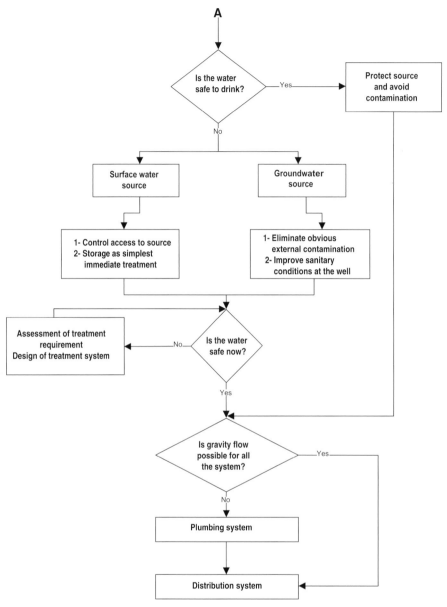

Reproduced, with permission, from: United Nations High Commissioner for Refugees (1999).

— for the general population: 15–20 litres per day per person;
— for operating water-borne sewerage systems: 20–40 litres per day per person;
— in mass feeding centres: 20–30 litres per day per person;
— in field hospitals and first-aid stations: 40–60 litres per day per person;
— in mosques: 5 litres per visitor;
— for livestock accompanying displaced persons and refugees: 30 litres per day per cow or camel, and 15 litres per day per goat or other small animal.

More recently, the Sphere Project has identified broadly agreed standards for emergency water supply (Sphere Project, 2000).

In addition to the 3–5 litres per person per day required for drinking and cooking, an ample supply of water is essential for controlling the spread of water-washed diseases

Figure 7.3 **Water demand under normal and emergency conditions**

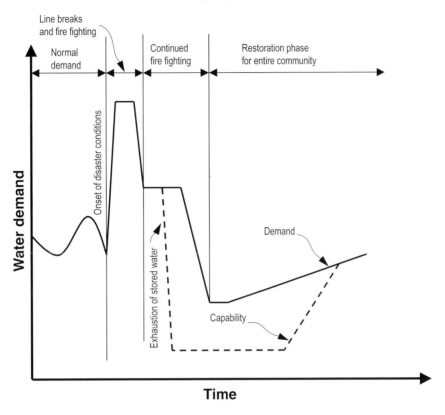

(diseases transmitted through lack of hygiene), even if the water supply does not meet WHO drinking-water quality guidelines or national standards.

The quantity of water needed by a community changes with time after the disaster. After a typical urban disaster, for example, there is a massive increase in water demand for fire fighting, and a gap between demand and supply capacity may occur when supplies of water stored in the treatment and supply system are exhausted (Figure 7.3).

7.4 Emergency water-supply techniques

7.4.1 Water sources

Site selection and water sources

A major factor in the choice of site for an emergency settlement should be the existence of reliable, good-quality water sources nearby. An inventory of the existing water sources should be made as part of the site-selection process. Permanent water-supply arrangements will depend on the length of time that the settlement is to be in use and the size of the population to be served. When existing water sources have been destroyed, new sources may also need to be selected.

Table 7.1 summarizes the characteristics of the principal water sources and options for extraction, treatment and distribution of water. Figure 7.4 shows a decision tree for choosing an appropriate water source for short-term emergency supplies.

Improving existing water sources

Steps should be taken to progress rapidly from the initial emergency supply of water by whatever means possible, to gradual improvement. In the longer term, it should be possible to improve and protect existing sources and to develop new ones, such as springs

Table 7.1 **Typology of water sources**[1]

Source	Treatment	Extraction	Distribution	Remarks
Rain	Unnecessary if catchment and receptacles clean	Channelling off suitable roofs and/or hard ground	Collection directly at household or institutional level	Useful as supplementary source of safe water in certain seasons
Groundwater:				
Natural spring	Unnecessary if properly protected	Simple gravity flow: preferably piped from a protective spring box	Individual collection directly, via storage tanks or gravity-fed distribution system	Source must be protected; yield may vary seasonally
Deep well (low water-table)	Unnecessary if properly located, constructed and maintained	Handpump possible if water-table less than 60 m deep and output required is low, otherwise motor pumps necessary	Individually pumped by hand, or motor pumped to storage tanks, possibly linked to distribution systems	Yield unlikely to vary much with seasons unless prolonged drought. Special construction equipment and expertise required. High yields often possible
Shallow well (high water-table)	Unnecessary if properly located, constructed and maintained	Hand pump or rope and bucket	Pumped or drawn directly from wells by individuals	Yield may vary seasonally; can be dug/drilled by local skilled labour. Care needed to avoid contamination
Surface water:				
Flowing (stream, river)	Always necessary: sedimentation, filtration and/or chlorination	Preferably pumped to storage and treatment tanks	Individual collection, preferably from storage/treatment tanks	Yield may vary seasonally; access to source should be controlled
Standing (lake, pond)	Always necessary, as above	As above	As above	As above

[1] Adapted from United Nations High Commissioner for Refugees (1992a).

and boreholes. The host population may give permission for their sources to be improved and shared. Figure 7.4 facilitates the selection of a water source and the identification of treatment options.

Water source protection

A minimum number of essential measures to protect water supplies should be taken immediately after a disaster, as follows:

- Consult and involve the people concerned in solving (and thus understanding) the problems associated with water supplies.
- Segregate water uses (drinking, bathing, livestock watering).
- Protect water sources from faecal contamination by fencing them in, and by arranging for the use of a defecation field or shallow trench latrines at a suitable distance from the source.
- Store water in large covered tanks or containers for a day or two, if possible, allowing sediment to settle out, as subsequent chlorination is more effective if the water

Figure 7.4 Choosing a water source and treatment options for a short-term emergency water supply[1]

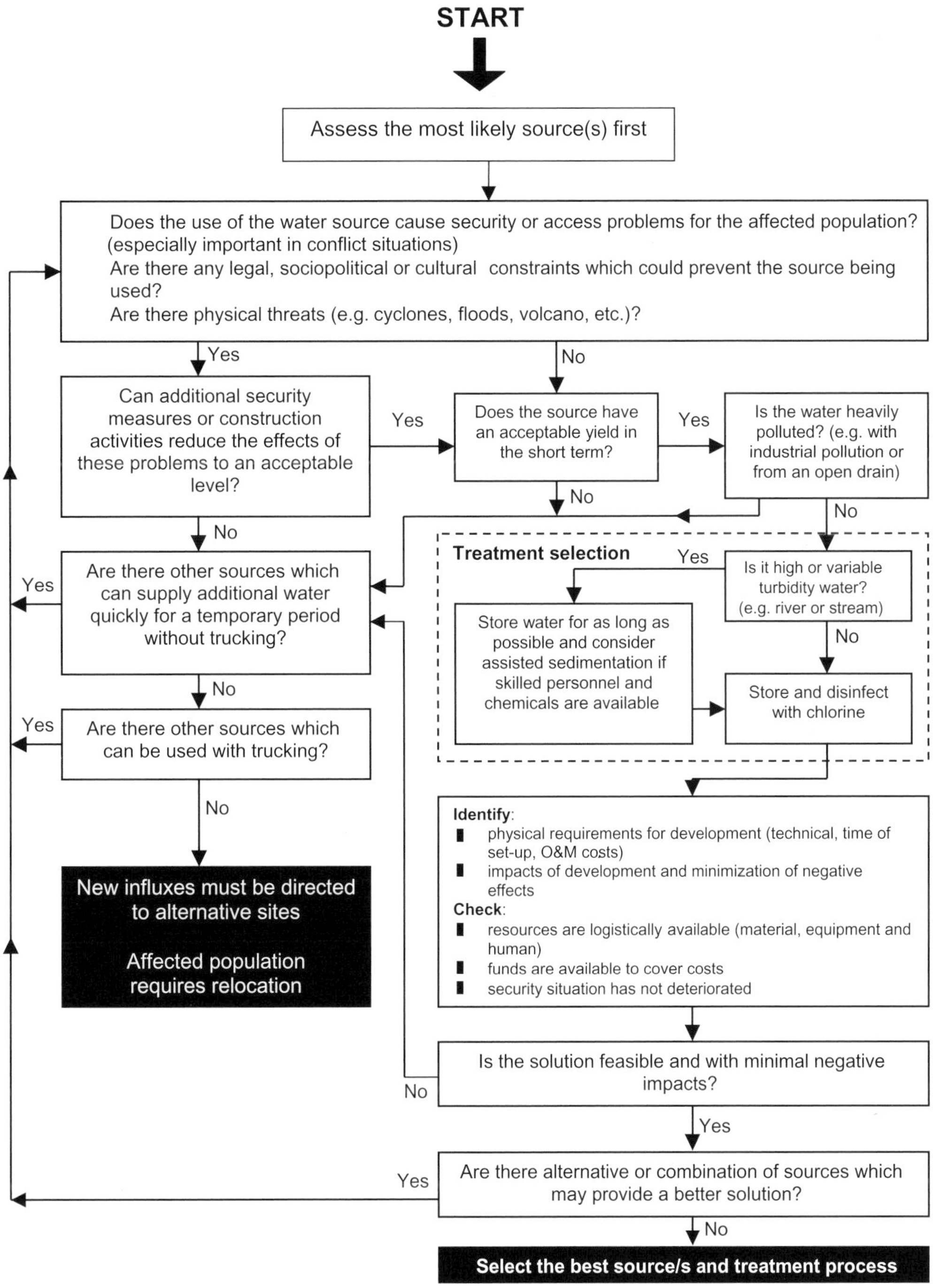

START

Assess the most likely source(s) first

Does the use of the water source cause security or access problems for the affected population? (especially important in conflict situations)
Are there any legal, sociopolitical or cultural constraints which could prevent the source being used?
Are there physical threats (e.g. cyclones, floods, volcano, etc.)?

Yes / No

Can additional security measures or construction activities reduce the effects of these problems to an acceptable level?

Does the source have an acceptable yield in the short term?

Is the water heavily polluted? (e.g. with industrial pollution or from an open drain)

Yes / No / Yes / No

Treatment selection

Is it high or variable turbidity water? (e.g. river or stream)

Store water for as long as possible and consider assisted sedimentation if skilled personnel and chemicals are available

Store and disinfect with chlorine

Are there other sources which can supply additional water quickly for a temporary period without trucking?

Are there other sources which can be used with trucking?

New influxes must be directed to alternative sites

Affected population requires relocation

Identify:
- physical requirements for development (technical, time of set-up, O&M costs)
- impacts of development and minimization of negative effects

Check:
- resources are logistically available (material, equipment and human)
- funds are available to cover costs
- security situation has not deteriorated

Is the solution feasible and with minimal negative impacts?

No / Yes

Are there alternative or combination of sources which may provide a better solution?

Yes / No

Select the best source/s and treatment process

[1] Source: House & Reed (1997)

is clear. After a few days, a better choice of locally-available water sources and more elaborate treatment may be possible.

- Give preference to groundwater rather than to surface water. Initially, it should be assumed that all surface water is contaminated.
- Use chlorine to protect water from contamination in the course of distribution and use, such that a free chlorine residual of 0.4–0.5 mg/l is achieved immediately after treatment (or 0.2–0.5 mg/l at the point of distribution).

Controlling direct use of sources

When people take water for a variety of uses directly from a source, the most rapid intervention to protect health is to segregate uses in time or space, to reduce the risk of contaminating drinking-water. Livestock should not be allowed to trample and defecate near human water sources, and water for livestock should be piped to watering troughs some way away from the source. Fencing maintained by local volunteers should be used to demarcate the human and animal watering places (Figure 7.5).

Environmental health staff should consult the people concerned, the village/community health or safety committee, and the primary health-care workers so that culturally acceptable methods of coordinating and segregating different types of use are adopted. There are usually socially established rules governing access, in terms of both time and space, to local water supplies, although in an emergency these may break down. They can, however, provide a basis for a constructive discussion of the problem with local people.

Roof-catchment systems

Depending on climate and weather conditions, roof-catchment systems can be used to supplement water supplies. Corrugated metal and tile roofs are best for this purpose, but even thatched roofs can provide good water, if debris is filtered out (Hall, 1990). Properly filtered and chlorinated, roof-catchment water can make a good independent or supplementary/reserve source for the camp kitchen or health centre.

Springs

Unprotected springs can be capped to prevent inflow of polluted surface waters (see Figure 7.6). The water can be piped into a covered reservoir, or to collection points convenient to both the host population and the camp.

Figure 7.5 **Use of fencing to demarcate human and animal watering places**[1]

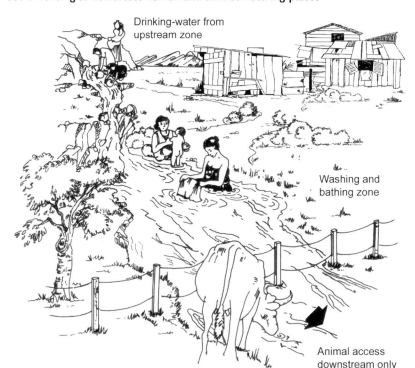

Drinking-water from upstream zone

Washing and bathing zone

Animal access downstream only

[1] Source: Chartier et al. (1991).

Figure 7.6 **A protected spring**[1]

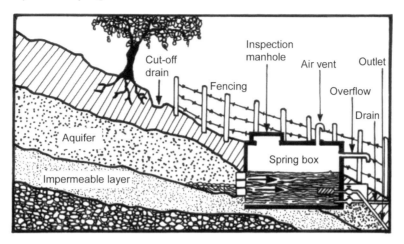

[1] Source: adapted from World Health Organization (1997a)

Figure 7.7 **Improvement of water hole with concrete caisson**[1]

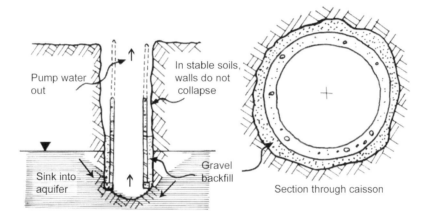

[1] Source: Watt & Wood (1979).

Crude water holes and shallow wells

Where there is an open water hole dug into the groundwater table (i.e. not simply a depression that accumulates run-off), concrete rings or caissons can be inserted into the well once it has been deepened (see Figure 7.7). Whether it is a well or an infiltration gallery, a crude water hole still needs further improvement to prevent contamination of the aquifer by surface water. The outside of the well may need to be sealed.

Where the existing source is an open, unprotected well, it can be improved by sealing the upper 3 metres of the walls and providing a cover, surface drainage and an improved low-maintenance pump (see Figure 7.8).

To seal the well, earth is excavated all round the existing well lining (as depicted) and refilled with "puddled clay", i.e. clay that has been thoroughly mixed with a little water and sand to the consistency of a thick paste, which is then compacted into position. The well should then be disinfected with 50–100 mg/l chlorine for 24 hours and flushed out. Water should be monitored for subsequent contamination. If contamination is detected (or if users are complaining of diarrhoea), water can be drawn from the well and chlorinated at the well, or at the household level (leaving a free residual chlorine of 0.4–0.5 mg/l after 30 minutes), until the source of contamination is found and removed.

Figure 7.8 **Improving an existing well with puddled clay**[1]

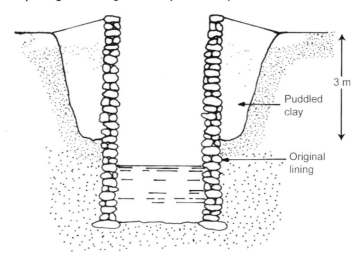

[1] Sources: adapted from United Nations Children's Fund (1986), Cairncross & Feachem (1978).

Figure 7.9 **A typical protected dug well installation**[1]

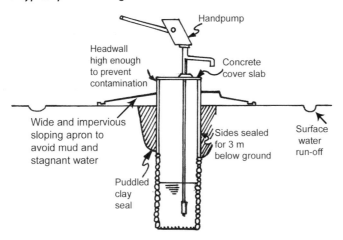

[1] Source: adapted from United Nations High Commissioner for Refugees (1992a).

These simple improvements are the first stages in the protection of a well. The most important improvements that can be made are providing a sloping surface around the well for drainage and raising the head wall high enough to block surface run-off. Other important features of a protected dug well are shown in Figure 7.9. Where possible, cover slabs and handpumps should be used, rather than buckets and windlasses, particularly when there is great demand from each well.

For information on safety precautions for digging wells, see Box 7.2.

Improving the yield of wells

Dug wells can be deepened and protected at the same time. They can also be extended laterally into the water-bearing stratum, which is especially useful if they cannot be deepened because of impenetrable rock. Figure 7.10 shows several possibilities: tunnels or adits constructed at the bottom of the well, porous pipes driven through the well lining, porous pipe driven or bored into the base of the well, etc. Care must always be taken to protect the well and the aquifer against the inflow of contaminated surface water. *Extreme caution must always be exercised to ensure that workers are not endangered* (see Box 7.2).

Figure 7.10 **Methods of improving the output of wells**[1]

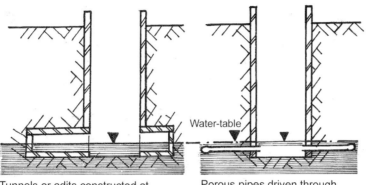

Tunnels or adits constructed at
bottom of well

Porous pipes driven through
well lining

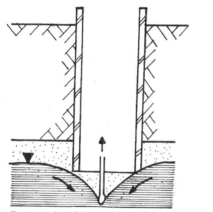

Porous pipe driven or bored
into base of well

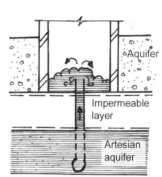

Penetrating down to an
artesian aquifer

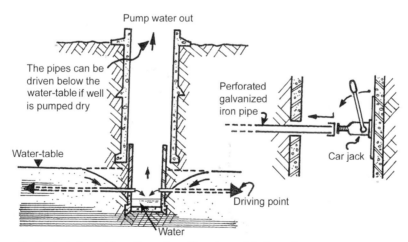

Perforated pipes driven through well's caisson into formations

[1] Source: Watt & Wood (1979).

Figure 7.11 **Connected wells**[1]

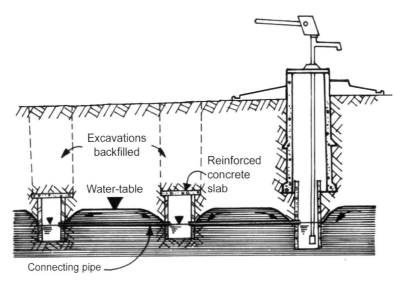

[1] Source: Watt & Wood (1979).

Box 7.2 Safety precautions for digging wells

Well-diggers should:

— not work in sections more than 1 m deep when deepening wells, without temporary shut-
    tering or well lining to prevent a collapse, unless the soil is known to be very stable (for
    instance from previous experience with unlined wells in the same locality);
— be aware of the risk of dangerous gases in deep wells;
— not allow building materials to fall into the well;
— exercise care while removing buckets of excavated earth and when entering or leaving the
    well (preferably using a harness or simple bosun's chair and never descending with one foot
    in a bucket);
— be provided with and wear hard hats and protective boots;
— ensure that electrical cables for dewatering pumps are properly protected and checked reg-
    ularly for damage;
— never lower diesel- or petrol-driven dewatering pumps into the well while deepening, as
    exhaust fumes are fatal.

For further information, see: Watt & Wood (1979), Oxfam (1990).

In some shallow aquifers, wells are constructed close together in a row and connected
with a tunnel or bored pipe. Only one is left open, and the remainder are backfilled,
thus saving lining material and time (see Figure 7.11).

In a variation on the well-established Iranian *qanat* (or *falaj*), a borehole can be
drilled horizontally into the hillside until the water-table is hit, providing an artificial
spring or, in the traditional way, a horizontal adit can be dug between a series of vertical wells until the water-table is encountered (Figure 7.12).

Boreholes

Over the past 40 years, a variety of well-drilling rigs have been developed, with different
designs now available for drilling through a range of geological formations, from unconsolidated alluvium to very hard crystalline formations. Some of this equipment is rela-

Figure 7.12 **Construction of a *qanat* or *falaj*[1]**

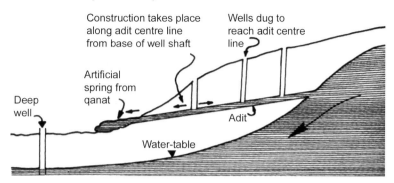

[1] Source: Watt & Wood (1979).

Box 7.3 Contracting out borehole drilling

Drilling will often be carried out by a specialized contractor hired by an NGO, health authority or municipality. The following should be considered when selecting a contractor:

■ Has the company a local or national reputation for good work? Can it provide details of similar drilling work that it has completed recently? Does it belong to a professional organization? Is it on a list of approved contractors for an organization employing drilling contractors?

■ Is there evidence that the company has the equipment to do the work? Is the equipment in good repair and well maintained? Does the company have maintenance and back-up facilities in case of plant breakdown? Is its depot close to the proposed drilling site, so that backup can be efficient? Is the depot kept in a clean and workmanlike state?

When contracting out for a more than 10 boreholes, it may be useful to hire two contractors, each with a clause in the drilling contract that specifies that if they do not meet time and quality requirements, the other contractor may be awarded the outstanding work.

Contracting out borehole drilling is a difficult exercise that requires considerable knowledge and experience. Having recognized this problem, UNHCR has published a suggested format for technical specifications for borehole drilling (United Nations High Commissioner for Refugees, 1992a).

---

tively cheap, portable, and simple to use. For instance, in an area with a high water-table, a well can be drilled with a hand auger, with a filter tube and filter pack of sand and gravel placed at the bottom; the entire well is sealed, protecting it from surface contamination. Other types of drilling equipment are expensive, large, and complex, requiring specialist teams of technicians to operate them. For a summary of drilling techniques, see United Nations High Commissioner for Refugees (1992a) and Davis and Lambert (2002).

Drilling boreholes is a skilled activity requiring specialist equipment and it is often contracted out (see Box 7.3).

Boreholes, deep wells and protected springs consistently yield the safest water from a bacteriological point of view. With deep boreholes in unfamiliar geology however, care should be taken to identify the chemical characteristics of the water by means of the appropriate tests in accordance with the *WHO Guidelines for drinking-water quality* (see also: United Nations High Commissioner for Refugees, 1992a).

Environmental health staff should provide information on water needs to help in the choice of drilling locations. They may be involved in sampling and testing water to ensure it is potable (see Section 7.4.3), and disinfecting boreholes before they are put into use.

Water harvesting

Various water-harvesting techniques are possible, ranging from roof catchments to more elaborate harvesting of rare, but heavy, rainfall. For example, Figure 7.13 shows the design of a Somali *hafir* routing run-off from rain into a ground reservoir and then to an outlet well.

Dust, animal manure, human excreta and other contaminants should be considered in all methods of water harvesting and, in an emergency, harvested water should be treated in the same way as surface water because of the likelihood of contamination during harvesting.

Rivers and lakes

It should be assumed that all surface water is contaminated and should be treated before consumption. It should only be used as a primary source if groundwater is unavailable or insufficient.

A wooden crib, anchored on the river bed with gravel or rocks, will protect the intake from physical damage (see Fig. 7.14A).

Surface water often needs some form of pretreatment to reduce turbidity before filtration and/or disinfection. Various methods are described in Section 7.4.3. The water

Figure 7.13 **Design of Somali *hafir*. A: overall plan; B: detail in perspective**[1]

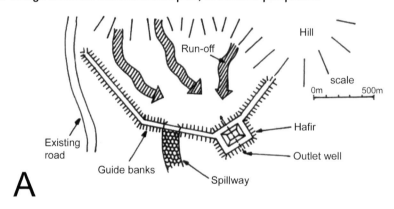

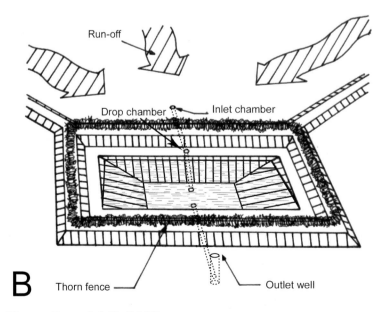

[1] Source: Pacey & Cullis (1986).

Figure 7.14 **Water intake systems for lakes or rivers: (A) Wooden crib at intake; (B) Lake or river-bed filter**[1]

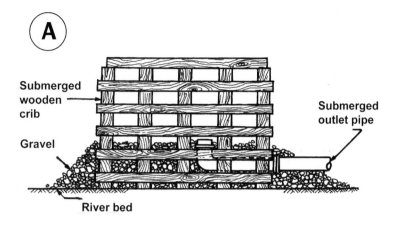

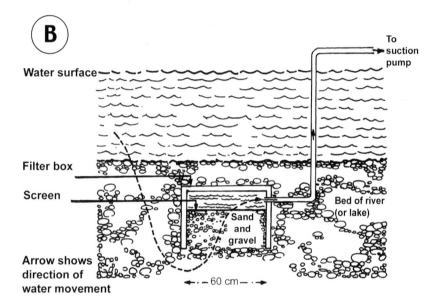

[1] Sources: A: Pickford (1977). B: United Nations Children's Fund (1986).

abstraction structure may incorporate a river-bed or lake-bed filter, as shown in Figure 7.14B. Water abstracted through such a sand and gravel filter (or even a crude screen) can then be stored and treated onshore.

Another method of pretreatment at source is the installation of an infiltration gallery leading to a protected well dug in the river or lake bank (see Figure 7.15). In low-flow rivers or streams that dry up seasonally, an underground dam may be constructed to impound underground water behind it.

7.4.2 Water quality and water testing in emergencies

Important quality criteria

The greatest water-borne risk to health in most emergencies is the transmission of faecal pathogens, due to inadequate sanitation, hygiene and protection of water sources. Water-borne infectious diseases include diarrhoea, typhoid, cholera, dysentery and infectious hepatitis. However, some disasters, including those involving damage to chemical and nuclear industrial installations, or involving volcanic activity, may create acute problems from chemical or radiological water pollution.

Figure 7.15 **Subsurface dam and infiltration gallery**[1]

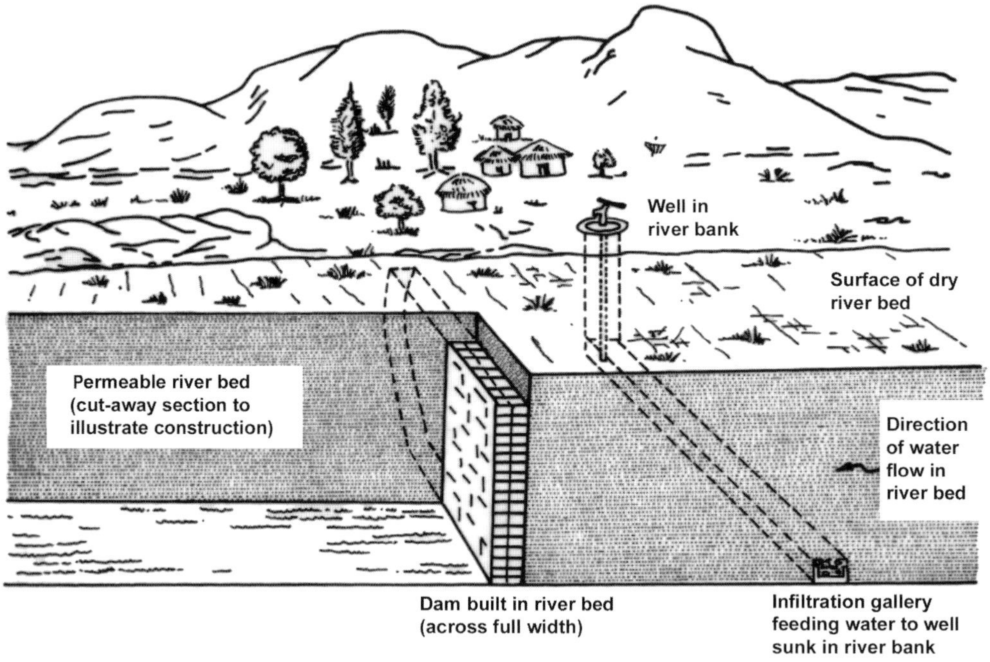

[1] Source: United Nations Children's Fund (1986).

Whatever the source and type of contamination, decisions on acceptable water quality in emergencies involve balancing short- and long-term risks and benefits to health. At the same time, ensuring access to sufficient quantities of water is vital for health protection.

Many chemicals in drinking-water are of concern only after extended periods of exposure. Thus, it is advisable to supply water in an emergency, even if it significantly exceeds WHO guidelines for some chemical parameters, if the water can be treated to kill pathogens and then supplied rapidly to the affected population. This will reduce the risk of outbreaks of water-borne and water-washed disease. When water sources are likely to be used for long periods, chemical and radiological contaminants of more chronic health importance should be given greater attention. In some situations, this may entail adding treatment processes, or seeking alternative sources.

Bacteriological testing

The principle of bacteriological testing is to identify a "faecal indicator" organism that is always excreted by warm-blooded animals, both healthy and unhealthy, and to take the degree of its presence as an indication of the degree of faecal contamination. Bacteria from the thermotolerant (faecal) coliform group are nearly always present in faeces, so their presence in water is a strong indication of faecal contamination. Typically, most thermotolerant coliforms are of the species *Escherichia coli*, which is always derived from faeces. The presence of any bacteria from the total coliform group is sometimes tested for, particularly as an indication of the effectiveness of a water-treatment system. Many members of the total coliform group are free-living and their presence does not depend on the presence of faecal contamination, but it can indicate that a treatment process has not removed or killed all bacteria. Other faecal indicator bacteria include faecal streptococci/intestinal enterococci.

Field kits for bacteriological testing usually employ the membrane-filtration technique, where a measured volume of water is filtered through a membrane, which retains the bacteria on its surface. The membrane is then incubated on a suitable medium, using a battery-powered incubator, for 18 hours. During this time, the thermotolerant coliform bacteria reproduce and form colonies. The number of colonies formed provides an index of the degree of faecal contamination in the original sample. This test is generally easy to perform. However, high turbidity caused by clay, algae, etc. (which may be suspended in large quantities after storms and floods) can interfere with the test, but as small volumes are often analysed in these circumstances, this may not be a significant problem.

The multiple-tube method is an alternative to membrane-filtration. Quantities of the water to be tested are added to tubes containing a suitable liquid culture medium and incubated, typically for at least 24 hours. The bacteria present in the water reproduce, and the most probable number of bacteria present is determined statistically from the number of tubes giving a positive reaction (colour change and/or gas production). This test can accommodate even turbid samples, containing sewage, sewage sludge, or mud and soil particles.

Bacteriological guidelines

Conventional bacteriological standards may be difficult to achieve in the immediate post-disaster period. The WHO guideline of zero *E. coli* per 100 ml of water should be the goal (World Health Organization, 1993a) and should be achievable even in emergencies, provided that chemical disinfection is employed.

Recognizing that achieving the guideline standards may be difficult in some emergency situations, it is practical to classify water quality results according to the degree of health concern (Lloyd & Helmer, 1991; Delmas & Courvallet, 1994). For example:

— zero *E. coli*/100 ml: guideline compliant;
— 1–10 *E. coli*/100 ml: tolerable;
— 10–100 *E. coli*/100 ml: requires treatment;
— greater than 100 *E. coli*/100 ml: unsuitable for consumption without proper treatment.

An indication of a certain level of a faecal indicator bacteria *alone* is not a reliable guide to biological water quality. Some faecal pathogens, including many viruses and protozoa, may be more resistant to treatment (such as by chlorine) than the indicator bacteria. More generally, if a sanitary survey suggests the likelihood of faecal contamination, then even a very low level of contamination measured by bacteriological analysis may be considered to be a risk, especially during an outbreak of a disease like cholera that may be water-borne.

The parameters most commonly measured to assess microbial safety are: *E. coli* (thermotolerant coliforms); residual chlorine; pH; and turbidity.

Residual chlorine

Chlorine content should be tested in the field with a colour comparator, generally used in the range of 0.2–1 mg/l of water. Taste does not give a reliable indication of chlorine concentration.

pH

It is necessary to know the pH of water because more alkaline water requires a longer contact time or a higher free residual chlorine level at the end of the contact time for adequate disinfection (0.4–0.5 mg/l at pH 6–8, rising to 0.6 mg/litre at pH 8–9, and may be ineffective above pH 9).

Turbidity

Turbidity, or cloudiness, is measured to determine what type and level of treatment is needed. It can be carried out with a simple turbidity tube that allows a direct reading in turbidity units (NTUs). Turbidity adversely affects the efficiency of disinfection (see Section 7.4.3.)

Sanitary surveys and catchment mapping

It is possible to assess the likelihood of faecal contamination of water sources by a sanitary survey. This is often more valuable than bacteriological testing alone, because a sanitary survey makes it possible to see what needs to be done to protect the water source, and because faecal contamination may vary, so a water sample only represents the quality of the water at the time it was collected. This process can be combined with bacteriological, physical and chemical testing to enable field teams to assess contamination and—more importantly—provide the basis for monitoring water supplies in the post-disaster period.

Even when it is possible to carry out bacteriological quality testing, results are not instantly available. Thus, the immediate assessment of contamination risk should be based on gross indicators, such as proximity to sources of faecal contamination (human or animal); colour and smell; the presence of dead fish or animals; the presence of foreign matter, such as ash or debris; and the presence of a chemical or radiation hazard, or a wastewater discharge point upstream. Catchment mapping that involves identifying sources and pathways of pollution can be an important tool for assessing the likelihood of contamination of a water source.

It is important to use a standard reporting format for sanitary surveys and catchment mapping, to ensure that information gathered by different staff is reliable and that information on different water sources may be compared. For an example sanitary survey format, see: World Health Organization (1997a), Davis & Lambert (2002). For more information on catchment mapping, see: House & Reed (1997).

Chemical and radiological guidelines

Water from sources that are considered to have a significant risk of chemical or radiological contamination should be avoided, even as a temporary measure. In the long term, achieving WHO guidelines should be the aim of emergency water-supply programmes based on the progressive improvement of water quality (Sphere Project 2000).

Testing kits and laboratories

Portable testing kits allow the determination in the field of water pH (acidity/alkalinity), free residual chlorine, faecal coliform bacteria count, turbidity and filterability. The use of such a kit in Nicaragua is described in Box 7.4.

When large numbers of water samples need testing, or a broad range of parameters is of interest, laboratory analysis is usually most appropriate. If laboratories at water-treatment works, environmental health offices and universities no longer function because of the disaster then a temporary laboratory may need to be set up. When samples are transported to laboratories, handling is important. Poor handling may lead to meaningless or misleading results.

Workers should be trained in the correct procedures for collecting, labeling, packing and transporting samples, and for supplying supporting information from the sanitary survey to help interpret laboratory results. For standard methods of water sampling and testing, see: World Health Organization (1997a), Bartram & Ballance (1996).

> **Box 7.4 Use of portable water-testing kits after hurricane Joan in Nicaragua[1]**
>
> Portable water-testing kits have been effectively used under disaster conditions, such as in Nicaragua after hurricane Joan blew away all the roof water-catchment systems in the town of Bluefields in 1988. People were forced to resort to old open, shallow wells that were normally used only for washing and cleaning, and that were located near latrines. The hurricane had also flooded these wells with filth. The least turbid and obviously contaminated ones were selected as emergency water sources and continuous chlorination was begun. Residents in each of the town's neighbourhoods were responsible for checking on free residual chlorine levels daily and adding daily doses of chlorine.
>
> [1] Catholic Institute for International Relations (1989).

7.4.3 Treatment of emergency water supplies

The processes required to render raw water potable depend on its physicochemical and biological quality. Surface water that is highly turbid and heavily contaminated usually needs some form of pretreatment to prepare it for disinfection or, in some cases, slow sand filtration. The pretreatment processes described below are storage and plain sedimentation, coagulation and flocculation, and roughing filtration.

Storage and plain sedimentation

Simply storing water for a number of hours improves water quality. Solid particles settle to the bottom of the storage tank, taking a proportion of the pathogens with them and reducing turbidity; there is a degree of improvement through natural bacterial die-off; and storing river water provides a buffer stock, allowing operators to avoid using raw water during peaks in turbidity after rains (Davis & Lambert, 2002). Water storage and plain sedimentation may be arranged at central level, as pretreatment for a piped supply. In such cases, samples of raw water should be taken and jar tests carried out to see how fast the solids settle, and to choose an appropriate storage time, storage capacity and dimensions of the storage tanks. In an emergency it is rarely possible to design and build tanks for specific situations, but an effective system may be improvised using a series of available water tanks in a configuration that takes account of the raw water quality, the degree of pretreatment required, and the quantity to be pretreated.

Plain sedimentation can also be organized at household level where centralized treatment is not possible. Water is allowed to settle in whatever large, clean, covered storage vessels are available. After 24 hours (or more if possible), the clear water is drawn or poured off the top. The sediment is discarded, or used for laundry if water is scarce. The resulting clear water should be chlorinated. Figure 7.16 shows a simple household storage system that allows settling to take place.

Coagulation and flocculation

Another method of reducing the turbidity of water uses coagulation and flocculation. In this process, colloidal particles such as clays, that do not readily settle in plain sedimentation, are encouraged to combine to form heavier particles that will settle by adding a chemical coagulant, such as aluminium sulphate (alum), ferric chloride, ferric sulphate, or natural coagulants. The dose of coagulant required depends on the nature of the raw water and the chemical used and has to be determined by carrying out jar tests with different doses of the coagulant. The effectiveness of coagulation and flocculation is strongly influenced by the pH of the water.

Figure 7.16 **Simple household storage system for removal of sediment[1]**

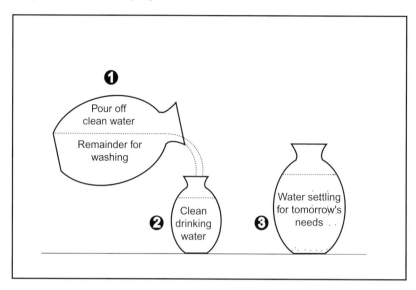

[1] Source: Chartier, Diskett & UNHCR (1991).

Once the dosage rate has been determined, a simple dosing system can be set up in an emergency, where the coagulant is rapidly mixed with the raw water as it is fed into a treatment tank. In a second stage, the mixture is gently stirred for 30 minutes, to facilitate flocculation. After this time, clear water may be drawn from the upper level of the tank, but in a batch treatment process (as opposed to a continuous flow process) it may take up to 8 hours for the particles to settle to the bottom of the tank and for the water to be ready for distribution. The rapidity of settling is greatest when initial mixing is done thoroughly. After a period, which depends on the turbidity of the raw water and the quantity being treated, the sludge at the bottom of the tank needs drawing off and disposing of. Care should be taken to ensure that sludge disposal does not contaminate water sources or agricultural land.

Roughing filtration

Roughing filtration is a process that combines filtration and sedimentation, that can be used to reduce the turbidity of water carrying large amounts of suspended solids. The clarified water may then be further treated by rapid sand filtration or slow sand filtration, or disinfected directly, if the turbidity is sufficiently reduced (to below 5 NTU preferably, but up to 20 NTU may be permitted). Roughing filters use relatively coarse media (5–25 mm diameter), and may be constructed to operate with horizontal flow or vertical flow. They have several advantages, including their simplicity, but they can take some time to install. Vertical-flow roughing filters may be made rapidly using Oxfam-type rigid tanks.

Rapid sand filtration and slow sand filtration

Rapid sand filters are commonly used in urban water-treatment systems, and they may need attention in an emergency because of changes in raw water quality or mechanical and electrical breakdowns. However, they are not recommended as an emergency water-treatment option because of a number of drawbacks, including the fact that they provide only partial treatment through a simple filtration process. Disinfection is required after rapid filtration.

Slow sand filtration, on the other hand, removes microorganisms and, if properly operated, produces water which is safe to drink. Slow sand filters may be designed and built following relatively simple procedures, on a large scale and on a small scale. A filter adequate for processing 60 litres per hour may be made in a few hours with only a metal drum and simple tools and fittings, though the need for careful operation makes this generally unsuitable for household level in an emergency. The method works best in warm climates at low levels of turbidity. Two major disadvantages of slow sand filtration is the relatively low yield for the size of the installation required, and the need for careful operation to ensure the top layer of sand with the trapped disease-causing organisms does not dry out. In addition, when there is a significant risk of water contamination in the distribution system or in the household, the treated water should still be chlorinated.

Disinfection

WHO endorses disinfection of drinking-water and in emergency situations drinking-water should be disinfected in all cases where population size and concentration, lack of sanitary facilities, or health information suggest a significant risk of water-borne disease. Disinfection should not be used as a substitute for protecting water sources from contamination. Water sources should always be protected to reduce the contamination of raw water and reduce the health risks associated with incomplete or unreliable disinfection procedures.

There are a number of different water disinfection methods used in stable situations, but the most common method in emergencies is chlorination. Important advantages of chlorine disinfection are that it is simple to dose and to measure, and that it leaves a residual disinfection capacity in the treated water, safeguarding against contamination in the home. This is particularly important when sanitation is inadequate. Chlorine gas is most commonly used in urban water-treatment works, but this requires careful storage and handling by well-trained staff, as well as dosing equipment. For emergency water-treatment installations, chlorine compounds in solid or liquid form are most often used, as these are simple to store and handle, and may be dosed using simple equipment, such as a spoon or bucket.

The chlorine compound most commonly used for water disinfection in emergencies is calcium hypochlorite, in powder or granular form. One form of calcium hypochlorite that is frequently used is high-test hypochlorite (HTH). Calcium hypochlorite should be stored in dry, sealed corrosion-resistant containers in a cool, well-ventilated place to ensure that it retains its strength. All concentrated chlorine compounds, such as HTH and concentrated chlorine solutions, give off chlorine gas. This gas is poisonous and may burn the eyes and skin, and can start fires or explosions. All concentrated chlorine compounds should be handled with care by trained staff wearing protective clothing.

Free residual chlorine levels of more than 0.3 mg/l for more than 30 minutes are required to kill bacteria and most viruses. Chlorination of stored water for direct consumption is best achieved using a 1% stock solution of chlorine made up according to the instructions given in Table 7.2. With this stock solution as base, water can be treated as described in Table 7.3. Minimum target concentrations for chlorine to point of delivery are 0.2 mg/l in normal circumstances and 0.5 mg/l in high-risk circumstances.

Chlorination is less effective in turbid water. If the raw water has a turbidity over 20 NTUs, then some form of pretreatment should be carried out. Ideally the turbidity should be less than 5 NTUs.

Contact time or free chlorine residual should be increased in water with a high pH (see Section 7.4.2).

Table 7.2 **Preparation of 1% chlorine stock solution[1]**

To make 1 litre of the stock solution, mix the quantity shown of one of the following chemical sources with water and make up to 1 litre in a glass, plastic or wooden container:

Chemical source	Percentage available chlorine	Quantity required	Approximate measures
Bleaching powder	35	30 g	2 heaped tablespoons
Stabilized/tropical	25	40 g	3 heaped tablespoons bleach
High-test hypochlorite	70	14 ml	1 tablespoon solution
Liquid laundry bleach	5	200 ml	1 teacup or 6-oz milk tin
Liquid laundry bleach	7	145 ml	10 tablespoons
Javelle water	1	Is itself a 1% stock solution	

A 1% solution contains 10 g of chlorine per litre = 10 000 mg/l or 10 000 ppm (parts per million).

1 tablespoon = 4 teaspoons

Avoid skin contact with any of the chemical sources or the stock solution, and avoid inhaling chlorine fumes.

This stock solution should be *fresh*, i.e. made every day, and protected from heat and light.

[1] Source: United Nations Children's Fund (1986).

Table 7.3 **Disinfecting water using a 1% stock solution[1]**

To produce an initial chlorine concentration sufficient to leave a free residual chlorine concentration of 0.4–0.5 mg/l after 30 minutes:

1. Prepare a 1% chlorine solution (see Table 7.2).

2. Take 4 nonmetallic water containers (e.g. 20-litre plastic buckets) and put 10 litres of the water to be chlorinated in each one.

3. Using a syringe, add progressively greater doses of 1% chlorine solution to the containers:

    1st container: 1 ml
    2nd container: 1.5 ml
    3rd container: 2 ml
    4th container: 5 ml

4. Wait for 30 minutes and then measure the residual free chlorine concentration, using a comparator or test strip.

5. Choose the sample with between 0.4–0.5 mg/l of free residual chlorine.

6. Calculate the amount of 1% chlorine solution needed for the quantity of water to be treated.

[1] Source: Delmas & Courvallet, 1994.

Designated individuals should be responsible for monitoring daily the free residual chlorine level in all distributed and stored supplies, including water in household containers. They can be recruited from the affected population and trained.

Chlorine-based tablets (containing trichloroisocyanuric acid) may be used for short-term emergency chlorination in floating plastic containers. These tablets are normally used for swimming pool chlorination, but may also be used in emergency situations for the continuous chlorination of water in wells or storage tanks, though the chlorine dosage is hard to control.

As indicated in Tables 7.2 and 7.3, a more reliable technique is to add the correct dose of chlorine to the water once it is drawn, at the collection point or at the household level, using a stock solution of a known active chlorine concentration (normally 1%). In an emergency, this may be organized by placing workers with a supply of chlorine stock solution at untreated-water collection areas, to add the correct dose of chlorine to water in buckets just after collection.

Disinfecting contaminated wells and tanks

A free residual chlorine level of 1–5 mg/l in a well or tank for 24 hours is sufficient to kill most pathogens once the well or tank has been cleaned of debris and protected. The well or tank should be pumped out, or flushed after disinfection, until the free residual chlorine concentration is below 0.5 mg/l. If there is an ongoing risk of contamination, then the source of contamination should be removed and/or the water should be disinfected continuously.

Other disinfection methods

Bringing water to a vigorous or rolling boil will kill most pathogens. Turbid water should be filtered through a clean cloth before boiling, to remove larger particles. The problem for most people in emergencies or disasters is the lack of facilities and fuel to do this. The boiling-point of water decreases with increasing altitude, so one minute of boiling time should be added for every 500 metres above sea level (United Nations High Commissioner for Refugees, 1992a).

In an emergency, individual households can treat a limited amount of water by storing it in clear glass containers and allowing it to remain in direct sunlight for a day to kill the pathogens. This method is more effective when the water has been oxygenated by leaving some space at the top of the bottle and then shaking it well (Reed, 1997).

Emergency decontamination processes may not always accomplish the optimal level of disinfection recommended by WHO, particularly with resistant pathogens such as viruses, and protozoan cysts or oocysts. However, implementation of emergency procedures may reduce the numbers of pathogens to levels where the risk of water-borne disease is largely restricted or even eliminated.

7.4.4 Water movement, storage and distribution

Water tankers

In the short term, water can be transported by purpose-built water-tank trucks (capacity typically 12 000 litres), water-tank trailers, or ordinary trucks carrying tanks, although this is an expensive option. Where purpose-built water tankers are not available, they may be improvised by securing rigid water tanks or flexible rubber/plastic tanks (also called pillow tanks or bladder tanks) onto the back of flatbed trucks. Flexible rubber or plastic tanks provide convenient storage on the ground for tankers to discharge into. However, they can be difficult to transport when filled with water, especially on poor-quality roads. Water delivered by tankers should be drawn from the safest possible sources and should be disinfected.

An element of contingency planning should be an inventory of tank trucks available locally, for instance in dairies, breweries and bottling plants, and those not being used by the fire service. Borrowed tankers must be thoroughly cleaned and disinfected before they are used for transporting water.

If water is carried in tankers, some arrangement should be made for filling them and for adequately storing the water at distribution points. Tankers should offload rapidly into small storage tanks at specified distribution points, rather than into individual water containers, which wastes a lot of time (see Figure 7.17). Water may be disinfected in tankers by adding the correct amount of chlorine as they are being filled, which allows time for chlorination during the delivery journey. The level of chlorine in the water at delivery should be monitored by independent staff, as well as by the drivers.

Water tankering is a costly option that requires very intensive management and monitoring. It should only be used as a temporary measure, unless there are no other suitable options.

Storage tanks

Water should be conveyed (possibly through pumping) to a storage tank of a suitable size, depending on the population to be served, the reliability of the water source, and the treatment system. As a general rule, for groups of fewer than 2000 people, storage volume should be equal to one day's demand. For larger groups, the storage volume per person may be smaller, but never less than one-sixth of the daily water demand (United Nations High Commissioner for Refugees, 1992a). However, the appropriate storage volume will depend on a number of specific factors, such as the reliability of the water source and pumping facilities (where relevant), security considerations, cost, and peaks in demand. If the tank can be raised to provide 10–20 metres head of water, final distribution to the settlement by gravity will be possible. Ready-made plastic/rubber pillow tanks and onion tanks, or steel section tanks with rubber liners should be used if available, as they are rapidly installed. For further details, see Section 7.4.5. Otherwise, ferrocement or masonry tanks may be required. A temporary water tank can be made by building a perimeter wall out of sandbags and lining it with plastic sheeting. However,

Figure 7.17 **A temporary water-distribution stand with three taps**[1]

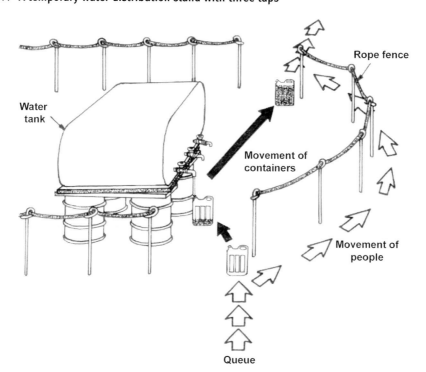

[1] Source: Davis & Lambert (2002).

skill is required to create a stable structure and to construct an effective outlet arrangement.

Water transmission and distribution

Both gravity flow and pumps are normally used for transmitting and distributing water. Gravity flow is preferable as it avoids dependence on pumps and power supplies, so reducing costs, workload, and the risk of supply cuts as a result of breakdowns or fuel shortages. If natural slopes are not available, storage tanks can be built on raised mounds of compacted earth, an adequate margin of earth being provided around the tank to avoid collapse due to erosion. If pumps are used for distribution, a back-up pump should always be available together with a fuel reserve in case fuel supply to the settlement is cut off.

Polyethylene pipe and uPVC pipe are usually used to distribute mains water in emergency settlements. They are both commonly used in diameters of 75–150 mm. Polyethylene pipe is also available in 50-metre or 100-metre coils, which can be laid rapidly. Polyethylene pipe also has the advantage of being very robust and flexible, so it may be laid on the surface for a short space of time. It is, however, considerably more expensive than uPVC pipe, and less readily available in some countries. Both types of pipe should be buried in a trench to reduce the risk of breakages (particularly uPVC pipe, which is more brittle), and to reduce exposure to sunlight, which causes them to deteriorate. When uPVC pipes with push-fit couplings are used for rapid laying in an emergency, they must be buried to avoid water pressure pushing them apart. Care should be taken to protect plastic pipes from being crushed by vehicles before they are buried. Gullies and areas where the pipe could be washed away or broken by a landslide should be avoided if possible. If they are unavoidable, these obstacles should be crossed by sections of steel pipe, suitably supported by cables or structures to protect them (see Figure 7.1).

Polyethylene pipe of 32 mm or 50 mm diameter can be used for final distribution to the taps. Water is directed to distribution points at regular intervals in the camp so that no one has to walk further than 500 metres to reach one. One tap is required for every 140–200 people. Typical distribution stands have multiple taps (e.g. six). Smaller and more evenly distributed water points are more accessible to the population, but may be more costly and take longer to install. Taps should be 0.6–1.0 metres above the ground, to allow containers to be filled easily, and should be self-closing. Distribution networks should normally be designed to provide a residual head of between 5–10 metres at the taps. A number of 50 mm valves can be fitted on distribution networks so that fire-fighting hoses can be connected. Regular supervision of the tap stand is desirable to avoid abuse and damage.

Washing clothes and bathing should not be allowed at taps used for drinking-water, but separate bathing and laundry areas should be provided. If these areas are not close to the water points, then they should have a piped water supply, otherwise people will tend to wash at the water points. Tapstands, and laundry and bathing areas, should be well drained and arrangements should be made with users to regularly clean the facilities and report leaks and damage. See Chapter 8 for information on drainage of wastewater.

Water containers

Families will also need containers, preferably with a narrow neck, to keep transported and stored water supplies free of mosquitoes and contamination. Rigid jerrycans are often available locally and are inexpensive. However, they are expensive to transport, which is a great disadvantage in situations where they need to be imported rapidly in large quantities. Many agencies have used collapsible models, which are smaller when folded and hence can be transported at greatly reduced cost. These are not very robust, however. Stackable water containers, with snap-on lids that include a small opening, are also used by some agencies.

7.4.5 Prepackaged water kits

Oxfam GB has designed a series of modular water kits, for use in emergencies, that are robust and easy to assemble. These have been widely used since 1982, both by Oxfam and by other organizations, mostly for supplying water to refugees and displaced people. The kits include a range of lightweight pumping, storage and distribution kits for rapid response; groundwater development kits; rubber-lined steel storage tank kits (commonly known as Oxfam tanks) in a range from $11\,m^3$ to $90\,m^3$; water-testing and treatment kits; and distribution kits based on industry-standard transmission and distribution pipe with distribution tapstands and self-closing taps.

Médecins Sans Frontières uses a range of lightweight prepackaged water kits for emergencies, including water-storage kits ($2\,m^3$ and $15\,m^3$); a water-transportation kit (collapsible tanks of $5\,m^3$ for truck platforms where tankers are not available); a water/sedimentation-coagulation kit; a water-filtration kit; a water-pumping kit (diesel and petrol motor pumps); a water-chlorination kit; and a water-distribution kit (standpipes with six self-closing taps).

IFRC provides emergency response units (ERUs), which are modular kits with trained personnel to meet the medical and sanitary needs of large numbers of people in emergencies. The IFRC specialized water-supply ERU produces 120000 litres a day of high-quality water suitable for hospitals and health institutions. Other IFRC ERUs include a mass water and sanitation ERU that can meet the needs of at least 40 000 beneficiaries. It provides chemical treatment, storage, transportation and distribution of 400000–600000 litres per day of clear water. IFRC has also had good experience with their basic health-care ERUs that provide basic essential, preventive and curative care in emergencies, based on WHO emergency health kits.

The kits mentioned above are light and transportable by road or air. They come complete and ready for installation, and are designed for installation within hours of arrival by a team of semiskilled workers with some supervision by an experienced engineer. They can easily be disassembled, moved and reassembled. The kits used by a number of different agencies are compatible, thanks to the inclusion of a range of types and sizes of pipe fittings.

Mobile water-treatment units, mounted on trailers or in shipping containers, usually combine coagulation, filtration and disinfection, or simply filtration and disinfection, and can provide anywhere from 4000–50000 litres an hour. They can rapidly produce water of high quality without the need to design and construct temporary water-treatment facilities. However, they are expensive to have on-hand for emergency use, and they require a water source near the affected area, as well as specialist technical expertise to operate them and provide adequate maintenance.

7.4.6 Facilities for personal hygiene

Communal facilities for maintaining personal cleanliness should be provided in shelters and camps. These may include showers, washrooms, laundries and disinfection rooms.

Proper maintenance and supervision of all these facilities is the responsibility of environmental health personnel and the users. Regular meetings are required to ensure this shared task is carried out correctly.

Soap is an essential aid to reducing disease in emergencies: regular hand-washing with soap is very important. People should have access to at least 250g of soap per person per month, for personal and domestic hygiene (Sphere Project, 2000).

Showers

Showers are preferable to baths, both for sanitary reasons and to conserve water. As a temporary measure before showers can be built, a specific place on a stream, lake or pond can be set aside for bathing, and screened for privacy. Different hours or separate places for men and women can be designated. Bathing areas must be separated from the drinking-water source. The number of showers to be provided should be determined through consultation with the users, as it may vary greatly, depending on climate and habits. Shallow basins should be provided for parents to bathe their small children.

Temporary bathing water should be checked to ensure that those using it will not contract water-borne diseases. If necessary, water should be filtered and allowed to settle before it is used. In some countries, mobile bathing facilities, mounted on trucks or rail cars may be available.

Overall water consumption for bathing is likely to be 30–35 litres per person per week at public facilities. Residents should have the opportunity to shower at least once a week and should be encouraged to bathe children frequently. If water supplies are limited, showers should be organized on an appropriate rota system, with records kept or tickets issued by the camp health committee.

While cold water can be sufficient in hot climates, hot water can be provided with the type of heater shown in Figure 7.18. This heater can be made from a 200-litre oil drum. The cold-water inlet, consisting of a pipe 4 centimetres in diameter, extends to approximately 5 centimetres from the bottom of the drum. The hot-water outlet is placed as close as possible to the rim so that no hot water is lost by overflow. The hot water in the drum is recovered by pouring in cold water. This forces the hot water upwards and though the outlet. The drum is placed on chimney bricks, approximately 6 bricks high, and a metal chimney is fitted at the rear of the drum. A gas, oil, wood or coal fire may be used, and the bricks act as a fire box to control ventilation. The entire heater can be covered by turf to insulate it.

Laundries

In temporary shelters, people may be expected to wash their clothes in tubs provided. In longer-term camps, however, communal laundry slabs or basins should be provided. When disinfection rooms are needed, clothes should be washed in them. Whenever possible, hot water should be provided. One washing stand should be provided for every

Figure 7.18 **Put-and-take water heater**[1]

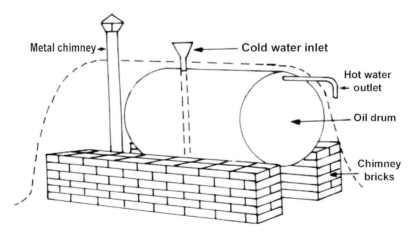

[1] Source: adapted from Assar (1971).

100 people, and a schedule for use established by the camp health committee. Soap should be used, rather than detergents. Proper drainage should be provided for wastewater, with traps for grease, soap and sand.

7.5 Operation and maintenance

When populations remain in one place for months or years after the disaster, longerterm measures can be taken. Health personnel can assist by designing a training programme for the community-based operation and maintenance of the water-supply system, or at least of the water distribution points and communal hygiene facilities of large systems (Arlosoroff, 1998; Shaw, 1998). This programme might also include sanitary inspection by local residents, especially women, and possibly gardening, which could be linked to child nutritional supplementation. On the whole, such integrated programmes for improving the health of communities are more effective than singlepurpose approaches based on water supply alone.

Environmental health staff should ensure that a monitoring programme is established so that water quality and availability are maintained at agreed standards and that problems are rapidly dealt with. It is useful to carry out periodic investigations of water consumption and water quality in the home, to find out if all the affected people have adequate access to the water supplied, and if there is a problem of water contamination in the home.

All mechanical equipment, as well as storage tanks, distribution systems and communal hygiene facilities need regular inspection, with an increasing need for repairs and replacement over time. Even if the water users contribute substantially to this work, the water-supply agency will usually need to take responsibility for the purchase of spare parts and materials.

7.6 Further information

For further information on:

— water sources, see: Watt & Wood (1979), Simmonds, Vaughan & Gunn (1983), Jordan (1984), van Wijk-Sijbesma (1985), Clark (1988), Kerr (1989), United Nations High Commissioner for Refugees (1992b), House & Reed (1997);
— water treatment, storage and distribution, see: Jahn (1981), Schultz & Okun (1984), Dian Desa (1990), United Nations High Commissioner for Refugees (1992b), Davis & Lambert (2002);
— water quality standards and water quality monitoring, see: Lloyd & Helmer (1991), World Health Organization (1993a), World Health Organization (1997a), Sphere Project (2000);
— managing water quality in the home, see: Sobsey (2002).

8. Sanitation

8.1 Human waste and health

8.1.1 Faeces

Human faeces may contain a range of disease-causing organisms, including viruses, bacteria and eggs or larvae of parasites. The microorganisms contained in human faeces may enter the body through contaminated food, water, eating and cooking utensils and by contact with contaminated objects. Diarrhoea, cholera and typhoid are spread in this way and are major causes of sickness and death in disasters and emergencies. Some fly species (and cockroaches) are attracted to or breed in faeces, but while they theoretically can carry faecal material on their bodies, there is no evidence that this contributes significantly to the spread of disease. However, high fly densities will increase the risk of transmission of trachoma and *Shigella* dysentery. Intestinal worm infections (hookworm, whipworm and others) are transmitted through contact with soil contaminated with faeces and may spread rapidly where open defecation occurs and people are barefoot. These infections will contribute to anemia and malnutrition, and therefore also render people more susceptible to other diseases. The intestinal form of schistomiasis (also known as bilharzia), caused by parasitic worm species living in the veins of the intestinal tract and liver, is transmitted through faeces. Its complex lifecycle requires the faeces to reach water bodies where the parasite larvae hatch, pass a stage in aquatic snails and then become free-swimming infective larvae. Infection occurs through skin contact (wading, swimming) with contaminated water.

Children are especially vulnerable to all the above infections, particularly when they are under the stress of disaster dislocation, high-density camp living and malnutrition. While specific measures can be taken to prevent the spread of infection through contamination by human faeces (e.g. chlorinating the water supply, providing hand-washing facilities and soap), the first priority is to isolate and contain faeces.

8.1.2 Urine

Urine is relatively harmless, except in areas where the urinary form of schistosomiasis occurs. This parasitic infection, caused by *Schistosoma haematobium*, is similar to the one described in the section above, except this parasite species resides in the veins around the bladder and its eggs are excreted with urine. In these areas, urinating in water courses should be prevented; otherwise, indiscriminate urination is not a health hazard.

8.1.3 Sullage

Wastewater from kitchens, bathrooms and laundries is called sullage. It can contain disease-causing organisms, particularly from soiled clothing, but its main health hazard occurs when it collects in poorly drained places and causes pools of organically polluted water that may serve as breeding places for *Culex* mosquitoes. This genus of mosquitoes transmits some viruses as well as the parasitic disease lymphatic filariasis. Mosquitoes that transmit malaria do not breed in polluted water.

8.1.4 Solid waste

Rats, dogs, cats and other animals, which may be carriers (reservoirs) of disease-causing organisms are attracted to discarded food, cloth, medical dressings and other components of solid waste. Small rainwater collections in solid waste may serve as the breeding places for *Aedes* mosquitoes, vectors of the dengue virus. Deep, compacted burial and, in particular, incineration of medical waste are essential to eliminate the associated health risks. Inorganic waste, such as fuel ash, can be hazardous to health. Items such as empty pesticide containers should be crushed and buried to ensure that they are not accidentally recycled.

8.1.5 The importance of hygiene behaviour

The links between sanitation, water supply, and health are directly affected by hygiene behaviour. It is important to bear this in mind when considering technical options, so that facilities provided in emergencies are acceptable to the users and can be used and maintained hygienically. See Chapter 15 for more information on hygiene promotion.

8.2 Strategy for excreta disposal in emergencies

Excreta-disposal techniques referred to in this section are described more fully in section 8.3.

8.2.1 Situations demanding an emergency excreta-disposal response

Disaster-affected urban areas

Major health risks due to inadequate excreta disposal after disasters arise in urban areas following damage to existing systems, or when parts of a city receive large numbers of displaced or homeless people, so putting increased pressure on facilities that may already be under strain. A rapid assessment of damage and needs is required to decide what emergency actions to take.

The immediate response may include establishing or reinforcing sewage tankering services, to bypass blocked sewers or to carry out intensive septic tank or latrine emptying in periurban areas. Every effort should be made to allow people to use their existing toilets, through temporary repairs to broken sewers and sewage treatment works. In extreme situations, it may be necessary, as a temporary measure, to discharge sewage directly into a river or the sea, or to hold it in a safe, isolated place. If this is done, the public must be informed, and any places used for this purpose should be fenced off.

When sections of the population can no longer use their toilets, public facilities may need to be provided, by allowing access to schools, community centers, etc., or by setting up temporary public toilets. If available, chemical toilets may be placed on street corners and emptied by municipal workers. Simple drop-hole latrines can be placed over open inspection covers, allowing excreta to drop straight into a sewer, if the sewer is still in operation and sufficiently flushed with sewage. If not, then water tankers can be used to flush them one or more times per day. Storm drains can also be used for this purpose, but only after careful consideration of the environmental risks.

Where bucket latrines are normally used, the collection of night soil may be disrupted by the emergency. Continued use of buckets should be encouraged and alternative arrangements made for collection and disposal (e.g. a common neighbourhood deep-trench latrine) until collection has returned to normal. The protection and health of the workers involved in bucket collection should be a major concern. The use of bucket latrines should be replaced by hygienic alternatives as soon as possible.

In general, defecation in rivers and streams should be discouraged unless absolutely necessary, and then only if an area downstream of other human use can be designated for the purpose. Similarly, defecation in the sea should also be discouraged, especially when the population density is high or when bays, lagoons, or estuaries are used for fishing. If the sea is to be used, the tides, currents and prevailing winds should be studied so that excrement does not wash back on shore, and a specific area set aside for defecation.

A neighbourhood health committee should be organized as soon as possible (or if it already exists, identified and mobilized) to liaise with the public-health authorities in making more permanent arrangements for human excreta removal and for supervising general waste disposal.

Previous training exercises should have revealed material needs, and the items concerned should be in stock, or obtainable on loan from another government department or the private sector.

Postemergency activities should focus on ensuring a return to, or improvement on, levels of service prior to the disaster.

Disaster-affected rural areas

Disasters affecting sparsely-settled rural areas are less often of great concern, because of the lower concentration of people and lesser risk of faecal contamination through inadequate sanitation. In such situations, a focus on the protection of water sources is usually the priority. However, protection of water sources often requires efforts to improve excreta disposal, at least in certain areas, and an emergency may provide the opportunity to raise awareness of sanitation generally, and start a longer-term process of improvement.

Displacement emergencies

In displacement emergencies, large numbers of people find themselves in crowded conditions, in transit, or in camps, with inadequate sanitary facilities. Initial sanitary arrangements can be very simple. As a minimum, defecation should not be allowed where it can contaminate the water supply or food chain. Defecation should be discouraged along river banks; in the beds of rivers or wadis (possible future water sources); within 30 metres of wells or boreholes; within 10 metres of taps; on or above the surfaces prepared for rainwater catchment; within 30 metres uphill of a spring or 10 metres downhill; or within 10 metres of any water-storage tank or treatment plant.

Open defecation should also be discouraged along public highways, in the vicinity of hospitals, feeding centres, reception centres, food storage areas, food preparation areas, and in fields containing crops for human consumption. When it is impossible to establish defecation fields, open defecation should be limited to specific, well-defined areas, which should be closed as soon as alternative sites for defecation are available.

Along displacement routes, between transit points, there may be a lot of open defecation by the side of the road. Faeces should be picked up, daily if possible, and buried nearby. If open defecation is inevitable and people also stop overnight by the side of the road, people should be encourages to use one side of the road for defecation and the other side for cooking and resting.

It is usually necessary to set up a more structured system, such as defecation fields, or defecation trenches, that ensure better separation and containment of excreta. These may be followed by longer-term, but intermediate, measures, such as public trench latrines when the transit center or emergency settlement is likely to remain in place for more than a few weeks. However, as emergency settlements are often likely to remain for at least a year, then construction of family toilets, usually simple pit latrines, should begin without delay.

Communal facilities should be regularly cleaned by staff who are rewarded for their work, and who are adequately trained and equipped. Clean latrines help to encourage proper use of the facilities; dirty latrines inevitably lead to carelessness and unsanitary defecation practices in and around them. Routine inspection by supervisors is necessary to ensure that cleaning standards are maintained and that repairs are carried out. Staff may need to meet with the users to encourage clean use of the toilets.

As far as appropriate, user families should be involved in latrine construction programmes. They should be involved in the choice of technology and materials, siting and orientation of latrines, pit digging, slab installation, and superstructure building. The implementing agency should work closely with user families to encourage latrine construction, provide advice on siting and construction, and ensure that pits and finished latrines meet standards for stability, capacity and hygiene. The agency may provide tools and materials, as well as advice and information.

8.2.2 Gradual improvement

Although people may be able to reduce their water use drastically for a short period following a disaster, they can do nothing about their production of excreta. Whenever environmental health staff travel to a disaster-affected location they find people who have already established a pattern of excreta disposal, using whatever means are available. The general strategy should be to gain a rapid understanding of existing practice and take temporary steps to improve it, if necessary, and then make further improvements, responding to areas of greatest need as defined by disease incidence and lack of access to facilities.

Subsequent steps in an emergency excreta-disposal response involve more detailed assessment of damage to existing facilities, in the case of urban-based disasters, or of likely population movements and the development of needs and resources in the case of displacement emergencies. This more detailed assessment should prompt a series of actions and reassessments that ensure a constant improvement in sanitary arrangements. The various options available need careful consideration and discussion with the population concerned, to produce a strategy that takes account of short- and long-term public-health risk, cost, time and user preferences. Technical options that may be used in a programme for gradually improving excreta disposal are presented in section 8.3.

8.2.3 Technology choice

Figure 8.1 provides a guide to technology choice for excreta disposal in emergencies that takes into account the difficulties posed by different types of ground condition. Where the opportunity exists for selecting and planning an emergency settlement site, environmental health staff should be closely involved in ensuring that sites are chosen and laid out in a way that provides suitable conditions for sanitation. See Chapter 6.

Any successful measure for managing human excreta includes the principles of separation, containment and destruction. A simple pit latrine, for example, separates excreta from humans; it contains it within the pit, beneath the slab; and the excreta is destroyed by a process of decomposition and die-off of pathogens. Whatever form of toilet is designed and built in an emergency, it must fulfill these three functions to minimize health risks.

Excreta disposal measures must be designed and built to avoid contamination of water sources that will be used for drinking-water.

Figure 8.1 **Decision tree for excreta disposal in refugee camps[1]**

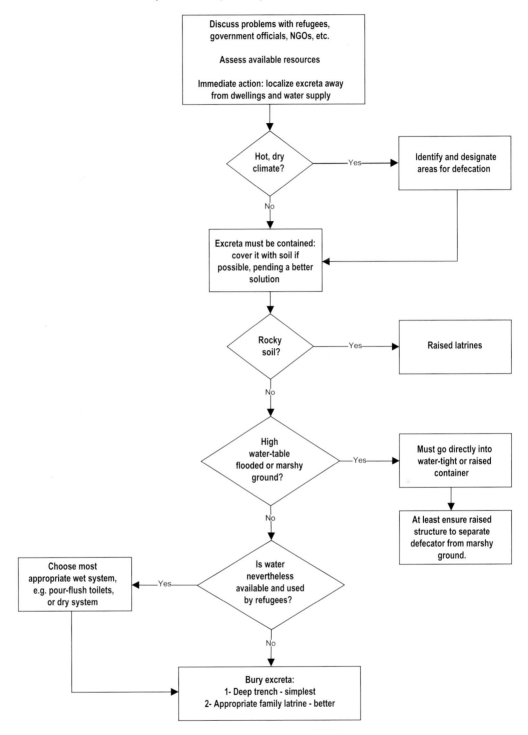

[1] Source: United Nations High Commissioner for Refugees (1999).

Consultation with the disaster-affected people is an essential aspect of technology choice. Whereas they are consumers with regards to water supply, they are producers with regards to excreta disposal and other aspects of sanitation. Sanitary arrangements and sensitivities vary a great deal between cultures, and different groups in the camp, such as men, women, or the elderly, may have special needs and wishes. A health committee is very important as a means of communicating with the disaster-affected people, for whom the living arrangements may be strange and disorienting. Sensitive and culturally-specific issues, such as arrangements for disposing of menstrual discharge, or for anal cleansing after defecation, can best be discussed with the health committee. For more information on consultation, see Chapter 15.

8.2.4 Assessment

Urban situations with existing facilities

A proper health assessment of the impact of damaged sanitation systems requires a sanitary survey. In particular, an assessment of the status of the sewage system is required as soon as possible after immediate disaster relief has been provided. Information should be gathered on the number of breaks or obstructions in sewer lines; the lengths and sizes of pipes that need to be replaced; and a list of the repair equipment required, such as pumps, bulldozers, excavating machinery, trucks, tools, construction materials, etc. An early estimate is also needed of the equipment, materials and labour necessary to restore sewage-treatment plants and pumping stations to working order.

In periurban areas where on-plot sanitation is likely to be the norm, assessments should identify the number of households without functioning toilets, the current arrangements made for excreta disposal by those households (including the use of neighbours' toilets), and requirements for immediate and postemergency action.

Displacement emergencies

In displacement emergencies, the assessment process is likely to be quite different, as the people concerned are likely to find themselves in situations they are not familiar with, with considerable loss of social cohesion. Key information includes the number of people currently affected and likely future population movements; existing excreta-disposal arrangements; predisaster excreta-disposal practices; ground conditions; availability of construction materials and tools; the workload and labour availability of the affected population; the water-supply and drainage situation; the general health of the displaced population; and the incidence and/or risk of excreta-related diseases.

8.2.5 Standards

UNHCR recommend one toilet per family as the best option, one per 20 people as the second best option, and one per 100 people, or a defecation field, as the third best; recommendations are given for the design and construction of facilities, to ensure they are appropriate and correctly used (United Nations High Commissioner for Refugees, 1999). The Sphere Project recommendations are similar to those of UNHCR, but provide more detailed advice on the quality of toilet facilities and their acceptability to users (Sphere Project, 2000).

8.3 Techniques for excreta disposal in emergencies

The techniques in this section are described broadly in order of increasing permanency and complexity. In some emergency situations, several of these options are used at different stages of the response as the situation develops. The first three techniques–defecation fields, shallow trench latrines, and deep trench latrines–have mostly been used in displacement emergencies, but may be useful in any situation where temporary toilets are needed rapidly. The other techniques are widely used in stable situations, but can be adapted to any long-term emergency settlement. Whatever the technical option chosen, consideration should be given to hand-washing facilities and night lighting. The needs of small children should be given special attention. See Box 8.1 for further information.

Figure 8.2 **Open defecation field**[1]

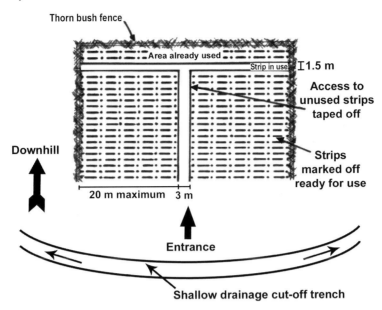

[1] Source: Reed (1994).

Box 8.1 **Excreta control and small children**

Children's faeces are generally more infectious than those of adults, and many children are unable to control their defecation, so preventing indiscriminate defecation by small children should be a high priority. In short-term relief centres, it may be possible to provide parents with disposable napkins. Usually, however, this is not possible, and parents should be encouraged to clean up and dispose of children's faeces rapidly and hygienically. Shovels, small spades, or home-made digging tools made from wood should be available to parents to enable them to bury children's excrement.

In Ethiopian relief camps in the mid-1980s, special defecation trenches for children were used successfully by the Save the Children Fund. Mothers sat on one side of the trench with their feet propped on the other side, and placed the children between their feet. When the children had defecated, they left via a hand-washing facility. Each time a mother left, a latrine guard shoveled earth over the faeces (Appleton & Save the Children Fund Ethiopia Team, 1987).

8.3.1 Defecation fields

A defecation field is illustrated in Figure 8.2. The area set aside should be of sufficient size to accommodate $0.25\,\text{m}^2$ per person per day excluding access paths. Separate areas for men and women are usually desirable. The field should be in a convenient place, but no nearer than 30 metres to other camp facilities. Ideally, it would be on land that slopes away from the camp and any surface water sources. The soil should be soft enough to dig easily in order to cover excreta.

Health education is required to obtain the cooperation and understanding of the user population. A defecation field requires an attendant, for providing information to users and for cleaning and maintenance.

Users should be directed to strips of land in the defecation field roughly 1.5 metres wide. They should use one strip until it is filled, usually entering by one access path and leaving by another. When a strip is filled, excreta is then covered by the attendant with at least 10 centimetres of soil and another strip is opened some metres away. The field is used systematically in this way, beginning with the strips furthest from camp. An improvement on this basic system is to dig shallow trenches (15 centimetres deep) in the strips, so that the excreta can be completely buried.

The active part of the field should be illuminated at night and demarcated with poles and pegs. Users should be guided to active strips by ropes or coloured tapes, as shown in Figure 8.3. A further improvement is the erection of walls of plastic sheeting, to divide the defecation field into smaller, more private areas, where this is culturally desirable.

8.3.2 Shallow trench latrines

Shallow trench latrines (see Figure 8.4) allow faeces to be buried and far better contained than in a defecation field. Approximately 3–5 metres length of shallow trench is needed for every 100 people, and it is preferable to have a number of shorter, shallow trenches. Trenches should never be used for more than a week before they are completely filled, compacted and replaced by new trenches. Shallow trench latrines should be sited in the same way as defecation fields.

Consultation with the camp health committee will reveal whether it is better to arrange for each family in a tent or shelter to dig and use its own shallow trench. A stock of shovels should be kept for use by residents.

After each visit, the user should shovel into the trench sufficient soil to cover the excreta. Boards can be placed along the edges of the trench to provide stable footing and prevent the sides from caving in. When the trench is filled to within 30 centimetres of the top, or after a week's use (whichever comes first), it should be completely filled, compacted and marked for future identification, and a new trench should be dug and used.

8.3.3 Deep trench latrines

A further improvement is the deep trench latrine, which is deeper, longer and wider than the shallow trench latrine. It can last 1–3 months and is constructed as shown in Figure 8.5. It can be constructed from a variety of materials, including wooden planks and plastic squatting plates for the floor and plastic sheeting, and wooden planks or

Figure 8.3 **A trench defecation field with guidance markers[1]**

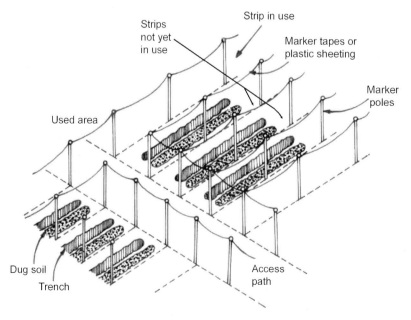

[1] Source: Reed (1994).

Figure 8.4 **Shallow trench latrine**[1]

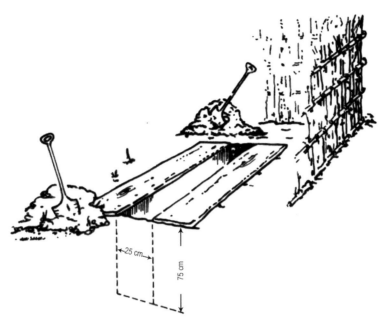

←25 cm→

75 cm

[1] Source: Rajagopalan & Shiffman (1974).

Figure 8.5 **Deep trench latrine**[1]

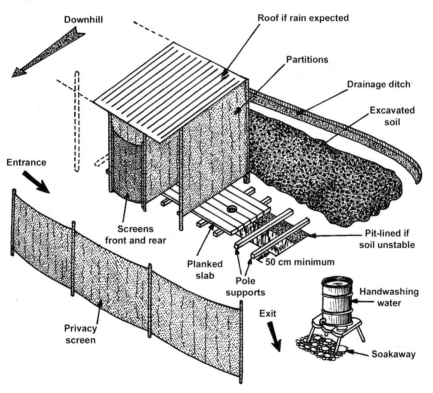

[1] Source: Reed (1994).

metal sheets for the superstructure. In the former Yugoslav Republic of Macedonia, during 1999, most Kosovar refugee camps had 10-metre-long deep trench latrines, each provided with 10 plastic squatting plates and superstructures with wooden frames and either metal or plastic sheeting.

In the example shown, each deep trench can accommodate up to six cubicles, screened for privacy as shown. Each cubicle measures 90 centimetres wide by 80 centimetres high. At peak usage, it is reasonable to use an estimate of 50 people per day per cubicle, or 240 each day for each deep trench. Soil is piled up and used to cover excrement, as in a shallow trench system. The simple arrangement of using boards across the trench as foot rests can easily be improved on as time and materials allow. Eventually, however, a wooden cover with either squatting plates or seats can be constructed. There may be carpenters among the residents, and volunteers should be mobilized to help; such improvements, and the use of ashes and soil to cover excreta, can help to control flies.

A number of agencies now use plastic latrine slabs that can be placed in line over a deep trench to form a row of toilets that are rapid to construct and easy to keep clean.

8.3.4 Simple pit latrines

Individual simple pit latrines, either hand-dug or drilled, may be an option in lower-density, longer-term emergency settlements (Figure 8.6). Family latrines are normally preferred as they are more hygienic than public facilities, and there are long-term benefits in terms of maintenance.

A family can dig its own latrine if given advice and provided with tools. Initial, simple screening to provide privacy can be improved to give protection from the weather as needed. It is important for the control of flies, mosquitoes and odours that tight-fitting lids for the squatting holes are provided and are always closed by users after each visit to the latrine.

The latrine slab can be made of sawn timber, logs (with or without an earth covering), concrete, plastic, or a combination of two or more of these. The latrine superstructure may be made of a wooden framework covered with plastic sheeting, grass, or other local materials. Temporary superstructures may be replaced by the users with more permanent materials after the emergency phase. The choice of materials for slabs and superstructures will depend on considerations such as cost, local availability, environmental impact, and ease of use for families constructing their own latrines.

Normally the pit should be designed to last at least a year, and its volume should be calculated on the basis of about $0.07\,m^3$ per user per year. In unstable soils, the top 50 centimetres of the pit, or the whole depth of the pit, may need to be lined to prevent collapse. Pit linings may be made of many different materials, including brick, concrete, old oil drums or bamboo. Pit linings should normally not be watertight below 50 centimetres deep.

8.3.5 Other types of latrine

The simple pit latrine is the basis for the design of a number of other types of latrine, described below. Some may be appropriate for specific soil or site conditions. Most require more time, materials and specialist knowledge for their construction.

Ventilated improved pit (VIP) latrines

The VIP latrine incorporates one-way ventilation through the pit to reduce odours and insect breeding. While nonventilated latrines should have lids to reduce these problems (Figure 8.6 A), the VIP latrine does not require a cover over the defecation hole if there is sufficient wind to create an air flow up the pipe (Figure 8.6 B). The end of the ventilation pipe should be covered with mosquito netting. Flies that breed in the pit and then fly up the pipe towards the daylight cannot then leave the latrine, and flies on the outside

Figure 8.6 **Various types of pit latrine: (A) nonventilated; (B) ventilated; (C) twin-pit, ventilated[1]**

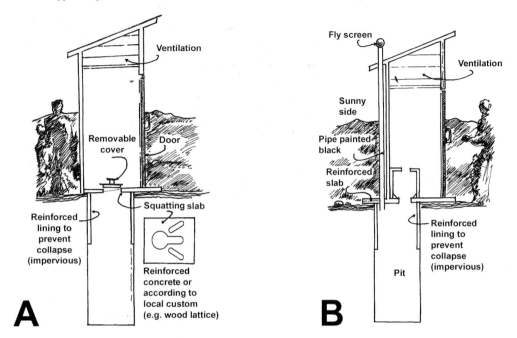

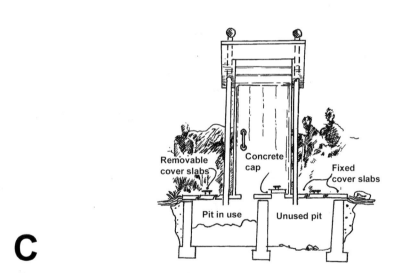

[1] Source: United Nations High Commissioner for Refugees (1999).

that are attracted by the smell coming from the top of the pipe are unable to enter the latrine. Pit design is as for the simple pit latrine.

Double-pit latrines

Double-pit latrines (Figure 8.6 C) are useful where there is limited room for digging new pits. The filled side can be emptied via an access hatch while the other side is being used. If the filling of one side takes sufficient time (at the very least, 6 months, better 2 years), emptying can be delayed until anaerobic decomposition has killed the pathogens. Double-pit latrines may be ventilated or nonventilated. A variation on this technique is the twin-pit latrine used with water-seal toilets. Two separate pits are used, joined to a water-seal toilet with a pipe with a Y-junction in an access chamber. Each separate pit is used in turn, as with the double-pit system, switching between pits being achieved by blocking one half of the Y-junction.

Raised or mound latrines can be used where there is a high water-table (Franceys, Pickford & Reed, 1992).

Composting latrines

The composting latrine can be used in lower-density, longer-term settlements, where the compost produced can be used in food production. It may take 12–24 months for the compost to become safe to handle, depending on the climate.

Water-seal latrines

Water-seal (or pour-flush) latrines are similar to simple pit latrines, but instead of having a squatting hole in the cover slab, they have a shallow toilet pan with a water seal. In the simplest type, excreta falls directly into the latrine pit when the pan is flushed with a small quantity of water. Pour-flush latrines can be connected at a later stage with either a septic tank, the effluent from which can be disposed of by means of subsurface-soil absorption, or a small-bore sewer system. It may be possible to install such latrines, depending on the lead time in setting up an emergency settlement; the length of its life (and hence the time available for incremental improvements); its location; and the availability of pour-flush pans.

8.3.6 Site selection for latrines

Latrines should be sited at least 30 metres from any water source. If the abstraction point is upstream of the latrine, the distance can be reduced provided that the groundwater is not abstracted at such a rate that its flow direction is turned towards the abstraction point (Franceys, Pickford & Reed, 1992). In heavily-fissured rock this distance may have to be increased substantially. Because pollution (faecal and chemical) tends to disperse downslope from its source, latrines should be sited *downhill* from any groundwater source, particularly if the bottom of the latrine is less than 2 metres above the water-table (see Figure 8.7).

Consideration should also be given to the pattern of usage of communal latrines. Such usage will probably not be uniform, but concentrated along lines of common travel (e.g. to and from feeding centres, schools, etc.). It may be necessary to close some latrines and open others at some stage, to adjust to demand.

Latrines should be sited no more than 50 metres from users' shelters, to encourage their use, but sufficiently far away (at least 6 metres) to reduce problems from odours and pests.

8.3.7 Management of excreta disposal facilities

One of the main reasons that sanitation facilities fail in emergencies is insufficient management. There are several reasons for this, including insufficient consultation with users at the design stage, leading to facilities that are not used as intended; insufficient resources provided for maintaining and cleaning public facilities; and inadequate supervision of self-build sanitation programmes, leading to incorrect siting and construction of latrines. Excreta disposal programmes in emergencies demand substantial resources and management support, from the assessment stage to decommissioning facilities or handing them over.

Figure 8.7 **Dispersal of pollution from its source**[1]
Key:
A. Pollution cone, spreading out about 1 metre all round, goes vertically downwards until the ground-water level is reached.
B. If the groundwater surface is less than about 3 metres deep, the pollution then spreads cone-wise, flowing with the groundwater. The groundwater can be diverted from its natural course if the area is within the circle of influence of pumping from a well. The bacterial content of the pollution spreads sideways and downwards, and becomes absorbed by the soil until, at about 10 metres from the source, it has virtually disappeared.
C. The cone of chemical pollution continues to spread until about 25 metres from the source, and then gradually reduces to almost nothing at a distance of about 100 metres.
L. Source of pollution at pit latrine, septic tank, or soakaway.

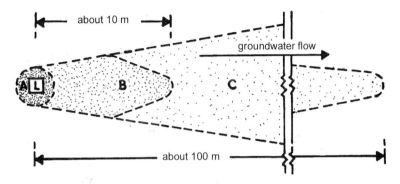

[1] Source: Pike (1987).

8.4 Disposal of wastewater (sullage)

8.4.1 Assessment of the problem and design of the response

The scale and nature of the wastewater problem should first be assessed. Important information includes: how much wastewater is produced, and by how much does production vary during the day and over longer periods; the nature of the wastewater, including whether it is likely to be contaminated with faeces, and characteristics pertinent to the disposal method to be used; the source of the wastewater; the location of risks or nuisances it may cause; and soil, topography, climate and other factors that may determine which disposal options are possible. In many emergency situations, it may be judged that the quantity and nature of the wastewater produced do not present a health risk sufficient to justify control activity. In others, efforts to limit the production of wastewater may be sufficient to keep the problem under control. In many situations, however, specific measures are needed to dispose of wastewater, and these are described below.

The response chosen should take the above factors into account, and be carried out in a way that complements concurrent activities in water supply and excreta disposal.

8.4.2 Wastewater disposal techniques

The main options for disposing of wastewater are to discharge it into water courses, with or without treatment, to infiltrate it into the soil, or to use it for irrigation (in which case most of the water is disposed of by infiltration, evaporation and evapotranspiration).

Disposal into water courses

If nearby water courses suitable for accepting the type and quantity of wastewater produced are available, the best disposal method may be to direct the wastewater to them through pipes or open channels. It may be possible to make a connection to an existing drainage network and thereby to treatment and discharge installations. It is important for staff to investigate the drainage system as far as the final discharge point, to avoid creating or contributing to environmental pollution and contamination of water supplies. But where relatively small quantities of slightly contaminated wastewater are produced (for instance, the water spilled at a water collection point), discharge into a water course may have no significant environmental impact.

Infiltration techniques

Infiltration into the soil should be facilitated where large quantities of spilled or used water will accumulate, e.g. under water-distribution tanks and taps, outside bath houses and laundries, and near communal kitchen areas.

The simplest technique is to construct a soakaway (or soakage pit). This is an excavation at least 1.25 metres deep and 1.25 metres wide, filled with stones, that allows water to seep into the surrounding ground. It is sealed from above by an impermeable layer (oiled sacking, plastic or metal) to discourage insect breeding. Wastewater is fed by pipe into the center of the pit (Figure 8.8).

Figure 8.8 **Unlined (A) and lined (B) soakage pits with effluent inlets[1]**

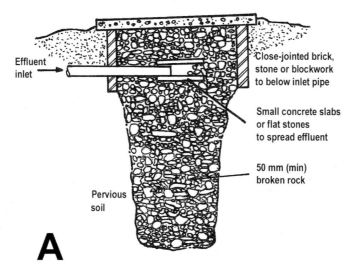

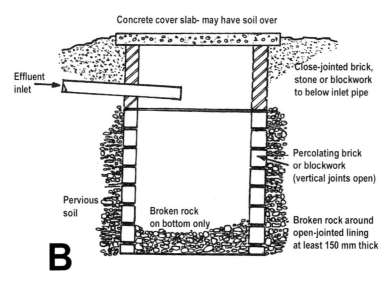

[1] Source: Assar (1971).

In emergencies, soakaways may consist simply of pits filled with small stones or gravel into which wastewater is directed. As long as the level of the water in the pit does not rise above the top of the ground, insect breeding is minimal.

Soakaways can only dispose of a limited amount of water because they provide a relatively small area of soil surface for infiltration. Infiltration trenches, which are commonly used for disposing of the effluent from septic tanks, overcome this problem through a series of parallel trenches in which perforated pipes are laid in a bed of gravel.

Evaporation and evapotranspiration techniques

Where infiltration methods do not work effectively because of low soil permeability, wastewater may be disposed of by using it for irrigation. Even when infiltration methods are possible, it may be appropriate to use wastewater for vegetable gardening if irrigation water is scarce. Such a system might be considered for longer-term use, for instance, adjacent to a nutrition rehabilitation centre, health centre or school.

Water is applied to garden plots by simple flood irrigation, or by allowing it to collect in basins from where water is carried to plots. Care must be taken to allow flood-irrigated beds and storage basins to dry out regularly to avoid mosquito breeding.

A simpler system that does not involve irrigation, is to allow water to flow into shallow pans, where it simply evaporates. Alternatively, soap-free wastewater from spillage at water collection points may be used for watering livestock, but care should be taken not to create muddy and contaminated areas near water points.

Grease traps

Whatever the disposal method chosen, wastewater from the kitchen and laundry area should first be put through a grease trap (Figure 8.9). If hot water containing fat is run into an adequate supply of cold water, the fat solidifies and rises to the surface, where it can be skimmed off. A strainer is fitted to the inlet to catch any large particles which might pass through the trap and choke the inlet to the soakage pit. The first baffle prevents the entering water from disturbing the layer of grease, the second keeps the effluent from carrying it off. Grease traps are also effective at reducing the amount of sand and soap in wastewater.

Figure 8.9 **Grease trap**[1]

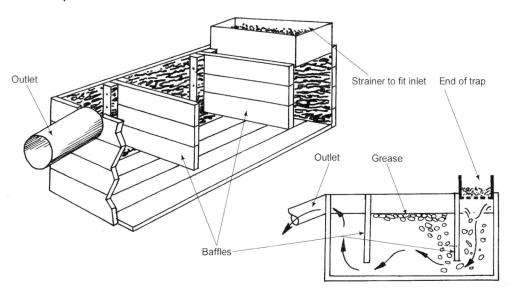

[1] Source: Skeet (1977).

8.5 Management of refuse

In many parts of the world, a disaster can cause transportation problems that disrupt waste-management systems that are inadequate even during normal times. Extra quantities of waste, or new forms of waste, such as rubble from destroyed buildings, or flood debris, may be generated by the disaster. Immediate problems that commonly follow disasters such as floods and hurricanes are blockage of roads and water courses and mixing of hazardous and nonhazardous wastes. The first priority is often the clearance of post-disaster debris to reduce health risks, open routes and lessen the psychological impact of the disaster.

8.5.1 Assessment of the problem and design of the response

As with wastewater, solid waste may not present a particular environmental health problem in emergencies. Where rural communities are displaced, for example, and they receive a dry ration of grain, pulses and oil distributed in bulk, there is likely to be very little solid waste produced. Assessments should seek to determine: the quantity of refuse produced by the affected population, and how that is likely to change over time (for example, as ration packaging changes, or as market activities develop or are reestablished); the density and composition of refuse produced; the composition of the refuse produced; existing patterns of refuse management, including storage and destruction; any collection, reuse and recycling activities already carried out; constraints on collection and transport, such as personnel reduction, the use of trucks for rubble removal in critical areas, and damaged or blocked routes. A population of 1000 people may commonly produce between 2–4 m^3 of solid waste per day (World Health Organization, 1991b).

The response chosen should take the above factors into account, and reflect knowledge about the possible duration of the emergency, the appropriate level of users' involvement, and the economic sustainability of different options. In some situations, it may be better to avoid launching a system of refuse collection and centralized disposal if it is unlikely that this can be sustained for more than a few months. In such cases, it may be better to focus attention on reduction, reuse and recycling of refuse, or stimulate local initiatives based on decentralized disposal methods.

8.5.2 Refuse storage

The number and size of refuse containers needed varies greatly from situation to situation, and can only be determined in practice through an assessment. But as a rule of thumb, one container of capacity 100–200 litres, preferably plastic or metal and with a tight-fitting lid, should be provided for every 10–20 families, placed not more than 15 metres from the shelter (United Nations High Commissioner for Refugees, 1999). Alternatively, one container of 50–100 litres may be provided for every 25–50 people (Pan American Health Organization, 1996). In some situations, large street-corner storage containers may be used, provided they have tight-fitting lids. In most cases, these recommendations will allow two days' worth of refuse to be stored.

In markets and commercial areas, large containers or collection bays may be needed. To control flies and rats, a market authority or committee should be established to manage cleaning of the market area and manage the refuse collection site. Certain wastes, such as waste from animal slaughtering, may need special containers to deal with the large quantities of liquids produced.

Arrangements for refuse storage, collection and transport should be made in consultation with the affected population and should aim to minimize nuisance and health risks.

8.5.3 Refuse collection and transport

Before starting the collection service, it is necessary to determine: the quantity of solid waste to be collected; how much waste will be generated; the frequency of the service; the quantity and size of collector trucks; the number of workers required; the final disposal method; and the disposal site.

For every 1000 residents, 2.5 workers should be appointed. Their tasks include cleaning streets and open spaces; collecting waste containers; cleaning facilities, markets, and the like; and transferring waste to the treatment or final disposal site. The number of workers will decrease as refugee services are organized (World Health Organization, United Nations Environment Programme, 1991).

Daily refuse collection is best, especially from kitchens, but collection not less than once a week is essential to minimize insect breeding (flies produce a new generation approximately every eight days in warm conditions).

One 5-ton truck will probably be sufficient for 10000 people, but this depends on the quantity and density of refuse collected, the ease of collection, and the time required to transport refuse to the disposal site. Although any kind of truck may be used for emergency responses, compactor trucks are always preferable if these can be afforded. Otherwise, the truck should be chosen on the basis of the volume and density of waste to be collected. Handcarts can also be used in large, densely-populated settlements.

Collection routes and frequency will be determined according to waste generation. This information should be communicated to the population as soon as possible.

8.5.4 Treatment and disposal

This section deals with disposal of household refuse and market waste. Disposal of medical waste should be managed completely separately (see section 8.5.6).

Burial

In low-density settlements where relatively small quantities of refuse are produced, small refuse pits may be dug by each family.

Alternatively, a communal trench 1.5 metres wide and 2 metres deep can be excavated by hand for the refuse. Each day, refuse should be covered with 20–30 centimetres of earth. When the level in the trench is 40 centimetres below ground level, the trench should be filled with earth and compacted, and a new trench dug. A 1-metre long trench for every 200 camp residents will be filled in about a week (Pan American Health Organization, 1996).

If time and available labour permit, refuse should be separated into material that is biodegradable (vegetable matter), which should be dumped in one trench, and other material (bottles, can, plastic, etc.), which should be dumped in another. The trench for biodegradable refuse can be dug out after 6 months and used as compost.

Bottles and cans may be cleaned and recycled, but care should be taken to segregate all containers used for dangerous chemicals, such as pesticides. Containers that have contained pesticides should be crushed so that they cannot be reused. They should be buried far from any water source.

Sanitary landfill

In most cases, the use of sanitary landfills will be the best option for final disposal. When existing landfills are inoperative or inaccessible, the construction of new landfills will be necessary. The landfill site should be:

— located away from the settlement;
— accessible;
— on vacant/uncultivated land;
— located in natural depressions with slight slopes;
— downwind from the settlement;
— sited and organized to avoid surface water and groundwater pollution;
— in an area that is not exposed to landslides or earthquakes.

The site must be carefully selected, as it may be used as a permanent place for final disposal.

Earthmoving equipment may be needed to modify the site and to manage the landfill operation. It has been estimated that an area of 0.4–0.5 hectares (4000–5000 m^2) can serve 10000 inhabitants (World Health Organization, United Nations Environment Programme, 1991).

Incineration

Incineration is a third possibility, but it is not usually suitable for the volume of domestic refuse produced by the general population, because it requires large incinerators and large amounts of fuel, and air pollution is almost inevitable. Incinerators should be located away from the settlement, on the opposite side from the direction of the prevailing wind. They should be built on an impervious base of concrete or hardened earth. Ash and any unburned refuse should be buried and covered with 40 centimetres of soil. In many countries, waste is partially burned at landfill sites. This has the advantage of reducing the volume of waste to be buried, but the smoke created is a nuisance and a hazard to health.

Waste recycling

It may be appropriate to encourage and facilitate recycling of refuse after collection and transport. Refuse can be sorted as an income-generating activity, producing paper, glass, metals and plastics for recycling, where these materials are present in significant quantities in the refuse. Measures should be taken to ensure that people sorting refuse for recycling are protected from health hazards, such as exposure to harmful chemicals, or cuts from sharps.

Composting is a practical way to treat the organic waste remaining after sorting. Simple methods produce good-quality compost for use in gardens. It may be possible to co-compost refuse and sludge from emptying latrines and septic tanks. In this case, special attention is required to ensure compost heaps attain and maintain adequate temperatures to kill pathogens. If there is any doubt about this, the compost should be stored for at least a year before use.

8.5.5 Disposal of rubble

Disasters often produce rubble from damaged buildings and other structures that far exceeds the capacity of solid waste management systems. This waste is not hazardous, but it hampers the emergency response by blocking roads and hiding the full extent of the damage, and blocks drainage channels, which leads to flooding and wastewater overflow.

It is necessary to take into account that all initial efforts are aimed at the rescue of buried people who may remain alive for up to seven days. Although quick and effective demolition methods are necessary, they should be carefully applied to prevent collapses that may produce even more damage.

After floods, accumulation of sludge both inside the house and outdoors may become a major problem. It is recommended that waste is removed manually from inside dwellings, mechanically from public roads, and then disposed of with other rubble. Ash produced by volcanic eruptions can be cleared by groups of workers, often from the affected community. New ash falls may need to be cleared every day or so.

Initial assessments of the affected areas and estimated tonnes of material to be cleared are crucial elements for demolition activities and waste management. These assessments should be rapid and general, as detailed research may usually be time-consuming, and a prompt response is required.

In highly developed urban areas, an average of 1.5 tonnes of building waste may be generated per square metre constructed (United Nations Environment Programme, International Environmental Technology Centre, 1992). In residential areas, this amount ranges from 0.5 to 1.0 ton per square metre constructed, depending on the materials used in each locality. Decisions on the demolition of damaged buildings are often difficult to make since costs, policies, structural risk and other factors must be first analysed.

The various components of rubble should be separated to facilitate recycling. Metals, mainly iron and steel, can be smelted for reuse. Concrete can be crushed for road-building, land reclamation, etc. Wood can be used as fuel. In many cases, the local population will spontaneously recover useful materials. This activity may need monitoring to reduce the risks of accidents and avoid legal problems. Final disposal may be in landfill sites.

8.5.6 Medical wastes

Special care must be taken with refuse from a field hospital or health centre. The main categories of waste of concern are: infectious waste; pathological waste; sharps; pharmaceutical waste; genotoxic waste; chemical waste; waste with high heavy metal content; pressurized containers; and radioactive waste (World Health Organization 1999c). Each type of waste requires specific measures for handling, storage, collection and destruction. In the case of simple health centers, particularly in rural areas, well-managed on-site burial may be appropriate. In larger centres producing a significant quantity of sharps and infected waste, incineration may also be required. When health facilities operate diagnostic laboratory services, radiological diagnosis and treatment facilities, pharmacies, etc., waste management is a specialized activity requiring trained and well-equipped staff, and the subject is beyond the scope of this book.

Waste management during triage and classification of victims

Triage and classification of victims generate potentially infectious waste. Since this is a rapid-response activity, it is highly recommended that all wastes generated during this stage, without exception, are stored in containers, preferably in red bags, that are properly labelled as "biocontaminated waste". Direct contact with such wastes must be avoided.

Waste management during routine medical activities

Management will be similar for permanent (existing hospitals and health centres) and provisional (field hospitals) health facilities.

Wastes should be segregated at the point of generation according to their type:

— biocontaminated wastes (including sharp materials);
— chemical wastes (drugs, chemical solutions, etc.);
— common wastes (paper, cardboard, glass, or the like; chemical product containers should be treated as chemical wastes).

For each hospital room, washable and easily disinfected PVC containers with a capacity of 40–50 litres should be used. Waste should be disposed of in coloured bags according to the following codification:

— red bags for biocontaminated wastes;
— yellow bags for chemical wastes;
— black bags for common wastes.

Hermetic plastic containers of 2–5 litre capacity or opaque glass bottles may be used to store sharp objects.

These wastes should then be collected separately every 12–24 hours. Small carts, preferably with lids, should be adapted to this end and the personnel assigned should be protected with aprons, masks, boots and gloves.

Treatment should be done according to the type of waste. Sharp materials should be disinfected with a 0.5% total chlorine solution before incineration or burial in a sharps pit. Biocontaminated wastes should be incinerated.

Burned biocontaminated wastes, disinfected sharp materials, and chemical wastes should be disposed of by burial on-site if possible. The burial area should be isolated and protected to avoid illegal recycling. However, this may not be possible in permanent health facilities, due to lack of space. In such cases, protected areas should be used at landfill sites to receive treated wastes. Common wastes may be managed by the municipal waste-collection service, as long as they do not contain hazardous material.

A temporary incinerator for medical waste can be made from an old 200-litre oil drum (Figure 8.10). However, this is unlikely to perform adequately, and although it may help reduce the volume of waste to be buried, it will produce a lot of black smoke and may only partially reduce the risk posed by the waste. In addition, the use of incinerators, as opposed to direct burial, creates an additional step in the disposal process, exposing workers to risk and increasing the chances of waste escaping into the environment. Brick-built incinerators, of sufficient performance, can be built, using designs that are readily available (e.g. Christen, 1996). A single-chamber brick incinerator

Figure 8.10 **Simple basket incinerator made from a discarded oil drum**[1]

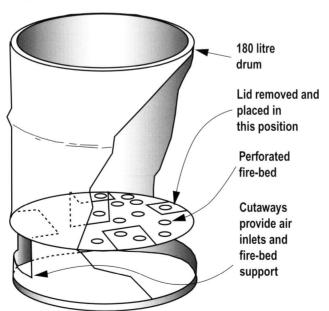

180 litre
drum

Lid removed and
placed in
this position

Perforated
fire-bed

Cutaways
provide air
inlets and
fire-bed
support

[1] Source: Skeet (1977).

Figure 8.11 **Balleul single-chamber incinerator**[1]

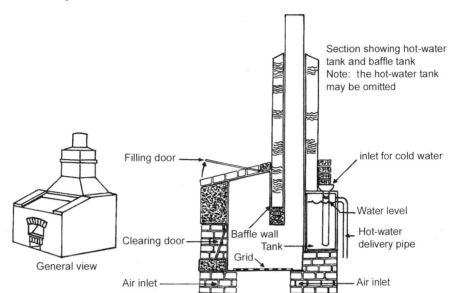

¹ Source: Christen (1996).

(Figure 8.11) that incinerates at 300–400 °C may destroy 99% of microorganisms and greatly reduce the volume and weight of waste (World Health Organization 1999c).

8.6 Further information

For further information on:

— sanitation assessment and programme design, see: Sphere Project (2000), Davis & Lambert (2002), Harvey, Baghri & Reed (2002);

— latrine designs, see: Feachem & Cairncross (1978), Winblad & Kilama (1985), Franceys, Pickford & Reed (1992), Cairncross & Feachem (1993), Pickford (1995), Davis & Lambert (2002);

— solid waste management, see: United Nations Centre for Human Settlements (1989);

— surface water and wastewater drainage, see: Davis & Lambert (2002), World Health Organization (1991c);

— management of medical wastes, see: Reed & Dean (1994), World Health Organization (1999c).

9. Food safety

9.1 The importance of safe food

Food may become difficult to obtain in an emergency or following a disaster. Crops may be destroyed in the fields, animals may be drowned, food supply lines may become disrupted, and people may be forced to flee to areas where they have no access to food. Moreover, the safety of whatever food there is may be affected, resulting in a greater risk of epidemics of foodborne disease.

Food safety problems vary in nature, severity and extent, and depend on the situation during the emergency or disaster. For example, during floods and hurricanes, food may become contaminated by surface water that has itself been contaminated by sewage and wastewaters. Flood waters often pick up large quantities of wastes and pathogenic bacteria from farms, sewer systems, latrines and septic tanks. The crowding of survivors after disasters may aggravate the situation, particularly if sanitary conditions are poor.

Any breakdown in vital services, such as water supply or electricity, also severely affects food safety. In the absence of electricity, cold storage may be more difficult, if not impossible, and foods may be subject to bacterial growth. This may happen at all stages of the food chain, from production to consumption. Lack of safe drinking-water and sanitation hampers the hygienic preparation of food and increases the risk of food contamination. Populations of pests and stray animals, such as dogs and cats, may also increase in the aftermath of disasters. Flies and other rapidly-breeding insects may increase dramatically in numbers. People may be tempted to eat drowned animals after floods, which carries a risk. Food is especially susceptible to contamination when it is stored and prepared out of doors or in damaged homes where windows and possibly even walls are no longer intact.

Fires or explosions may result in foodstuffs becoming contaminated with dangerous chemicals or microorganisms, as well as being damaged by water. Food may be damaged by smoke, chemicals used in fire fighting, or by other chemicals originating from the accidental release or improper use of insecticides, aerosols, rodenticides and other toxic substances.

Disaster-affected people eating food from centralized kitchens that are not properly equipped or run are extremely vulnerable to outbreaks of foodborne disease. The combination of environmental contamination and improper handling of food increases the risk of epidemics of diseases such as cholera and shigellosis.

In emergencies and disasters, food safety authorities should review all stages of the food supply, from production, processing and manufacturing, transport, distribution, and sale, to preparation in food service and catering establishments and households. It is essential to assess in what way the food supply may have been adversely affected, and to identify the priority measures (including education of the public) needed to protect consumers. The measures that should be considered are detailed in Sections 9.2 and 9.3, but most of them require planning and preparedness before emergencies or disasters occur. For example, suitable locations for mass feeding, such as school kitchens, as well as equipment, supplies and training facilities, should be identified as part of emergency preparedness planning.

9.2 Food control

9.2.1 Food control measures

Following a disaster, an assessment should be made of its effects on the quality and safety of food. Food safety authorities should ensure that foods that have not been affected are adequately protected, are not exposed to other sources of contamination, and are not kept under conditions in which bacterial growth may occur (see Table 9.1). For example, in warehouses that have been flooded, high humidity favours the growth of moulds and bacteria in foodstuffs. Whatever intact foods remain should be moved to a dry place, away from the walls and off the floor.

The extent and type of damage to food should be assessed, and a decision made regarding the separation and reconditioning of salvageable food. Unsalvageable food should be disposed of properly, either by using it as animal feed, if appropriate, or by destroying it. In addition, before they resume their activities, food businesses should be monitored to ensure they have regained the ability to ensure food safety.

If crop fields have been contaminated by human excreta, such as following floods or damage to sewerage systems, an assessment should be carried out rapidly to assess the contamination of crops and to establish measures, such as delayed harvesting and thorough cooking, to reduce the risk of transmitting faecal pathogens. Attention is also needed when pigs or cattle graze on contaminated land, to avoid the transmission of tapeworms. If water bodies used for fishing or for harvesting water vegetables have been contaminated, assessment and analysis of risk should be undertaken to decide what special measures may be needed to prevent the spread of fish tapeworms or parasitic flukes, or of diseases such as salmonella and cholera.

9.2.2 Salvageable and unsalvageable foods

Public health and food safety authorities may be asked to examine food and advise on its fitness for human and/or animal consumption and, whether food is salvageable or unsalvageable.

Salvageable foods are those that have been damaged, but that can be rendered safe through reprocessing. Unsalvageable foods are those that are irremediably damaged by microbiological, chemical or physical contaminants, or that have been exposed to conditions making such contamination likely; they should be destroyed.

The necessary precautions should be taken to ensure that all foods that have been contaminated (or are likely to have been contaminated) and that cannot be made safe by reprocessing are properly disposed of. Contamination may occur without visible signs (e.g. bottles and jars can become contaminated by seepage through crown caps and screw tops), hence the guiding principle is: if there is any doubt as to the safety of the food, it should be destroyed (New Zealand Ministry of Health, 1995).

However, food is a valuable commodity, particularly in emergencies. Faced with severe shortages, people may consume food that is unfit or not intended for human consumption. For example, in 1971–1972 in Iraq, bread prepared from seed grain treated with methyl mercury caused an outbreak of poisoning. Thousands of people were affected and several hundreds died. Any decision taken by the health authorities should therefore be based on a risk–benefit assessment: where there is a risk of a shortage, the salvaging of food should be considered, provided it does not endanger public health. In disasters and emergencies, people are likely to suffer from malnutrition as a result of food shortages, and malnourished people are more vulnerable to foodborne hazards, i.e. they may be harmed by lower doses of pathogens or toxic chemicals than healthy people. In general, foods chemically contaminated as a result of pollution, chemical spills or other secondary accidents involving toxic waste are difficult or impossible to salvage and may need to be destroyed.

Table 9.1 **Control measures for ensuring food safety**

Step	Hazard	Action
Supply/purchase	Contamination of raw foodstuffs	Obtain foods from a reliable supplier.
		Specify conditions of production and transport.
	Contamination of ready-to-eat foods	Purchase foods from reliable supplier.
		Request application of the HACCP[1] system during food preparation.
Receipt of food	Contamination of high-risk foods with pathogens	Control conditions of transport (temperature and time).
Storage	Further contamination	Store foods wrapped or in closed container.
		Control pests.
	Growth of bacteria	Control temperature and duration of storage, rotate stock.
Preparation	Further contamination, via hands or in other ways	Wash hands before handling food.
		Prevent cross-contamination via surfaces, cooking utensils.
		Separate cooked foods from raw foods.
		Use boiled water, particularly if the food is not subject to subsequent cooking.
	Growth of bacteria	Limit time of exposure of food to room temperature.
Cooking	Survival of pathogens	Make sure that food is cooked thoroughly (i.e. all parts have reached at least 70 °C, particularly the thickest parts and/or centre).
Cooling and cold holding	Growth of surviving bacteria or their spores, production of toxins	Cool food as quickly as possible to temperatures below 5 °C, e.g. place foods in shallow trays and cool to chill temperatures.
		Avoid overfilling the refrigerator or cold storage room. During long periods of cold storage, monitor the temperature fluctuations and, when necessary, take measures.
	Contamination from various sources	Cover food properly, avoid direct or indirect contact with raw foods and non-potable water.
		Use clean utensils to handle cooked food.
Hot holding[2]	Growth of surviving bacteria or their spores, production of toxins	Ensure that food is kept hot (i.e. above 60 °C).
Reheating[3]	Survival of bacteria	Ensure that the food is thoroughly reheated.
Serving	Growth of bacteria, spores, production of toxins	Ensure that food is thoroughly reheated.
	Contamination	Prevent contact with raw foods, unclean utensils and non-potable water.
		Do not touch food with hands.
		Serve food when it is still hot.

[1] HACCP: hazard analysis critical control point. See (Bryan, 1992).
[2] Alternative step to cooling.
[3] This step is necessary for foods that have been prepared in advance, as well as leftovers.

The disposal of food deemed unfit for human consumption should be confirmed and documented. It should be carried out in a manner that prevents the deliberate or accidental diversion to the human food supply. The condemned food may be compacted and buried, incinerated, or denatured by adding obviously inedible substances, such as used motor oil, diesel fuel, etc. (World Health Organization, 1992a).

9.2.3 Inspection of food businesses

After a disaster has occurred, food industries and catering establishments should be inspected. Steps should be taken to ensure that foods that have been adversely affected are not marketed. Businesses should resume their activities only when the necessary conditions for safe food production or preparation are met, i.e. when the premises used for food production or preparation have been cleaned and disinfected; electricity, water supplies and sanitation have been restored; equipment is operating; properly trained staff are available; etc. Slaughterhouses should also be inspected.

Markets usually recover or develop quickly in emergencies and provide a valuable means of access to food for the disaster-affected population. However, markets should be regularly inspected and the cooperation of stallholders should be sought to ensure that safe food preparation and handling is carried out.

Controls should be in place to ensure that irredeemably damaged foods are not marketed and that food distributed through markets, retailers or street food vendors has not been subject to time–temperature abuse or otherwise contaminated. When salvaged foods are sold, they should be labelled accordingly and consumers should be clearly informed of measures they need to take to render them safe.

9.2.4 Control of donated or imported food

During food relief operations, the authorities responsible for food and health should monitor the condition of donated or imported food from its port of entry onwards. Food that is found on inspection and/or laboratory analysis to be unfit for human consumption should be condemned and rejected. Where there is a large demand for food, and the defect is such that safety is not seriously compromised, the conditional acceptance of substandard food may be considered.

9.3 Food safety and nutrition

9.3.1 General considerations

General principles for the safe handling and preparation of food apply to all contexts, including the household, mass-feeding centers for disaster-affected people, and targeted-feeding centers, such as therapeutic-feeding centers. Box 9.1 presents a modified version of WHO's golden rules for safe food preparation (World Health Organization, 1991d).

9.3.2 Providing dry rations for household cooking

After a disaster, as soon as families have reestablished their capacity to cook, any food they may be given is usually distributed in dry form to prepare and consume in their homes or temporary shelters. In addition to safe water for food preparation, a means of washing hands and utensils will be needed. People may not always be familiar with all kinds of dry foods, especially when the foods have been supplied by international food aid programmes. When necessary, they should be shown how to prepare any unusual foods. A shortage of fuel for cooking may also be a major constraint, and this may need to be supplied to ensure adequate cooking and reheating of cooked food. Otherwise, common cooking facilities may need to be provided for every block of shelters. With

Box 9.1 Golden rules for safe food preparation[1]

1. **Cook raw foods thoroughly.** Under normal circumstances raw foodstuffs and water may become contaminated with pathogens, but in times of disaster the risk of contamination is even greater. Thorough cooking will kill the pathogens, which means the temperature of all parts of the food must reach at least 70 °C. Uncooked fruits or vegetables should not be eaten, unless they can be peeled. If milk has not been pasteurized, it should be boiled before use. Cooking will not necessarily destroy biotoxins.

2. **Eat cooked food immediately.** When cooked foods cool to room temperature, bacteria begin to grow. The longer the wait, the greater the risk. To be on the safe side, eat cooked foods as soon as they come off the heat.

3. **Prepare food for only one meal.** Foods should be prepared freshly and for one meal only, as far as possible. If foods have to be prepared in advance, or if there are leftovers, they should be stored cold, i.e. below 5 °C (in a refrigerator or in a cold box), or hot, i.e. above 60 °C. This rule is vitally important when it is planned to store food for more than 4–5 hours. Cooked foods that have been stored must be thoroughly reheated before eating, i.e. all parts reheated to at least 70 °C. Thorough reheating of foods is essential if refrigerators have ceased to operate for some hours due to power cuts.

4. **Avoid contact between raw foods and cooked foods.** Safely cooked food can become contaminated through even the slightest contact with raw food. This cross-contamination can be direct, e.g. when raw fish comes into contact with cooked foods. It can also be indirect. For example, preparing raw fish and then using the same unwashed cutting surface and knife to slice cooked food should be avoided, or all the potential risks of illness that were present before cooking may be reintroduced. Cross-contamination may also occur in a freezer when the power has been off for some time and this should be checked for. The juice of raw meat and poultry may drip onto other foods.

5. **Choose foods processed for safety.** Many foods, such as fruits and vegetables, are best in their natural state. However, in disasters and emergencies, they may not be safe and should be peeled before consumption if eaten raw. Foods that have been processed (e.g. canned food and packed dried food) and that have not been affected by the disaster may be safer. Dry rations may be easier to keep safe, as they do not need cold-storage, but they do need to be kept dry.

6. **Wash hands repeatedly.** Hands should be washed thoroughly before preparing, serving or eating food and after every interruption, especially after use of the toilet or latrine, changing a baby or touching animals. After preparing raw foods, especially those of animal origin, hands should be washed again before handling cooked or ready-to-eat foods.

7. **Keep all food preparation premises meticulously clean.** Since foods are so easily contaminated, any surface used for food preparation must be kept absolutely clean. Scraps of food and crumbs are potential reservoirs of germs and can attract insects and animals. The immediate surrounding of the temporary shelter, especially the kitchen and food storage areas, should be cleaned and sullage and solid kitchen waste should be disposed of properly. Food should be stored in closed containers to protect it from insects, rodents and other animals. Fly and rat traps should be used if necessary.

8. **Use safe water.** Safe water is just as important for food preparation as for drinking. If the supply of safe/potable water has been disrupted, the water intended for drinking or food preparation should be boiled. For example, condensed or powdered milk must be reconstituted with potable water only. Ice made from unsafe water will also be unsafe and may be a source of food contamination.

9. **Be cautious with foods purchased outside.** Sometimes food served in restaurants and by street food-vendors is not prepared under hygienic conditions. In times of disasters or emergencies, the risk that such foods are contaminated is greater. Therefore, caution must be exercised in the choice of food: only food that has been thoroughly cooked and is still hot when served should be eaten. Food bought from street food-vendors should be thoroughly cooked in the presence of the customer. Apart from fruits and vegetables that can

be peeled, raw or undercooked foods should be avoided. Only water that has been boiled, or disinfected with chlorine or iodine, should be drunk. Beverages such as hot tea or coffee, wine, beer, carbonated water or soft drinks, packaged fruit juices and bottled water are usually safe to drink, if not damaged by the disaster. Ice should be avoided, unless it is made from safe water.

10. **Breast-feed infants and young children.** Breast milk is the ideal source of nourishment for infants during their first months of life. It protects infants against diarrhoea through its anti-infective properties, and minimizes their exposure to foodborne pathogens. In times of epidemics and disaster situations, when foods may be contaminated or scarce, breast milk will ensure a safe and nutritionally adequate food for infants from birth up to the age of 4–6 months. Continued breast-feeding after this age can also contribute to the prevention of foodborne infections in older infants and young children.

[1] Source: World Health Organization (1991d).

decentralized cooking, accidental fires are a hazard, and fire-fighting equipment should be placed at strategic locations. Responsible volunteers should look out for fires and should be able to control them.

The advantage of providing dry rations is that recipients have more independence. Individual dry rations also avoid the risk of widespread intoxications or infections, which increases when mass cooking is done under unhygienic conditions. Nevertheless, with the appropriate safeguards listed above, centralized cooking may sometimes be necessary, especially if water and fuel supplies are scarce and sanitation is unsatisfactory.

9.3.3 Mass-feeding centres

A general feeding programme, based on the distribution of cooked food, may be necessary for a short initial period in situations where people do not have the necessary resources to prepare their own meals hygienically, or in some conflict situations where they risk having dry rations taken from them. However, mass preparation of cooked food has a number of disadvantages, including the risk of food-borne disease transmission (World Health Organization, 2000b). As soon as conditions allow, general feeding programmes should be based on the distribution of dry rations. In some cases, as an alternative to mass feeding, it may be possible to help households by providing dry rations that do not need cooking or by setting up temporary shared neighbourhood kitchens where people can prepare food for their own families or in groups.

Large-scale preparation of cooked food may also be done in supplementary-feeding centres that provide vulnerable and moderately malnourished individuals with a cooked supplement to the daily diet. The measures recommended in this section are also relevant to therapeutic-feeding centres. Additional precautions required in therapeutic-feeding centres are described in section 9.3.4.

Where mass food preparation is necessary, it is essential to supervise food handling practices and ensure strict adherence to food safety rules to minimize the risk of mass food intoxication or epidemics of foodborne infections. Basic rules of hygiene are given in World Health Organization (1995b). The general recommendations given in Box 9.1 and Table 9.1 are valid for most operations.

It is essential that food-handlers and supervisors who oversee the preparation of food in mass-feeding centres are trained in safe food handling (Jacob, 1989) and in HACCP, the hazard analysis critical control point system (Bryan, 1992). The latter will help them to think critically, analyse the prevailing conditions and potential hazards, and adapt their food safety measures to the situation. The HACCP system can be applied to each specific food-preparation activity, and the hazards related to foods or operations can be identified and control measures determined.

It is of the utmost importance that employees and volunteers who are preparing foods should not be suffering from an illness with any of the following symptoms: jaundice, diarrhoea, vomiting, fever, sore throat (with fever), visibly infected skin lesions (boils, cuts, etc.), or discharge from the ears, eyes or nose.

All personnel should therefore be made aware of their responsibilities and of the importance of observing the rules for safe food handling. All food-handlers should be instructed to report to their supervisor anyone suffering from an illness with any of the symptoms mentioned above. Posters aimed at reminding staff about the rules of safe food handling may be helpful, and should be placed at strategic places in the food preparation area. Illustrations will be particularly useful if food-handlers are illiterate. The local health committee has an important role in facilitating safe community feeding activities.

Where centralized catering is required, one kitchen should be set up for every 200–300 families (1000–1500 people), with a supervisor appointed to ensure food safety in all centers. Kitchens and eating areas should be sturdy, well-roofed and well-ventilated structures, in areas of the settlement with good access and space for users to wait for meals.

Box 9.2 outlines the facilities that should be available in mass-feeding centers and therapeutic-feeding centers.

9.3.4 Therapeutic-feeding centres

Food safety is perhaps most important where therapeutic or intensive child feeding is under way (World Health Organization, 2000b). Children fed in this way are very vulnerable to infections, and specific measures are required (see Box 9.3), in addition to those required generally for food safety in centralized catering centres (see Box 9.1). Cooking and feeding for therapeutic-feeding patients should be done in a building specifically allocated for this. To ensure optimal sanitary conditions, the maximum size for such a feeding unit should be sufficient for about 50 children and their parents or guardians. If more space is needed, additional units should be provided.

9.3.5 Breastfeeding and breast-milk substitutes

WHO recommends full and exclusive breastfeeding of infants until 4–6 months of age, with continued breastfeeding with adequate complementary feeding for up to two years if possible (World Health Organization 2000a). Aid workers should be able to encourage breastfeeding practices if they understand and follow the guidelines given below:

- Support all mothers in breastfeeding in accordance with WHO recommendations.
- If a mother is sick or malnourished, give her extra food and support so that she can continue breastfeeding her baby.
- If a mother has stopped or reduced breastfeeding, help her to relactate or reestablish exclusive breastfeeding.
- If an infant's biological mother is not available, arrange for another mother to breastfeed it.
- If no other woman is available to provide breast-milk, provide a suitable substitute, e.g. infant formula or animal milk, while taking the necessary precautions, such as:
  — the infant formula to be used must be in generic packaging, and must not display the brand name;
  — clear instructions must be given on how to prepare the formula hygienically;
  — the formula must be freshly prepared for each feed: no left-overs must be kept;
  — parents and guardians must be advised to feed infants by cup, and to avoid the use of feeding bottles, teats and pacifiers.

For infants 6 months and older, infant formula is not needed.

Box 9.2 **Facilities needed at mass-feeding centres**

■ **Water supplies.** Only safe water should be used for all purposes in the feeding premises. Piped water may be suspect, especially after certain disasters. Water should be tested as soon as possible (see section 7.4.2), and if in doubt, water supplies should be chlorinated in the centre.

■ **Toilets for staff and users.** Separate, safe excreta-disposal facilities for staff and people being served should be provided at the mass-feeding centre. At least one toilet should be provided for every 50 people working or eating at the centre. Toilets and latrines must be kept clean at all times. Anal cleansing materials should normally be supplied.

■ **Hand-washing facilities.** A sufficient number of basins, each with soap, nail brush and a clean towel, must be provided for the food-handlers. They should be located in or near the toilets.

■ **Facilities for dealing with liquid wastes from kitchens.** If not discharged into public sewers, kitchen wastewaters should be disposed of by other sanitary methods, such as a soakaway or covered cesspool. A grease trap or strainer must always be provided and properly maintained to prevent clogging (see Section 8.4.2).

■ **Facilities for dealing with solid wastes from kitchens.** Solid kitchen wastes must be deposited immediately in rubbish bins. Filled bins should not be left in the preparation and cooking areas, but should be tightly covered and taken outside for collection and disposal.

■ **Basins, tables, chopping blocks.** All furniture and equipment must be kept as clean as possible. Surfaces in contact with food during preparation and serving should be thoroughly cleaned and disinfected with a strong chlorine solution (100 mg/l) after each meal.

■ **Facilities for dish washing.** Separate basins must be provided for washing, eating and cooking utensils. Any grease or food scraps on the utensils should be scraped into a rubbish bin; the utensils should then be washed in a basin with hot water and detergent, and rinsed. They should then be laid on wire baskets or trays and immersed in boiling water for disinfection for 5 minutes; alternatively they may be immersed in a sterilization solution, preferably hot, (e.g. sodium hypochlorite or calcium hypochlorite solution at 100 mg chlorine/litre for 30 seconds). Wiping dry is unnecessary, and undesirable if clean cloths are not available. The baskets or trays should be dried in a dust-free place.

■ **Adequate and appropriate materials for cooking/refrigeration.** When refrigeration is not available, damaged or perishable foods should be bought on a daily basis and cooked and served as soon as possible. Centrally produced ice may allow the use of improvised cool chests for the short-term storage of some perishables. It may also be possible to use a kerosene-powered refrigerator, or a portable generator for electric refrigerators. Staff should aim to prepare food sufficient only for each meal, to avoid the need to store cooked food.

■ **Layout to prevent cross-contamination**. The space inside the food preparation premises should be arranged so as to prevent cross-contamination of prepared food from sources of contamination, such as raw food and especially animal products.

■ **Adequate and appropriate materials for eating.** Common cups, plates and cutlery are acceptable if they are thoroughly washed and/or disinfected after use. Disposable plates, cups, etc., may be appropriate, especially when disaster victims are in transit.

■ **Control of rodents and other pests** Effective ways to combat flies include, trapping flies, properly screening kitchen areas, and disposing of waste and sullage. Spraying against flies is not necessary. If rodenticides are used in food-storage areas and kitchens, they should be labelled and their use should be carefully monitored. They should never be placed on surfaces used for food preparation, or where they could accidentally fall into food being prepared.

■ **Food safety information.** Food safety educational material, such as posters, should be provided in accessible places in the food preparation areas.

Box 9.3 Specific measures required in therapeutic-feeding centres

- Ensure that dry feeds are not reconstituted in advance and that the leftovers are not stored for the next meal.
- Make sure that foods prepared from raw ingredients are thoroughly cooked and, after preparation, given immediately they are cool enough to eat.
- Make sure that safe water is given to infants and children, and is used to prepare complementary food (or reconstituted feed). If in doubt, boil the water before use. Store water so that it is safe from all sources of contamination, e.g. hands during serving.
- Make sure that helpers or parents feeding and attending to infants and children wash their hands before feeding them and are aware of the principles of safe food handling. Cups, plates and spoons should be washed after every meal.
- Equip the therapeutic-feeding unit with a large boiled or chlorinated and well-monitored water supply (at least 30 litres per person); a facility for helpers or mothers to wash their hands before assisting children; a separate facility for washing the cups and other utensils; and latrines.
- Install showers or other facilities so that patients and helpers who stay in the centre overnight can bathe.
- Provide a screened, shaded area protected from dust, flies, etc. with sufficient floor space covered with matting or plastic for mothers or helpers to sit with weak children who need to be fed. Feeding weak children with a cup and spoon can be very time-consuming.

HIV and infant feeding

HIV infection can be transmitted through breastfeeding. Nevertheless, breastfeeding should be encouraged among mothers who are HIV-negative or of unknown HIV status. During the emergency phase following a disaster, it may not be possible to provide testing facilities for pregnant women and mothers, or to provide drugs to reduce transmission. In the postemergency phase, the possibility of reducing transmission through breastfeeding with voluntary testing, drugs and alternative feeding practices for HIV-positive mothers should be considered.

9.4 Public education and information

While education of the public in food safety is important at all times, in disasters and emergencies it becomes vital. In such circumstances, the possible contamination of raw foodstuffs, the pollution of the environment, and the disruption of basic health services increase both the risks of epidemics of foodborne diseases and the severity of their health consequences. It is then necessary to intensify health education activities and extend the channels for communication with the public.

The WHO golden rules for safe food preparation, adapted to emergencies and disasters (see Box 9.1), can provide a basis for public education on food safety.

Special attention should be drawn to the importance of breastfeeding and, in particular, the grave risks of using breast-milk substitutes under the unhygienic conditions that may prevail during emergencies, particularly if sanitation is compromised, safe water is scarce, and facilities for sterilization (i.e. for heating or boiling) are unavailable to mothers.

It is therefore necessary to:

— remind the public of the rules of safe food handling whenever the contamination of water or raw foodstuffs could give rise to epidemics of microbial foodborne diseases, such as after hurricanes, floods and earthquakes;
— advise the public to avoid the types of food that are likely to be contaminated following an explosion in a chemical plant situated near home garden plots, or a nuclear accident that contaminates pastures or crops with radionuclides.

Ideally, households should be prepared in advance and have access to alternative facilities for safe food storage and preparation, and agents for disinfecting water. This preparation may include bottled gas or wood for cooking food and boiling water, and ice-boxes and ice for cold storage, whenever electricity, gas or water supplies are disrupted.

9.5 Safe and hygienic warehouse management

Storage structures should have good roofs and ventilation. Bags must not lie directly on the floor—pallets, boards, heavy branches, bricks, or clean, dry plastic bags or sheets should be placed underneath them. Products should be kept at least 40 centimetres from walls and 10 centimetres from the floor. Damaged bags should be rebagged and stored apart from undamaged ones. A reserve of good-quality empty bags should be kept for this purpose. Spilled food should be swept up and disposed of promptly to discourage rats. Bags should be piled two-by-two cross-wise to permit ventilation. Wet bags should be allowed to dry in the sun before storing them.

Spills of cooking oil in the warehouse should be immediately cleaned up to prevent workers slipping and injuring themselves. Similarly, bags should not be piled too high and piles should be stable so that workers are not injured by falling bags.

Fuel, pesticides, chlorine and other chemical stocks should never be stored in the same place as food.

9.6 Further information

For further information on:

— food safety procedures, see: World Health Organization (1984a), World Health Organization (1989b), World Health Organization (1991d), Bryan (1992), World Health Organization (1992a);
— supplementary and therapeutic feeding, see: Sphere Project (2000), World Health Organization (2000a);
— breastfeeding and breast-milk substitutes, see: United Nations High Commissioner for Refugees (1989), Savage-King (1992), World Health Organization (2000b), Sphere Project (2000);
— food storage, see: Walker (1992).

10. Vector and pest control

10.1 The importance of vector and pest control in disasters and emergencies

Some disasters give rise to increases in the populations of vector or nuisance species, usually insects or rodents. Floods may create new mosquito breeding sites in disaster rubble and stagnant pools. A general breakdown of sanitation may favour the multiplication of houseflies and rodents. People living in partially destroyed houses or primitive shelters may have lost the normal protection afforded by screened windows or mosquito nets.

Serious infection hazards may arise when massive migrations bring people of different origins together in temporary camps infested with disease vectors. Under such conditions, people who are relatively immune carriers of parasites can set off a disease-transmission cycle to which weaker people and people who are not immune fall victim. Examples of disease outbreaks observed in such situations include malaria (transmitted by *Anopheles* mosquitoes), epidemic typhus (transmitted by lice) and dengue fever (transmitted by *Aedes* mosquitoes).

Malaria is one of the five leading causes of mortality in emergency situations, and in endemic areas its control is likely to be one of the main health priorities. The implication of flies in the transmission of diarrhoeal disease is open to some debate, but fly control is likely to have a positive impact on health in most postdisaster situations, particularly when sanitary conditions are poor and diarrhoea, *Shigella* dysentery, or typhoid prevalence are high. Other vectors may be important in specific locations, depending on the prevalences of the vector and the disease before the disaster, and the susceptibility of the population.

In addition to the disease hazards presented by vector species, many insects and other arthropods can constitute a major nuisance in disasters. The impact of nuisance further adds to the stress and psychosocial instability from which disaster victims usually suffer. Standing water rich in organic matter can produce massive numbers of biting midges (*Culicoides* spp.) which do not transmit any disease, but cause extreme nuisance and often trigger allergic reactions in sensitive people. Several mosquito species can also be a great nuisance without presenting a direct risk to health. On the other hand, some of the most serious disease vectors are hardly considered a nuisance in many areas as their bites are almost painless (e.g. *Anopheles* mosquitoes, the vectors of malaria).

When wild or domestic host animals have been killed or driven away by disaster, ectoparasites, such as ticks, bugs, lice and fleas, may invade a community and produce a serious additional risk of zoonotic vector-borne disease. Another, related, vector-borne disease risk may arise when refugees enter territory formerly occupied only by wildlife and accompanying parasites. Examples of diseases that may then emerge include plague (from rats) and Lyme disease (from ticks).

When action against such pest organisms is considered during disasters, a distinction must be made between *disease control* and *nuisance control* (see Section 10.2).

The vectors likely to be present in emergency settlements and the diseases they carry are shown in Box 10.1.

> **Box 10.1 Vectors and diseases likely to be present in emergency settlements**
>
> | *Vector* | *Main diseases* |
> |---|---|
> | Mosquitoes | Malaria, yellow fever, dengue, viral encephalitis, filariasis. |
> | Houseflies | Diarrhoea, dysentery, conjunctivitis, typhoid fever, trachoma. |
> | Cockroaches | Diarrhoea, dysentery, salmonellosis, cholera. |
> | Lice | Endemic typhus, pediculosis, relapsing fever, trench fever, skin irritation. |
> | Bedbugs | Severe skin inflammation. |
> | Triatomid bugs | Chagas' disease. |
> | Ticks | Rickettsial fever, tularaemia, relapsing fever, viral encephalitis, borreliosis. |
> | Rodent (mites) | Rickettsial pox, scrub typhus. |
> | Rodent (fleas) | Bubonic plague, endemic typhus. |
> | Rodents | Rat bite fever, leptospirosis, salmonellosis, melioidosis. |

10.1.1 Assessment

At an early stage in the emergency response, and in planning for possible emergency settlements, an assessment should be made of vector-borne disease risks and pest nuisance, and the scope for their control using the techniques available. Special measures for vector and nuisance pest control (as distinct from general environmental health measures, such as wastewater disposal and excreta disposal) may be expensive and time-consuming, so it is important to know that they are worth carrying out in an emergency, when there are many other health priorities demanding action. As vector-borne disease risk is a function of the presence of the vector, the prevalence of the disease organism, and the susceptibility of the population, these three conditions need to be assessed to justify a major environmental management activity. The assessment of vector-borne disease risk and patterns requires specialist expertise and cooperation between the sectors of health, water supply and sanitation, and site selection and planning.

10.2 Disease control and nuisance control

10.2.1 Disease control

The control of a vector-borne disease can be achieved by various means. In emergencies, these include, in order of priority:

1. Diagnosis and treatment.
2. Vector control.
3. Environmental hygiene.
4. Personal protection.

10.2.2 Nuisance control

In emergencies, nuisance control will not be the most important priority, so targeted applications of pesticides will seldom be justified. The measures to be taken should aim at medium- and longer-term environmental improvement, in the following order of priority:

1. Identification of the causative agent.
2. Environmental hygiene.
3. Personal protection.

10.3 Available control measures

This section is concerned primarily with the control of insect vectors. For information on rodent control, see United Nations High Commissioner for Refugees (1997).

Appropriate diagnosis and treatment of patients are possible only in the presence of adequately trained medical and/or paramedical personnel. Most vector-borne diseases require a microscopic diagnosis by trained laboratory personnel. Some parasites (e.g. *Plasmodium falciparum,* which may cause cerebral malaria) may be resistant to most or all available drugs. Serious cases of viral vector-borne infections, such as dengue and yellow fever, require careful clinical management, combined with symptomatic treatment. If these are not available, vector control becomes even more important.

The success of vector control will depend on reducing the density and longevity of the species responsible. In the context of an acute emergency, longevity reduction is generally the more cost-effective option. In contrast, nuisance control is exclusively a matter of density reduction.

10.3.1 Density reduction

Reducing the population density of vectors and nuisance species is achieved by measures directed at the breeding sites: environmental management (drainage, filling, levelling of depressions and borrow pits, etc.) or the use of insecticides (larvicides). In the latter case, the target organisms must be susceptible to the chemical. In addition, this chemical should not kill nontarget organisms (such as fish) or present a hazard to people drinking water from the same source. For further information on density reduction by environmental management, see Section 10.4.

10.3.2 Longevity reduction with pesticides

Longevity reduction depends on the use of insecticides that kill the adult vectors. Although environmental management is the preferred strategy for reducing vector density (Section 10.4), the use of insecticides for longevity reduction is often called for in emergencies, due to the urgent nature of the problem and the risk of epidemics of vector-borne disease among susceptible populations.

Insecticides for killing adult vectors must be applied in places where the vector will rest, such as the inside surfaces of houses in the case of *Anopheles* mosquitoes, or cracks in walls and other hiding places in the case of triatomid bugs. In addition, the target species must be susceptible to the chemical and the chemical must not be a health hazard to the population or personnel carrying out the spraying. The design and implementation of these measures must therefore be the responsibility of specialized personnel.

The following questions must be answered before insecticides are used to control larvae or adult forms of disease vectors:

- What is the vector species responsible for disease transmission among the population?
- To which insecticides is it susceptible?
- Where does it breed?
- Where does it rest?
- Which is expected to be more cost-effective and rapid: killing larvae or killing adults?
- Can the required pesticide be obtained in the correct formulation?
- Is the use of this pesticide to control the target vector compatible with national strategies for vector control?
- Is the correct equipment available?
- Are trained personnel available or can they be made available?

■ What precautions must be taken to protect human safety?

■ Will it be possible to adopt more permanent measures (such as personal protection, environmental management, etc.) at a later stage?

It is risky and inadvisable to use insecticides unless these questions can be answered satisfactorily. Environmental health staff should obtain advice from vector specialists to answer many of these questions, via the Ministry of Health, WHO or other organizations with expertise in this field.

Box 10.2 provides information on methods of pesticide application. For further information on the choice of pesticides, equipment for applying pesticides, and instructions for their safe use, see: Chavasse & Yap (1997), Rozendaal (1997), United Nations High Commissioner for Refugees (1997).

Certain pesticides, e.g. the persistent organic pesticides such as DDT, are banned or subject to restrictions in many countries. It is necessary to determine which pesticides can be used for vector control in a country affected by a disaster. A pesticide banned for agricultural purposes may be permitted for use in disease control (and vice versa). Most legal restrictions are based on assumed or proven hazards to the environment, but some are related to proven human toxicity hazards associated with short exposures. In general, appropriately registered pesticides should not pose an unacceptable risk if properly used. Under the conditions prevailing in emergencies, there is usually no need to use persistent insecticides; vector susceptibility is a more critical criterion when selecting an insecticide.

With specific reference to DDT, the text of the Stockholm Convention on Persistent Organic Pollutants, agreed in May 2001, contains the following paragraphs that are relevant if indoor residual spraying is part of an emergency response:

1. The production and use of DDT shall be eliminated except for Parties that have notified the Secretariat of their intention to produce and/or use it. A DDT Register is hereby established and shall be available to the public. The Secretariat shall maintain the DDT Register.

. . .

Box 10.2 Pesticide application methods and equipment for emergencies

Dusting	Hand-held dusters, manually operated or mechanized.
Residual insecticide spraying	Knapsack sprayers with special nozzles.
Ultra-low volume spraying	Low-dosage applications to large areas from fixed-wing aircraft or helicopters.
Space spraying	Interior or exterior applications with pesticide aerosols dispersed under pressure from vaporizers or fogging machines.
Impregnation	The treatment of materials such as bedding, clothing and mosquito nets with pesticides in emulsion or solution (by dipping and drying, or by spraying with knapsack sprayers).

3. In the event that a Party not listed in the DDT Register determines that it requires DDT for disease vector control, it shall notify the Secretariat as soon as possible in order to have its name added forthwith to the DDT Register. It shall at the same time notify the World Health Organization.

Rapid procurement of DDT may be the main obstacle to using DDT in an emergency. Should it be decided to use DDT, then WHO guidelines should be strictly adhered to (World Health Organization, 1995c).

If it is decided to use pesticides for the control of epidemics in a post-disaster situation, the order of priority from the point of view of safety should be as follows:

1. Spray personnel (applicators, loaders, drivers, pilots).
2. The population to be protected.
3. Supplies of food and drinking-water.
4. Domestic animals and livestock.
5. The wider environment.

Spray personnel are listed first because they are likely to be the most vulnerable, both because of their greater exposure risk and because of the likelihood that, in disasters, such personnel may be relatively poorly trained in safety precautions. Pesticides of low human toxicity in the concentrate formulation needed are to be preferred. A comprehensive classification of pesticides by hazard has been made by the International Programme for Chemical Safety and WHO (World Health Organization, 1998a). For advice on accidental poisoning by pesticides, see Annex 3.

Information on common types of insecticide formulations suitable for use in disasters, their characteristics and advantages, is given in Box 10.3.

Chemical vector control is an immediate priority in many disasters. In the aftermath of a disaster and over the longer term, environmental hygiene and personal protection are more cost-effective in reducing vulnerability. This is equally true for the management of nuisance organisms.

Box 10.3 Characteristics and advantages of common insecticide formulations used in disasters

Dusts and granules
Composed of the active ingredient and an inert carrier. This type of formulation is used mainly to control lice and fleas. When used to control pests in vegetation, granules provide better penetration than dusts.

Water-dispersible powders
Composed of the active ingredient, a wetting agent, and an inert carrier. Before being used, the powder must be mixed with water to obtain a suspension. This type of formulation is usually relatively cheap. For public health use, these powders should contain no more than 200–800 g of active ingredient per kg (20–80%). Suitable for residual applications, e.g. to achieve long-lasting control of mosquitoes in buildings.

Emulsifiable concentrates
Composed of the active ingredient, a solvent and an emulsifier. Must be mixed with water before use.

Slow-release formulations
The active ingredient is microencapsulated and made into briquettes or strands, to provide controlled release of insecticides for controlling mosquito larvae.

10.4 Environmental management for vector and pest control

WHO defines environmental management as the modification or manipulation of environmental conditions, or of their interaction with the human population, with a view to preventing or minimizing vector propagation and reducing human–vector–pathogen contact (World Health Organization, 1980). This definition can easily be extended to include the management of nuisance pests.

10.4.1 The benefits of environmental management

Even if the most appropriate immediate response to vector or pest outbreaks is chemical control, sustained spraying is generally not recommended unless there are no other, more sustainable alternatives. A procedure such as environmental management, which has more long-lasting effects, will contribute to a healthier environment and thus to vulnerability reduction in the population concerned. The timing of the switch from chemical control to other methods will depend on many factors: environmental management may not be the preferred choice as long as life-threatening hazards exist. It is often advisable to pursue the two approaches at the same time. For instance, insecticides may be used for rapid reduction of the adult fly population during a *Shigella* dysentery outbreak, at the same time as refuse control and excreta control measures are taken to reduce opportunities for fly breeding. Such an integrated approach requires clear decision-making criteria and procedures adapted to local conditions.

The advantages of environmental management over pesticides are: (1) there are no problems of pesticide resistance; (2) there is no risk of intoxication or environmental contamination from the inappropriate management of chemicals; and (3) the results are often longer lasting and will contribute to vulnerability reduction and improvements in public health. Environmental management is not necessarily cheaper than control with chemicals and seldom provides "quick fixes". To be successful, it requires good cooperation with other sectors (public works, agriculture, water supply and sanitation). Choosing the mix of most cost-effective environmental management methods in post-disaster health programmes is difficult and demands fairly high-level technical skills and experience.

10.4.2 Environmental management measures for vector and pest control

Environmental management generally requires an understanding of the biology of the vector or pest organism. It is equally important to have a solid understanding of the role of human behaviour in vector-borne disease transmission. Even if there is no man-made determinant underlying the problem, there is always a need for community involvement in implementing the solution.

Most disease vectors are insects, such as mosquitoes, midges and flies. Mosquitoes require water for their immature stages, but not all kinds of water are suitable for all kinds of mosquitoes. Some require relatively small pools of clean, stagnant water (e.g. the *Anopheles* malaria vectors). Others prefer water in containers such as jars, bottles, tanks, etc. (e.g. the *Aedes* vectors of dengue and yellow fever). Large bodies of water, such as reservoirs or flooded land, will usually not be acceptable to mosquitoes unless there are floating mats of debris or vegetation. Environmental measures for the control of mosquito breeding can therefore range from levelling land, filling borrow pits and draining flooded areas etc., to covering/mesh screening of water containers and removing floating debris and plants from lagoons.

Human activities, particularly those that concern food production, eating, drinking, sleeping, defecation and laundering, can promote the propagation of vectors and pests or affect contacts between humans and vectors. Defecation fields, for example, should always be kept at a distance from cooking areas, because of flies and possible surface rainfall run-off. In most of tropical Africa, they should also be situated away from rainfall run-off to bathing or fishing waters, because of the risk of contamination with schistosomes. Another example is the promotion of animal production and farming to reduce dependence on food distributions. If well managed, the presence of animals near emergency settlements may keep mosquitoes away from people. On the other hand, animals may be reservoirs of vector-borne and other infectious diseases unless they are properly treated or vaccinated.

Environmental engineering intended to improve the quality of life may have negative health impacts if the biology of disease vectors or parasites is not taken into account. For instance, if hand pumps are installed in poorly drained locations, the resultant water-logging may result in mosquito breeding habitats, produce puddles containing water snails, or increase soil moisture sufficiently for hookworm transmission to become possible. Run-off water should therefore be drained some distance away or allowed to percolate into the ground in soakaways.

Environmental management should also extend to the environment of human settlements, both indoors and outside. To prevent mosquitoes resting around houses, weeds and shrubs should be regularly cut down. Rubbish should be removed or burned at least once a week to avoid the build-up of housefly populations, and food stocks should be kept in rat-proof buildings. In Latin American countries, shelters should be constructed in such a way as to avoid providing hiding places for the triatomid bugs that carry Chagas disease. In large parts of Asia, ponds and pools should be regularly cleared of water hyacinth and other floating vegetation as these harbour the larvae of *Mansonia* mosquitoes, the major vectors of Brugian filariasis (elephantiasis).

Competent authorities in the local health department and relevant literature should be consulted before the most appropriate environmental management method is chosen.

10.5 Hygiene and personal protection

10.5.1 The importance of hygiene and personal protection

Whereas environmental management aims to protect *populations* from the risks of vector-borne disease transmission, hygiene and personal protection are measures intended for *individuals*. Population-based interventions will do much to protect each individual in a disaster-stricken community if undertaken properly. However, some vulnerable groups, such as the sick and wounded, children, the elderly, pregnant women and people who lack immunity (including relief workers), may need additional protection.

Information on both hygiene and personal protection should be provided to the public in the same way as any other health education message. Personal protection measures that involve the use of vaccines, drugs (e.g. for prophylaxis) or pesticides (e.g. in impregnated mosquito nets) should be promoted by qualified health staff and used under their guidance. Table 10.1 gives examples of hygiene and personal protection methods for use against some target vectors or pests.

10.5.2 Repellents

In many societies accustomed to nuisance pests and vectors, people use a variety of substances as repellents. When these practices are effective and harmless, they should be encouraged in emergency situations, and it may be locally popular and effective to provide repellents of proven efficacy to the affected population. However, there is insufficient evidence of the effectiveness of repellents in reducing vector-borne disease at a population level to make this a general recommendation.

Table 10.1 **Examples of hygiene practices and personal protection methods against selected disease vectors, diseases, and nuisance pests**

Target species	Disease(s) carried	Personal protection methods		Vector hygiene methods
		Vaccine[1]	Other methods	
Anopheles mosquitoes	Malaria	–	Chemoprophylaxis, mosquito nets (impregnated)	Residual indoor spraying, burning mosquito coils at night, space spraying before retiring (bedroom needs to be screened for effectiveness)
	Lymphatic filariasis	–	Mosquito nets (impregnated)	
Culex mosquitoes	Lymphatic filariasis	–	Mosquito nets (impregnated), repellents	Elimination of breeding sites on compound
	Japanese encephalitis	+	Mosquito nets (impregnated), repellents	
Aedes mosquitoes	Viral encephalitis	±	Repellents	Elimination of breeding sites in and around house
	Dengue/DHF[2]	–		
	Yellow fever	+		
	Lymphatic filariasis	–		
Cockroaches	Diarrhoeal infections	±		Kitchen hygiene, all food leftovers removed at night
Houseflies	Diarrhoeal infections	±		Kitchen hygiene, proper (re)heating of cooked food, daily rubbish removal
	Eye infections	–		
Tsetse flies (Glossina)	Sleeping sickness	–	Repellents, impregnated clothing	Avoiding riverside laundering and defecation, installation of tsetse traps in human settlements.
Bedbugs	None	n.a.[3]	Mosquito nets (impregnated)	Regular airing and washing bedding materials and beds
Jigger fleas	None	n.a.	Wearing shoes	Pig control in residential areas, chemotherapy of dogs and cats, pesticide treatment of adjacent land
Lice	Epidemic typhus,	+	Chemoprophylaxis	Body hygiene, including use of shampoos, laundering clothes
	Relapsing fever	–	–	
	Trench fever	–	–	
Rodents	Plague	+		Rat-proofing of houses and storage facilities, rubbish removal, kitchen hygiene
	Leptospirosis	±		

[1] –: no operational vaccine available; +: operational vaccine available; ±: operational vaccine available for some.
[2] dengue haemorrhagic fever.
[3] n.a.: not applicable.
N.B.: Relief workers and health personnel should wear protective clothing (often impregnated with pesticide), or take other precautions in accordance with existing WHO and ILO guidelines.

10.5.3 Impregnated materials for malaria control

There is growing experience with using insecticide-impregnated mosquito nets, curtains and wall fabrics for providing protection against mosquitoes in emergency situations. The most effective of these methods is the use of impregnated mosquito nets, which have been shown in trials in several countries to be effective in reducing malaria transmission and nuisance biting by mosquitoes. In addition, they can also reduce the prevalence of sandflies, bedbugs, and head and body lice (Thomson, 1995).

The preferred insecticides for impregnating nets, curtains and fabrics are pyrethroids, such as permethrin and deltamethrin, in emulsifiable concentrates (United Nations High Commissioner for Refugees, 1997). Mosquito nets may be purchased already impregnated, or may need to be impregnated before use. All materials need to be reimpregnated after six months, and should not be washed during that period. Reimpregnation should be carried out immediately before the main malaria transmission season, when there is a seasonal pattern (Thomson, 1995).

There are a number of operational difficulties associated with the use of impregnated materials in disasters and emergencies that have to be resolved if these measures are to be effective. These include ensuring that the majority of the population actually keeps the mosquito nets and uses them correctly; ensuring that nets are not frequently washed, which reduces the concentration of the insecticide; and ensuring that nets are reimpregnated when needed.

10.5.4 Disinfection and disinfestation

Some disease vectors may be controlled by disinfestation, which is the process of removing from the body and clothing, or killing, animals that transmit disease (lice, mites, fleas, ticks, etc.) and their eggs.

Disinfestation by mass dusting people and their clothing with insecticides is humiliating, usually unnecessary, and dangerous if done incorrectly. It is better, if possible, to use a disinfection unit for this purpose. If mass dusting is considered necessary (e.g. because of an epidemic of flea-borne or louse-borne disease), the process must be explained to the population concerned, and the least toxic effective dust used.

Disinfection methods (for destroying disease organisms) can also be used for disinfestation, though the reverse is not true. Methods of disinfection effective against disease vectors and nuisance pests on clothing include the use of physical agents, such as ultraviolet light, dry heat, boiling water and steam, or chemical agents such as sulfur dioxide, ethylene oxide, formaldehyde, formol, cresol, phenol and carbolic acid. *Some of these agents are dangerous and should be used only under expert supervision.*

All articles not likely to be damaged may be disinfected by steam. Leather goods, clothing with leather facings or strapping, furs, rubber and other material that may be spoilt by steam can be sprayed with a 5% formol solution.

A simple steamer for clothing is illustrated in Figure 10.1. To kill lice and fleas, clothing should be steamed for 15 minutes, in combination with insecticide treatment. The process may need to be repeated every month.

10.6 Further information

For further information on:

— pesticides for vector control, see: Chavasse & Yap (1997);
— pesticide poisoning, see: World Health Organization (1998b), Group of Agricultural Pesticides Manufacturers (1993), Keifer (1997);

Figure 10.1 **Simple steamer for clothing**[1]

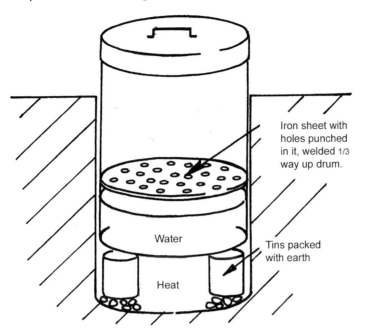

Iron sheet with holes punched in it, welded 1/3 way up drum.

Water

Tins packed with earth

Heat

[1] Source: Appleton & Save the Children Fund Ethiopia Team (1987).

— vector and pest control in displacement emergencies, see: Thomson (1995) and United Nations High Commissioner for Refugees (1997), Sphere Project (2000);

— environmental management, see: Cairncross & Feachem (1993);

— protection at the community or household level, see: Rozendaal (1997).

11. Control of communicable diseases and prevention of epidemics

11.1 The importance of communicable diseases in emergencies and disasters

The five most common causes of death in emergencies and disasters are diarrhoea, acute respiratory infection, measles, malnutrition and, in endemic zones, malaria. All except malnutrition are communicable diseases directly related to environmental health conditions, and even malnutrition is greatly exacerbated by communicable disease.

Disaster-affected people are particularly vulnerable to communicable diseases when the disaster and its immediate consequences reduce resistance to disease because of malnutrition, stress, fatigue, etc. and when post-disaster living conditions are unsanitary.

The control of communicable diseases depends on a healthy environment (clean water, adequate sanitation, vector control, shelter), immunization, and health workers trained in early diagnosis and treatment. Thanks to effective environmental health measures, epidemics following disasters are no longer common. Exceptions are the epidemics occurring in chronic emergencies triggered by drought and civil strife, such as those that occurred in Africa in the 1980s and 1990s, and the epidemics of communicable diseases that have swept refugee camps in Africa and other parts of the world. Functioning disease surveillance systems and intact environmental health services are crucial in protecting public health and in responding to these outbreaks when they occur in times of disaster.

The conditions leading to an epidemic are caused mostly by secondary effects and not by the primary hazard, except in the case of flooding, which can cause an increase in waterborne and vector-borne diseases (see Box 11.1). Other hazards may leave standing water or pollute, or interrupt drinking-water supplies. High winds, coastal storms, mud slides and even earthquakes can all result in standing water, especially where a "cascade" of physical effects occurs. For instance, in the Andes it is not uncommon for a volcanic eruption to melt ice and snow, creating floods, mud flows and rock falls. Earthquakes can trigger landslides that block rivers, causing flooding. In all these cases, excess standing water can promote the breeding of insect disease vectors, or contaminate water supplies with waste or sewage.

Both natural disasters and armed conflict may result in the breakage of water mains or the interruption of electricity supplies required to pump water. Sewer pipes and sewage treatment works may also be broken or rendered inoperable.

Besides waterborne and vector-borne disease, there may also be major epidemics of highly contagious diseases—those spread by personal contact. These are most commonly the result of crowding survivors living in crowded temporary accommodation without adequate ventilation or adequate facilities for personal hygiene and laundry.

The length of time that people spend in temporary settlements is an important determinant of the risk of disease transmission. The prolonged mass settlement of refugees in temporary shelters with only minimal provision for essential personal hygiene is typical of a situation that may cause epidemic outbreaks of infectious diseases (see Box 11.2). Camps established to provide food relief during famine are a special case, as large numbers of people who are already weak and possibly ill are likely to remain in such camps for a long time.

Box 11.1 **Flooding in the Czech Republic**[1]

Eastern areas of the Czech Republic were severely flooded in the summer of 1997. A total of 438 towns and villages were affected, and 2151 homes were destroyed. More than 200 000 people were left without electricity and 30 000 without gas. About 3500 wells and other water sources were contaminated and wastewater-treatment plants were rendered inoperable. The Centre of Microbiology of the Czech National Institute of Public Health took immediate action, in collaboration with the regional hygiene stations. All reports of outbreaks of typhoid fever, sal-monellosis, shigellosis, acute diarrhoea, viral hepatitis A, tularaemia, invasive meningococcal disease, toxoplasmosis, leptospirosis and Lyme disease were evaluated, and a special hepati-tis A vaccination programme was launched among 3–15-year-olds in selected areas. Postdis-aster analysis showed that leptospirosis had increased threefold, but that there had been no demonstrable flooding effects in the other diseases targeted. No viral hepatitis A was reported from the populations vaccinated. Recommended follow-up measures included monitoring and controlling rodents.

[1] Source: B. Kriz, unpublished data, 1998.

Box 11.2 **Monitoring mortality among refugees in eastern Zaire**[1,2]

During the emergency phase of a relief operation, death rates should be expressed as deaths/10 000 per day to allow for the detection of sudden changes. In general, health workers should be concerned when crude mortality rates (CMRs) in a displaced population exceed 1/10 000 per day, or when under-five mortality rates exceed 2/10 000 per day.

In eastern Zaire in July 1994, the CMR among one million Rwandan refugees ranged from 34.1 to 54.5/10 000 per day, among the highest ever recorded. Between 6 and 10% of the refugee population died during the month after arrival in Zaire. This high mortality rate was almost entirely due to an epidemic of diarrhoeal diseases and inadequate water supply.

By the third week of the refugee influx, relief efforts began to have a significant impact. Routine measures, such as measles immunization, vitamin A supplements, standard disease-treatment protocols and community outreach programmes, were established in each camp, and the water-distribution system began to provide an average of 5–10 litres per person per day.

[1] Source: International Federation of Red Cross and Red Crescent Societies (1997b).
[2] Now the Democratic Republic of the Congo

A comprehensive overview of the public health consequences of various forms of disasters may be found in Noji (1997). Table 11.1 presents an overview of the disease problems most often encountered following disasters. Such problems are more likely to occur where predisaster conditions, such as those in many densely populated mega-cities, are unsanitary. Steps taken in advance to reduce poverty, increase the level of awareness and organization, and extend normal health and sanitary services will provide additional protection for the community if disaster strikes.

11.2 Measures for controlling communicable diseases and epidemics

11.2.1 Preparedness and prevention

Preparedness measures taken before a disaster can greatly increase the ability to control communicable diseases and prevent epidemics. Such measures include: training health and outreach staff in the identification and management of specific diseases considered

Table 11.1 **Diseases affecting displaced populations in disasters**

Disease	Symptoms	Environmental risk factors	Health hazards
Acute upper respiratory tract infections	All symptoms of the common cold, fever and heavy coughing. Chest pain and pain between shoulder blades in pneumonia.	Crowding, poor hygiene	Influenza and pneumonia may cause severe complications, especially in groups at risk
Diarrhoea	Watery stools at least three times a day, with or without blood or slime. May be accompanied by fever, nausea or vomiting.	Contaminated drinking-water or food, or poor sanitation	Dehydration, especially in children, shown by dark colouration of urine, dry tongue or leathery skin
Measles	A disease of early childhood, characterized by fever and catarrhal symptoms, followed by maculopapular rash in the mouth.	Crowding, poor hygiene	Severe constitutional symptoms, high case fatality rate
Malaria	Painful muscles and joints, high fever with chills, headache, possibly diarrhoea and vomiting.	Breeding of *Anopheles* mosquitoes in stagnant water bodies	Disease may rapidly become fatal, unless medical care is provided within the first 48 hours
Meningococcal meningitis	Infected persons may show no symptoms for a considerable time. When an epidemic is in progress, headache, fever and general malaise will suggest the diagnosis, which must be confirmed by lumbar puncture.	Crowding	Often fatal if untreated at an early stage; neurological problems in survivors
Shigella dysentery	Diarrhoea with blood in the stools, fever, vomiting and abdominal cramps.	Contaminated drinking-water or food, or poor sanitation, poor hygiene	Case fatality rate may be high
Viral hepatitis A	Nausea, slight fever, pale-coloured stools, dark-coloured urine, jaundiced eye whites and skin after several days.	Poor hygiene	Long-term disabling effects
Louse-borne typhus	Prolonged fever, headache, body pains.	Unhygienic conditions leading to lice infestations	May be fatal without treatment
Typhoid fever	Starts off like malaria, sometimes with diarrhoea, prolonged fever, occasionally with delirium.	As for diarrhoea	Without appropriate medical care, may lead to fatal complications in a few weeks
Cholera	Modest fever, severe, but liquid diarrhoea (rice water stools), abdominal spasms, vomiting, rapid weight loss and dehydration.	As for diarrhoea	As for diarrhoea
Dengue and dengue haemorrhagic fever (DHF)	High fever, headaches, pain in muscles and joints, red spots on skin.	Breeding of *Aedes* mosquitoes in natural or artificial containers, filled with water	Dengue usually runs a mild course. DHF, however, is often accompanied by heavy haemorrhages, which may be fatal
Diphtheria	Inflamed and painful throat, coughing.	Crowding, poor hygiene	A secretion is deposited in the respiratory tract, which can lead to asphyxiation

Table 11.1 **(continued)**

Disease	Symptoms	Environmental risk factors	Health hazards
Tetanus	Muscle spasms, starting in the jaws and extending to the rest of the body over several days	Poor hygiene, injury	Fatal
Rabies	Fatigue, headache, disorientation, paralysis, hyperactivity	Bite from infected animal host	Fatal if untreated
Relapsing fever (louse-borne or tick-borne)	Acute high fever at intervals	Unhygienic conditions leading to lice or tick infestations	Often fatal in untreated persons, depending on immunity levels
Heat stress	Elevated body temperatures, nausea, vomiting, headache	Excessive temperatures	Risk of coma

to be a threat; creating local stocks of supplies and equipment for diagnosis, treatment and environmental health measures in case of disease outbreaks; strengthening health-surveillance systems and practicing protocols for managing information on certain diseases; raising awareness among the population likely to be affected by a disaster on communicable diseases and the need for early referral to a health facility.

Acute respiratory infections and diarrhoea are most often the major killers in emergency situations. To prevent them, hygiene promotion, the provision of adequate quantities of safe water, sanitation facilities and appropriate shelter are absolutely necessary. Measles outbreaks are a common hazard in emergencies, often with a high case fatality rate. Early vaccination campaigns should be considered before any cases appear.

11.2.2 Public-health surveillance

Public-health surveillance is the collection, analysis and dissemination of health information to enable appropriate action to be taken. This is particularly important in disasters and emergencies because of the particular vulnerability of the affected population, the sudden changes that can occur in health due to the unstable nature of the situation, and the need to share quantitative data rapidly with a range of partners to enable rapid and effective action to be taken (Médecins Sans Frontières, 1997a).

It is important to designate specific health staff for public-health surveillance. Neighbourhood and community health workers, as well as the personnel of temporary relief centres and hospitals, should be alert to patients presenting with any of a list of diseases, including typhoid or paratyphoid fever, cholera, typhus, plague, encephalitis or meningitis, as well as to excessive numbers of poisonings (including food poisoning) or cases of malaria. Histories should be taken from these patients, contacts identified, and the source of the disease isolated. Surveillance of public-health problems may be possible to some extent even under the worst conditions of large-scale population movement. Existing reporting systems can be extended to create an area-wide surveillance system that covers priority diseases, including serious water- and sanitation-related epidemic diseases.

Figure 11.1 is a specimen weekly surveillance summary sheet to report results from health-care centres to a central epidemiological surveillance unit. This may need to be adapted for specific emergencies.

Active surveillance of population movements can provide data for planning emergency interventions and for general disease surveillance. A system will be required for tracking the locations of large, dense settlements and for surveillance of population

Figure 11.1 **Specimen weekly surveillance summary sheet**[1]

WEEKLY MORBIDITY/MORTALITY SURVEILLANCE FORM

District/Town/Settlement/Camp:

Health clinic:
Reporting period:
Name and signature of reporting officer:

Reported main cause of illness/death (final diagnosis)	<5 YEARS		5 YEARS AND OLDER		Total	
	CASES	DEATHS	CASES	DEATHS	CASES	DEATHS
Acute watery diarrhoea						
Bloody diarrhoea						
Suspected cholera						
Severe RTI/pheumonia						
Suspected malaria/fever of unknown origin						
Malnutrition						
Measles						
Meningitis						
Trauma						
Acute jaundice syndrome						
Other/unknown						
Total						

Average crude mortality rates (deaths/10 000 total population/day) _____
Average under five year old mortality rates (deaths/10 000 total under fives/day) _____

[1] RTI = respiratory tract infection.

movements. Small teams of observers at key transport nodes—bridges, passes and major junctions—can help to provide detailed information on movement patterns, e.g. the numbers and demographic profile of people moving on foot, the numbers and types of vehicles, their occupants and average loading, the types of possessions carried, and the stated destinations. This information can help staff to anticipate future patterns of settlement. Aerial surveillance can also assist. The most effective approach is usually to extend the routes and patterns of reporting used by existing administrative structures in the areas where people are arriving.

11.2.3 Outbreak control

Suspected disease outbreaks, indicated by information from a health surveillance system, should be rapidly investigated using standards protocols for assessment (Médecins Sans Frontières, 1997a; World Health Organization, 1999b). The assessment should enable decisions to be taken on how to control the outbreak.

The two main strategies for controlling outbreaks of communicable disease are to reduce the number of cases through preventive activities and to reduce mortality due to the disease through early case detection and effective treatment. These measures should be put into place rapidly, and should not be delayed while waiting for laboratory confirmation of the disease in question. They key to effective outbreak control is a rapid response, before the outbreak develops into a major epidemic. Mass immunization is a priority in emergency situations, where people are displaced, there is disruption of normal services, there are crowded or insanitary conditions and/or where there is widespread malnutrition, regardless of whether a single case of measles has been reported or not. One confirmed case of cholera should prompt all diarrhoea cases to be treated as cholera.

Preventive and curative measures work together to reduce the sources of infection by rapidly isolating and treating patients and controlling animal reservoirs; to protect susceptible groups through immunization, nutritional support and possibly chemoprophylaxis (e.g. to protect vulnerable individuals in the case of a malaria outbreak); and to reduce transmission through improvements in hygiene conditions and hygiene behaviour.

The role of outreach workers in these three activities is important. They can inform people about the disease and encourage early referral of patients to a treatment/isolation centre; identify vulnerable families and individuals requiring particular support or protection; and encourage improvements in hygiene conditions and hygiene behaviour by identifying areas where facilities need to be improved and protective hygiene behaviours need to be promoted.

11.3 The control of cholera: an example

Cholera is used as an example because the disease remains endemic in many parts of Africa, Asia and Latin America. In the early 1990s, cholera epidemics affected millions of people in Africa and Latin America. Its prevention and control in emergencies provide examples of general approaches to be adopted with other epidemics.

"Healthy" cholera carriers (i.e. people carrying *Vibrio cholerae* with no manifest disease) are now common in the general population of many developing countries. Although most cases of cholera are mild and treatable with simple measures, the disease can rapidly progress and result in death from dehydration. It can also spread easily where there is rudimentary sanitation and crowding, as in a refugee camp. It is therefore important to plan ahead in order to prevent cholera by the proper management of the water supply, sanitation and food hygiene in camps.

Those responsible for routine health surveillance should be alert to the possibility of cholera, should be familiar with the signs of the disease and should report suspected cases promptly to the authorities. Plans should also be made for the necessary steps to be taken if cholera does break out. These should specify the additional health and environment measures to be taken, as well as how to treat cholera patients.

A case of cholera should be suspected when:

— in an area where the disease is not known to be present, a patient aged 5 years or more develops severe dehydration or dies from acute watery diarrhoea;
— in an area where there is an outbreak of cholera, any patient aged 5 years or more develops acute watery diarrhoea, with or without vomiting (World Health Organization, 1993b).

Although cholera can be treated, it cannot be controlled by vaccinations or by mass chemotherapy, but only by redoubling efforts to safeguard water supplies; maintaining a high free residual chlorine level (preferably 0.4–0.5 mg/l) in water supplies; disposing of faeces so as not to contaminate water or food; encouraging hand washing with soap or ashes; and encouraging hygienic preparation and storage of food. The role of hygiene education in these control measures is critical.

Patients suspected of suffering from cholera should be treated in a place set aside for this purpose. One arrangement for dealing with cholera in a refugee camp is described in Box 11.3. In areas where an outbreak of cholera is possible, supplies and equipment for outbreak control and treatment should be stored locally to deal with the first stages of an outbreak; staff should be trained in case management; and the population should be made aware of the risk of an outbreak, the need for early referral of patients with diarrhoea, and preventive measures they can take. For further information on clinical treatment of cholera see: World Health Organization (1993b).

11.4 Further information

For further information on:

— the control of communicable diseases in emergencies, see: Benenson (1995), Perrin (1996), Médecins Sans Frontières (1997a), Sphere Project (2000);
— planning medical supplies, equipment and drugs, and handling donated drugs in general, see: United Nations Development Programme, Inter-Agency Procurement Services Office (1995).

Box 11.3 Epidemic cholera in refugee camps[1]

Cholera can spread very quickly in overcrowded living areas. If an epidemic breaks out:

Control
- An emergency treatment facility should be established.
- Apart from patients, people visiting the facility should be limited to those giving care.
- Stored drinking-water should be purified with at least 0.2 mg per litre of free residual chlorine.
- Sodium hypochlorite or calcium hypochlorite should be added to water at the following chlorine concentrations:
  0.05% (0.5 g per litre) for washing;
  0.2% (2 g per litre) for cleaning walls and floors;
  1% (10 g per litre) for disinfecting contaminated bedding and clothes, and for cleaning latrines.

Public-health measures
- Treat wells in the affected area; cover them if possible. Appoint someone to treat each collected bucket of water with sodium hypochlorite or calcium hypochlorite. Ideally this should done at every well when the water is collected.
- Health workers should regularly visit households to detect cases.
- Gatherings of people should be restricted.
- Carry out precautionary measures to reduce contamination of food sold in markets.
- Test samples of water for the presence of *Escherichia coli*. This indicates faecal pollution and the possible presence of bacteria that cause diarrhoea.
- Send stool samples for laboratory testing, if possible, to confirm the presence of cholera.
- Good record keeping (number of cases and deaths) at clinics and treatment centres will help in assessing whether the epidemic is getting worse, or whether public-health measures are having a positive effect.
- Use patient records to plot outbreaks on a map of the camp.
- Disinfect homes of patients if resources are available.

[1] Source: Chartier, Diskett & UNHCR (1991).

12. Chemical incidents

12.1 Types of chemical incident

A chemical incident has been defined as "an unexpected uncontrolled release of a chemical from its containment". A public-health chemical incident has been defined as "where two or more members of the public are exposed (or threatened to be exposed) to a chemical" (World Health Organization, 1999d). In the majority of cases, this is an acute release, where the exposure dose is rising or is likely to rise rapidly. When the release is chronic, the exposure and dose do not rise quickly and public-health measures do not have to be taken so rapidly, though the public-health concern may emerge suddenly and acutely. This chapter is concerned with acute releases. It is not concerned with incidents involving attacks with chemical weapons.

12.2 The health effects of chemical incidents

Chemical incidents affect people in a number of ways, including:

— the effects of explosion;
— the effects of fire;
— the toxic effects of the chemicals.

12.2.1 Toxic effects of chemicals

Chemicals enter the body through the skin, eyes, lungs or digestive tract. The rate of absorption via these paths is different for different chemicals, and is also affected by the concentration of the chemical in contact with the body (the concentration may change over time), the length of time that the chemical is in contact with the body, the air temperature, humidity and the person's age.

Within the body itself, the effect depends upon the actual toxicity of the chemical and on the biologically effective dose (i.e. the quantity of chemical taken into the target tissue). The way the dose is accumulated in the target tissue can make a difference to its impact. Even if the exposure is short, the peak level might be high enough to cause toxic effects. When the exposure is prolonged and the dose rate low, it may be the total cumulative dose that causes toxicity.

Effects can be local (e.g. burning or blistering of the skin, eyes or respiratory tract) or systemic, and the pattern may be influenced by age, gender, immune state, concomitant exposures and general fitness. Some effects (e.g. eye and respiratory irritation or central nervous system depression) can occur within minutes or hours of the exposure. Other effects (e.g. congenital malformations or cancers) may take months or years to appear.

12.2.2 Public-health effects of chemicals

Stress and anxiety

The occurrence of major chemical incidents has shaped the way members of the public perceive exposure to chemical substances. Such incidents are fear-inducing because they

Fig. 12.1 **Pathways of exposure**[1]

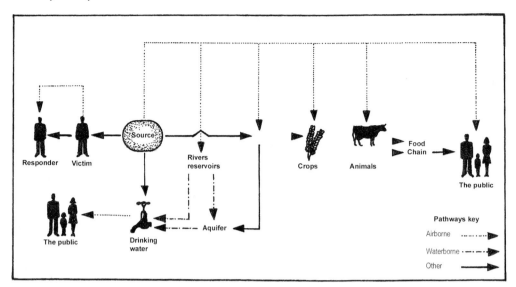

[1] Source: World Health Organization, 1999d.

have the potential to cause large numbers of deaths and illness and because they raise questions about the fragility of technologies over which the public may have little or no control.

Deaths and illness

Large incidents cause considerable numbers of deaths (e.g. the explosion at Bhopal, India in 1984). However, there are many more less-serious incidents which cumulatively have a large health impact (Bowen et al., 2000). These chemical incidents remain unreported unless a specifically designed and targeted reporting system is in place.

Societal and economic costs

Significant economic costs relate to livelihoods, inward investments, and other costs such as closures of health care facilities, schools, factories, etc., litigation and compensation, and helping affected communities recover.

12.3 Operational planning and preparedness

As with responses to all types of disaster, careful planning and thorough preparedness are prerequisites for an effective response to a chemical incident. At the national level, government needs to set up procedures and organizations to ensure that the public-health management of any chemical incident is effective and comprehensive. A national plan should be circulated and discussed widely until agreement has been reached. At the local level, public-health authorities need to identify situations where chemical incidents could occur, and assess the likely health risks to exposed people, property and the environment. The public-health sector needs to be fully involved in the planning and preparedness process, including emergency plan development and implementation. Many organizations will be involved in the planning and response phases of chemical incident management (see Table 12.1).

Table 12.1 **Organizations and groups involved in planning for, and managing, chemical incidents**

Public-health/environmental-health departments and institutes	Public and community groups
Poisons centres	Emergency services/civil defense
Toxicology laboratories	— fire
Local hospitals	— police
Specialist hospitals	— ambulance
Occupational health services	— transport
	— emergency medical responders
Food safety organizations	Military
Local government	Specialist environment agencies
Central government	— rivers
Major local chemical industries	— ocean/sea
Environmental groups, pressure groups and watchdogs	— wildlife
	— transport
Nongovernmental organizations /Red Cross/Red Crescent	— agricultural
	— air quality
	Pollution control agencies
	— factories inspectorates
	Weather services

12.3.1 Multidisciplinary public-health working arrangements

Establishing a multidisciplinary chemical incident team is usually the best way of achieving the necessary tasks, in both the planning and response phases. In addition, if the team enhances their skills with training during the planning phase, the resulting teamwork during an incident is likely to be greatly improved. The geographical area covered by the team needs to be decided, and a coordinating mechanism should be established.

The chemical incident team may be comprised of staff from a number of agencies concerned with health, civil defense and disaster management. The team should also draw upon scientific expertise and should build up good relationships with experts, so that during an incident, help and assistance are speedily obtained.

12.3.2 Vulnerability assessment

Vulnerability assessment, also known as community risk assessment (CRA) in the field of chemical incident management, is an assessment of the potential effects of a chemical incident in the local area. It is comprised of four steps:

— the identification of hazardous chemical sites, pipelines and transport routes;
— the identification of possible incident scenarios and their exposure pathways;
— the identification of vulnerable populations, facilities and environments;
— an estimation of the health impact of potential chemical incidents and the requirements for health-care facilities.

CRA is a complex process and involves a wide range of expertise and agencies. A coordinated approach to data requests and collection is required to produce valid and complete data that meet the needs of the various agencies and experts involved. The public should also be involved. Not only can they provide local knowledge, but their understanding will increase and their anxiety will be reduced when findings are shared. Conducting a CRA develops and strengthens the relationships between the emergency services, the public health services, the chemical industry and the general public. It also helps to identify training requirements.

The identification of hazardous sites in the local community is an important means of recognizing possible emergency situations. Once they are identified, it is possible to check the availability of appropriate expertise, site emergency plans and evacuation, procedures, materials, decontamination equipment and antidotes. There are, however, no generally accepted guidelines for doing this, and it is best to pool ideas and experience from all members of the team.

Ideally, a local inventory should be collated and kept up to date because chemical use may change frequently. For example, chemicals such as fertilizers, swimming pool disinfectants and fireworks are only transported and stored locally at certain times of the year.

12.3.3 Local incident surveillance and environmental monitoring.

For each site identified, the chemicals present (current and planned) are identified and scenarios of possible releases are developed for each one. For each site and substance, the exposure pathways and vulnerable zone (the area to which the contaminants might be transported through air or water) are estimated and mapped out. This can often be done using computer models. It requires a thorough knowledge of the topography of the area, the waterways, the reservoirs and the prevailing climate.

The populations that could be affected within the vulnerable zone are then identified, with an emphasis on any particularly vulnerable groups (children in schools, the elderly in residential facilities, hospital patients, etc.). In addition to the residents of the vulnerable zone, other people in the area at certain times could also be affected, such as workers (both inside the plant and in its vicinity), motorists and visitors to entertainment facilities. Factors that affect vulnerability include the amount and quality of shelter, the access into and out of the site, and people's awareness of risks and response measures.

Facilities and structures in and around the vulnerable zone that provide essential services (e.g. hospitals) and which could be disabled by an incident should be identified. Areas where contamination would have significant effects, such as farmland, water bodies used for leisure activities or wildlife support, and ecologically important sites should be considered.

Assessing vulnerability around chemical transport routes presents greater difficulties, but is extremely important. Highly toxic chemicals are often transported by rail, which passes through densely populated areas, and by inland waterways.

12.3.4 Baseline health assessment

To measure the impact of a chemical release on health, it is necessary to know the background levels of illness in the community before the release.

In most countries, health data are only available at population levels greater than that likely to be affected by a chemical incident. This can make it more difficult to identify any changes in the health of the affected population. To overcome this difficulty, routine data should be collected from populations around the chemical sites. This can be expensive, but should be considered for very high-risk sites. If routine data are not available to produce a baseline measure, a one-off survey may be considered.

In addition, it is helpful to take baseline measurements of chemical biomarkers from the people most likely to respond first to an incident, because they have a long-term risk of exposure. Ideally, these measures should be conducted by the occupational health services. The samples may be frozen and analysed after an incident, together with a post-incident sample, to measure the influence of the chemical incident.

12.3.5 Health impact assessment

This brings together assessment of exposure pathways and degrees of vulnerability in different scenarios to calculate the number and distribution of casualties expected, and the type and severity of possible injuries. The assessment identifies evacuations required in case of acute exposure and considers the effects of secondary contamination. Air dispersion modelling programmes may be used during this process.

It is important to determine the capacity of the local health-care facilities, including toxicology laboratories. Facilities need to be assessed for their patient capacity, medical equipment, decontamination equipment, drugs and antidotes, and number of staff and their level of training. This assessment can be compared with the casualty estimates from the various scenarios, to determine when to call in additional help, or to refer patients to facilities out of the area. These estimates are imprecise, but can help identify the links that need to be established with health facilities in other areas.

12.3.6 Baseline environmental assessment

Air, water, soil, sediment and food in the vicinity of chemical plants should be sampled and tested for the full range of chemicals (or their by-products) being manufactured, used or stored. Laboratory services should be identified for this task. Priority areas may need to be selected from the CRA and targeted. It may be helpful to carry out a complete environmental assessment, to predict the levels of environmental contamination from a variety of likely release scenarios. There are various computer dispersion models available for this purpose, though many of these models are unable to take sufficient account of all the relevant variables.

12.3.7 Liaison with the local community

The people who live and work in the area that could be affected by a chemical release should not only be informed about the plans for a chemical incident, but should also be involved in drawing them up. Community members who help with these preparations must represent their local community.

Large public meetings

This is the most common and familiar way of initiating face-to-face discussions with the public, though it is often one of the least effective ways to institute a dialogue. However, public meetings can be beneficial if the officials involved are knowledgeable about the local risks and skilled in risk communication.

Public availability sessions

Although time consuming and resource intensive, a personal and confidential discussion between a concerned individual or family and a health professional is perhaps the most effective way to discuss risk issues. Public availability sessions are publicized and hosted by public-health agencies in the local community; experts are available to talk with all interested individuals, either by appointment or on a first-come, first-served basis.

Community advisory panels

Community advisory panels (CAPs) provide the opportunity for an effective dialogue between community representatives, health officials and chemical industry representatives. They help ensure continuity over a period of months or years, and the opportunity for mutual education.

CAPs typically comprise 12–15 community representatives, chosen either by self-nomination or by community organizations. The panels, whose members represent the widest possible spectrum of community interests, usually meet every 3 months in a public forum. Rules regarding the conduct of meetings and issues to be covered are agreed upon at the outset.

Public warning systems

Once an incident has occurred, there is a need for robust warning systems for informing the public of the incident and of any protective measures they should take. For example, a warning system may involve sounding a siren, so the public know they should listen to the radio for information and instructions. This can be very effective and is appropriate for high-priority areas, though the public need training and updating in the process.

Other mechanisms for public interaction

Site visits can help the community to understand the measures taken by the industry to protect the workers and the public. Mass mailings are an efficient way to notify residents of a concerned community about new scientific findings, planned activities or upcoming meetings. These are most effective when they are done in a one-page, "fact sheet" format with bulleted information. Information sheets are also helpful in providing information about the priority sites and their chemicals, warning formats and protective actions to be taken. Radio and television can be very effective media, depending on local availability.

12.3.8 Public-health plans for chemical incidents

Planning for major incidents and disasters has been comprehensively developed throughout much of the world. In most countries, there is a general plan covering major incidents and disasters. In addition, there is often a general plan covering the roles of the emergency services in chemical incidents. There are usually also major incident plans in hospitals that cover most types of incidents. However, public-health plans to deal with chemical incidents are usually nonexistent or poorly developed.

The public-health chemical incident plan needs to take account of four different scenarios:

— a release from a fixed site: this will usually be a registered hazardous site;
— a detected release of a known chemical from a non-fixed site such as a road tanker (which may not be clearly labelled as carrying hazardous material);
— a detected release of an unknown chemical: typically, this will occur in releases from sites not on the hazardous site inventory, or with unknown combustion products from a chemical fire;
— a silent release, where the release is unknown or suspected from other routes.

The plan will also be significantly improved if key members of the local community are involved throughout the process. Extensive evaluation of the plan and its implementation should be carried out after every incident or training exercise.

12.3.9 Databases

At the time of an incident, it is vital to have rapid access to data about the chemical. It is important therefore that the chemical databases are purchased and installed, or that uninterrupted access to databases is established well before an incident. The data required include:

— the physical characteristics of the chemical (these influence the way it disperses in the environment and how it enters the body);

— the biological tests available to detect exposure and/or adverse health effects;

— environmental sampling techniques and equipment needed;

— lists of antidotes and decontamination procedures;

— medical signs and symptoms and methods of treatment.

12.3.10 Reducing the probability of incidents

The CRA may have identified sites and procedures where improvements could lessen the probability of an incident occurring. Often, some of these improvements can only be made by the company producing, storing or transporting the chemical, and it may require a multi-agency team to negotiate these changes.

12.3.11 Reducing the health risks of incidents

Common measures to reduce the health risks of chemical incidents include:

— locating chemical sites away from centres of population;

— registering all chemicals in commercial establishments with a hazard inventory to ensure rapid identification of the released chemical;

— regularly evaluating plans and their implementation;

— storing reduced amounts of chemicals;

— clearly labelling all chemicals in transit;

— rapidly notifying the chemical incident emergency services in the event of a chemical release;

— regularly surveying and standardizing the reporting of incidents, including small "routine" ones;

— decontaminating land or water already contaminated by waste disposal;

— preventing or containing water run-off from fire-fighting;

— constructing drainage ditches or holding tanks to contain leaked liquid chemicals.

12.3.12 Establishing routine procedures

Routine procedures to be established are described in this section.

Recognizing chemical incidents

Detection can occur in the following ways:

■ The polluter informs the emergency services, who inform the public-health services.

■ The release itself is observed—often as a major event, such as an explosion or oil tanker disaster.

■ The public provide information about environmental indications (e.g. colour, smell or eye irritation).

■ There is an ad hoc observation of a rise in an environmental contaminant.

■ Routine environmental monitoring data show a rise in a contaminant.

■ Clinicians and others (e.g. poisons information centres) are presented with a sudden rise in an unusual health problem.

■ Routine health monitoring data show a rise in a sentinel health event or other health measure.

A programme for recognizing chemical incidents therefore requires the public, local institutions and organizations, and all members of the emergency, environmental and health services to be regularly alerted to the possibility of chemical incidents, and to be educated on the means of communicating rapidly with each other and with the chemical incident team. It also requires a surveillance and monitoring system, a chemical incident network coordinator who is always available, and a well-publicized, twenty-four hour incident telephone line.

Conducting population health surveillance

Routine population health surveillance related to chemical incident management is the ongoing and systematic collection, analysis and interpretation of health data in order to do the following:

— identify a health event that may be related to an unknown, acute release of a chemical;
— monitor trends in health status markers;
— stimulate epidemiological research likely to lead to control or prevention;
— permit assessment of control measures.

General health statistics

Data from a wide variety of routine sources need to be collated and presented in a way that allows trends to be identified and comparisons to be made. This requires data that are reasonably accurate, comprehensive, up-to-date and easily accessible. To calculate incidence rates and exposure rates it is essential to first define the population. In an emergency, a rapid estimate of the population by direct counting, or sampling and extrapolation, is usually more reliable than census figures or other established data.

Mortality statistics

Most countries have systems for registering deaths, usually with information about cause of death. However, inaccuracies may occur at any step in the chain of procedures leading to the production of mortality statistics, and staff should ascertain the degree and type of inaccuracies associated with the data they use. Nevertheless, trends in mortality figures may indicate a health event related to an unknown chemical incident.

Health centre data

In many countries, hospital admissions are the main source of data about illness and disability. Usually, however, the data about patients are not related to geographical areas. For medical conditions of particular concern, the population admission rates need to be calculated by searching the records of all the hospitals that the patients might have been admitted to.

It is also important to set up links with outpatient services, private practice, accident and emergency care, and other primary-care facilities, so that in the event of a chemical incident, rapid contact can be made to ascertain numbers of people attending for primary care.

Cancer registration

Cancer registries have been useful in identifying spatial and temporal clusters of cancers and sometimes in allaying public fears about the existence of clusters surrounding chemical plants. However, there are significant problems in using cancer as a potential end point for environmental health assessments. There is a long latency between exposure and disease onset, 30 years or more, which makes it difficult to conduct follow-up studies on exposed populations long enough to detect cancer onset. This is usually compounded by a lack of accurate information on the exposures of people with cancer. Cancer data have been useful for assessing chronic exposures, but their usefulness in identifying acute exposures has yet to be demonstrated.

Congenital malformations

Population-based registries have been set up in some countries both for research into the cause of congenital malformations and to detect changes in the frequency of different classes of congenital disorder. Experience with the use of these registries, however, has shown that recognition and registration of the malformations is quite a slow process, and it is not feasible to use them to identify chemical incidents. Congenital malformations registers may be more useful for prospective assessment of the population health effects after known incidents of exposure, by linking new entries in the congenital malformation register with the population of exposed people.

12.3.13 Conducting exercises and training

Training and education play an important part in preparedness for, and response to, chemical incidents. The emergency services, other relevant health professions, local chemical plants, etc. need to train their personnel to properly manage occurrences that might grow to become chemical incidents, as well as chemicals incidents themselves, to understand the responsibilities of other professionals, and to minimize the risks to the workers and members of the public.

It is important that all those with specific responsibilities in a chemical emergency response should receive joint theoretical and practical training in the use and implementation of jointly agreed emergency response plans. This will enable them to become familiar with taking part in a broad cooperative effort to respond to a chemical incident.

Core training for the response team is an important mechanism for the various agencies' staff to get a good understanding of their own and others' needs. Public-health elements that should be included in the core training are:

— risk and exposure assessment;
— epidemiology and toxicology;
— emergency actions and procedures to reduce risk to responders and the public;
— the use of protective equipment;
— shelter and protective measures and procedures;
— biological and environmental sampling;
— the key components of a major chemical hazard control system;
— risk communication techniques;
— regular exercises.

Public-health and environmental-health staff require specialist training to a higher level in the relevant core areas. Countries need to review how to establish access to comprehensive training for all health professionals concerned. This may be organized through public-health training centres, poisons information centres, national information and advisory centres, or local response units.

Exercises should be used to maximize the effectiveness of training. There are four main types of exercise: orientation, tabletop, functional and full-scale simulations. Individual agencies may also consider holding preliminary orientation exercises to introduce participants to their responsibilities under the chemical incident plan, and to prepare them for the exercise.

Orientation exercises

An orientation exercise acquaints staff in a single discipline with policies and procedures in the chemical incident plan, and provides a general overview of the plan provisions. It is particularly effective in ensuring that personnel understand their roles and responsibilities and how to access background information and specialist advice. It also helps to clarify any complex or sensitive elements of the public-health chemical incident plan.

The orientation exercise does not generally involve any direct simulation, but is used to review procedures and informally apply them to potential emergency situations, preferably those involving priority sites and chemicals.

Tabletop exercises

A tabletop exercise is more formally structured and often involves more than one sector with responsibilities under the plan. Prepared situations and problems are combined with role-playing to generate discussion of the plan, its procedures, the resources that can be called on, and the policies to be adhered to when making decisions. Tabletop exercises are a good method of familiarizing individuals and groups with their roles and demonstrating proper coordination. They provide a good environment within which to reinforce the logic and content of the plan and to integrate new principles into the decision-making process. Participants are encouraged to act out critical steps, recognize difficulties, use the expertise of the other sectors represented and resolve problems. Tabletop exercises usually take 2–4 hours and require specially trained facilitators.

Functional exercises

A functional exercise is an emergency simulation designed to provide training and evaluation of integrated emergency operations and management. More complex than a tabletop exercise, it focuses on the full-scale interaction of decision making and agency coordination involving a typical incident. All field operations are simulated; information about activity is transmitted using communications equipment, including radio and telephone. It permits decision makers, off-site incident coordinators, on-site incident managers, and operations personnel to practise emergency response management in a realistic situation with time constraints and stress. It generally includes several organizations and agencies, practising interaction of a series of emergency functions. These may include: initial information gathering from the incident hotline; deciding the make-up of the core team; direction and control off-site; communications to be made with those on-site; and access to databases and mobilization of specialists, to provide advice, public warnings and decisions on evacuation.

Full-scale simulation exercises

A simulation exercise focuses on several components of an incident response and management system simultaneously. It includes the interactive elements of a community emergency programme, similar to the functional exercise, but also uses a detailed scenario to simulate an emergency. The exercise includes practicing on-site direction and operations, and also includes coordination and policy-making roles at the incident coordinating centre. Direction and control, mobilization of resources, communications, assessment, decontamination, treatment, triage and other special functions are commonly exercised.

An audit of the various exercises will enable the chemical incident plan to be updated and improved, and for training requirements to be identified. An audit should ask the following questions:

- **Plans:** did the plans work and are there any improvements to be made?
- **Teamwork:** how did the individual team members act in the group, and interact with each other?
- **Decisions:** did the team reach the right conclusions and make the right recommendations in light of available data?

12.3.14 Conducting national chemical incident surveillance and contributing to international chemical incident surveillance

Important public-health lessons can be learned from an analysis of an actual incident and any epidemiological study conducted following it. In the same way, important lessons can be learned from collating data about the range of incidents that occur within a country and around the world.

The data should make it possible to do the following:

— map the production, storage, transport and use of chemicals;
— detect trends in the occurrence of different types of chemicals commonly involved in incidents;
— provide estimates of the scale of morbidity and mortality related to the chemical incidents;
— stimulate epidemiological research likely to lead to control or prevention;
— identify risk factors associated with the occurrence of chemical incidents;
— permit assessment of control measures;
— improve the practice of staff who manage the surveillance system;
— pinpoint additional expertise, training, resources and facilities needed to deal with incidents in the area;
— stimulate governments to initiate proper incident control mechanisms at the international level.

12.4 Dealing with chemical incidents

In any chemical incident, there are essential steps to take as part of the chemical incident plan. These are described below in approximate chronological order.

12.4.1 Alerting the health-care services

Public-health/environmental-health professionals are in a good position to assess the extent of the casualties and to alert and activate local and more distant health-care facilities. This will involve providing accident and emergency departments with information about the nature of the chemical(s) and any precautions to be taken, and information about secondary contamination and how to decontaminate casualties, staff and equipment.

12.4.2 Best outcome assessment/estimation

Once a chemical incident has occurred, there are a number of courses of action or management options that can be taken at different points in the sequence of events. A management option can be any choice available to the emergency responders, such as whether to extinguish a fire or let it burn out, whether or not to use a chemical dispersant following an oil spill, or whether to evacuate people from an affected area or recommend sheltering.

Each of these management options may end up with a different outcome on the health of the public, the responders and the environment. Chemical incident response staff, for example, will be primarily concerned with containing the chemical, while hospital doctors will be dealing with the casualties, and neither will be able to view the incident from a distance or in the long term. The function of the chemical incident team is to try to work out the management option that arrives at the best outcome for the health of the public and the environment. The accuracy with which this can be done depends on the amount of information and data that arrives from the incident site, and the amount of time available before a decision is required.

12.4.3 Information and public warnings—communication skills

The public often needs information about:

— the incident;
— measures being taken to contain the release;
— who is currently under threat;
— the health effects of exposure;
— what the public can do to protect themselves;
— when, where and how further information will be made available.

Public warnings and directives must be clear and repeated. Often this is done through the media, but may also be conducted through public-address systems. All public information must be consistent, and should be provided by a small number of people with strong communication skills and training.

12.4.4 Advice on protection

Proper assessment during the incident can determine whether individuals or a population are likely to be exposed, and the possible health effects of short-term, acute and chronic exposure. This assessment may be done by the emergency services for populations near the incident site, or by the chemical incident team for more distant populations.

12.4.5 Sheltering or evacuation/removal.

For the public, usually the most feasible protective measure is sheltering—i.e. staying in a building, closing all the windows and doors, and shutting down any ventilation or air-conditioning systems until the chemical (usually in a cloud) has passed. This procedure will usually protect the population for about 2 hours, which is more than enough for the majority of incidents.

Evacuation often involves complex arrangements for providing transport, shelter, food, water and appropriate medical care. It may also require ensuring the security of the properties left uninhabited. See Section 4.2 for further information on evacuation.

Evacuation may be the better option in one or more of the following cases:

— the chemicals are widely dispersed and contamination is extensive;
— toxic chemicals are suspected, but cannot be identified readily;
— the chemical is highly hazardous;
— the air will be hazardous for a prolonged period.

The decision on whether to evacuate people or encourage them to seek protection by sheltering must be based on a balance of the risks of the two options, with the primary consideration being the risk of exposure (both level and duration).

12.4.6 Other restrictions to protect health

If soil is contaminated, it may be necessary to restrict movement through the contaminated area. People should be kept upwind of an air-contamination site, or away from any plume of smoke or dispersion cloud. Modelling and monitoring should be carried out to determine whether groundwater movement has dispersed the contamination over a wider area or contaminated water supplies. Other measures include restricting the distribution or use of contaminated crops, livestock or drinking-water. Alternative supplies need to be identified and provided in this case.

12.4.7 Organizing registers and samples

There are three important steps that have to be taken to organize a register of data on exposure to the chemical(s) of concern:

— entering details of all the exposed people into a register;
— taking samples from the people in the register;
— taking samples from the contact medium (e.g. the soil, water or air) these people were exposed to.

Environmental modelling or rapid environmental sampling may make it possible to ascertain the media that have been contaminated and their geographical distribution, and the populations likely to have been exposed.

By collecting these data it will be possible to:

— ascertain when the risk of exposure in certain areas falls below the threshold for protective action;
— ascertain the populations and individuals requiring further follow-up and treatment;
— supply baseline data for long-term follow-up studies;
— assess the success of mitigation efforts;
— add to the understanding of the incident and exposure effects;
— uncover continuing problems;
— provide estimates for planning and resource allocation, using data on the distribution and severity of health effects, and on the environmental effects;
— support environmental and community remediation efforts;
— develop reference background material for future similar incidents and add to toxicological databases;
— refine the theoretical models of assessment;
— provide information for litigation and compensation.

Ideally, all named registers should contain details of the person, exposure time, exposure route, portal of entry, symptoms and biomarkers. Named registers require a set of agreed definitions, permission from the individuals concerned, confidentiality assurance, an updating mechanism, and a commitment of time and resources, which can be considerable.

12.4.8 Collection of samples—biomarkers of chemicals and their effects

Biological measurements, both of exposure and of the effects of exposure, can be an important tool. Unfortunately, and contrary to widespread misconceptions, no single blood test will identify which of the thousands of chemicals in the world an individual has been exposed to. Testing for biomarkers of exposure and biomarkers of effect requires specific sampling and handling techniques for each chemical or class of chemical, and many of the tests can only be carried out in specialist toxicology laboratories (World Health Organization 1993c).

Biomarkers of exposure

These are measurable levels of the parent chemical or its metabolites found in one or more body fluids or tissues in an exposed population. Sensitive, replicable assays for the human body burden of many contaminants are available, but often must be performed soon after exposure.

If elevated levels could be caused by factors other than exposure to the agent of concern, it is important that information be gathered on hobbies, secondary occupations, source of water supplies, and any other determinants with elevated levels. It may be possible to compare the target population to a reference population that resembles the exposed population, except for the exposure. Reference levels exist for many tests.

A preliminary exposure survey should test samples from the subgroup most likely to be highly exposed to contaminated environmental media (exposure biomarkers), or most vulnerable to exposure (effect biomarkers). If samples from these groups do not show measurable levels, it is unlikely other individuals in the wider population will have been exposed, and further investigation of other exposed people is unlikely to be fruitful.

Biomarkers of effect

For many contaminants or situations, it is not possible to study biomarkers of exposure. In some cases, this is because the half-life within the human body is short. In other cases, it is because laboratory tests are not available, or that the chemical does not enter the body and has only a local effect. In such circumstances, it may be possible to measure intermediate health effects of exposure by using physiological measurements known to change with exposure.

If biomarkers have not been taken or are not available, levels may need to be inferred from:

— occupation, and specific place and type of work;
— special features of exposure, such as working in a confined space or the level of ventilation;
— whether indoors or outdoors at the time and the level of physical activity;
— the volume of chemical used in a process (e.g. volume of paint containing mercury used in a home);
— immediate symptoms, such as burning or itching, that may indicate the level to which an individual has been exposed to the chemical;
— time from exposure to onset of symptoms—a rapid onset may indicate a high dose;
— special features that may affect absorption within the body (e.g. smoking, exercise or abrasions);
— measures taken to reduce contamination of the individual (e.g. washing skin and clothes immediately);
— scorching of vegetation or animal sentinels.

12.4.9 Environmental monitoring

Monitoring at the source of contamination should continue well beyond the moment at which the release is thought to have been controlled, to ensure that it has indeed been controlled.

It may be that some modelling of the likely distribution of the chemical has already been done. If so, it may be useful to check its accuracy by sampling outside the predicted contaminated zone. This is particularly important if there are reports of health effects in these areas.

It is also important to assess the concerns of the community about the possible contamination of their environment and their own exposure. These may point to areas for further study or remediation, and may also guide the presentation of the results of the investigation, to demonstrate how community concerns have been addressed.

12.5 Assessing the impact on public health

The main objectives of assessing the health effects of a chemical incident on the public are as follows.

■ *To offer advice about exposure and protection*: information is needed from the incident on the source and type of chemical, and on the likely exposure pathways; and information is needed from databases about the type, frequency and severity of the health effects of the chemical (ideally, at different concentrations of environmental contamination).

■ *To offer advice about treatment*: all those exposed, or suffering from acute health effects need to be identified and followed up for as long as necessary.

■ *To contribute to the public health toxicological information base*: it is important to set up epidemiological studies for gathering data on the health effects of chemical concentrations seen in acute exposures, since the evidence base is limited.

12.5.1 Health impact assessment

The methods used to assess the impact on public health vary depending on the stage of the incident.

Stage 1. Preparedness

During the planning and preparation stages, public-health/environmental-health professionals should become familiar with the sources of data on exposure and health risk and effect.

Stage 2. Rapid health-risk assessment

During the acute stage of an incident, a rapid health-risk assessment must be conducted. Initially this can be done using models to predict health effects, based on information gathered from other exposures.

Stage 3. Exposure assessment

The next method is to start assessing the exposure levels. This involves four principle methods (United Kingdom Department for Environment, Food and Rural Affairs, 1999):

— environmental and personal/biological monitoring;
— questionnaires of activity and movement in relation to the contaminant;
— modelling the incident source, chemical dispersion from the source and population exposure;
— assessing markers, often using other indicators, such as animal sentinels.

Stage 4. Assessment of acute health effects

The next stage is to start assessing the acute health effects. This involves gaining data on toxic and stress-related effects and their functional, physical, morbidity and mortality outcomes. Advice can be given on protection, treatment and follow-up.

Stage 5. Assessment of longer-term health effects

Similar data on the longer-term health effects can be collected, although this demands considerable commitment and resources from both the agencies and the public.

Stage 6. Epidemiological studies

The short- and long-term health effects can be identified using epidemiological studies correlated to the causes. Large-scale analytical epidemiological studies are expensive in time and resources. Descriptive studies requiring fewer resources can be used to assess

Table 12.2 **Different types of epidemiological study**

Analytical studies	Descriptive studies
Panel studies	Ecological studies
Cohort studies	Cluster investigations
Case-control studies	Disease and symptom prevalence studies
	Cross-sectional studies

the feasibility of a major study, address the concerns of the public, and generate hypotheses for further studies. Different types of analytical and descriptive epidemiological studies are listed in Table 12.2.

12.6 Further information

For further information on chemical incidents and health, see: United States Environmental Protection Agency (1990), World Health Organization (1990), United Nations (1991), Organisation for Economic Co-operation and Development (1992), Sullivan & Krieger (1992), Olson & Mycroft (1994), Organisation for Economic Co-operation and Development/United Nations Environment Programme (1994), United States Federal Emergency Management Administration (1994), van Leeuwen & Hermens (1995), European Commission (1996), Organisation for Economic Co-operation and Development (1996), United States Department of Transportation (1996), Ackermann-Liebrich et al. (1997), Lillibridge (1997), United Nations Environment Programme (1998), World Health Organization (1999d), Berglund, Elinder & Järup (2001).

13. Radiation emergencies

13.1 Health consequences of radiation

Radiation can kill or damage living cells, but as many of the billions of cells in the human body are replaced every day, minor exposures to radiation may have little or no effect on an individual. Major exposures to radiation, however, can have health effects which can be divided into *deterministic*, or **acute** effects, and *stochastic*, or **late** effects. Deterministic effects include skin burns, radiation sickness and death. Stochastic effects, on the other hand, include cancers and inheritable defects that result from damage to the genetic material in cells.

Radiation emergencies can have severe psychological effects on the victims, as the fear of an unfamiliar, invisible and potentially terrible danger causes acute stress. Such stress and its associated problems can arise even when radiation exposure is low or insignificant.

13.2 Radiation from nuclear incidents

There are several ways in which a person can become overexposed to ionizing radiation. In peacetime, the more likely ways are accidents in nuclear power plants or research institutions dealing with radioactive materials; and undue exposure to radioactive waste or radioactive source used in industry, medicine and research laboratories. More recently, the threat of terrorist acts that involve nuclear facilities, or the theft of radioactive substances, has become more prominent.

The medical and health responses to a radiation emergency depend on its magnitude. The International Nuclear Event Scale (INES), with eight levels, is used to inform the public about the severity of events at nuclear facilities (see Table 13.1).

13.3 International and local response to a major nuclear accident in compliance with the Convention on Early Notification and Assistance Convention

In the case of a nuclear accident, the level of radiation hazard for the population depends upon: the quantity and type of radionuclides released into the environment; the distance of the populated areas from the source of radioactive release; the type of buildings; the population density; the meteorological conditions at the time of the accident; the season of the year; the character of agricultural development in the area; water supplies; nutritional habits; and the nutritional status of the population.

In nuclear reactor accidents that release radioactive material into the atmosphere, the following routes are expected to result in radiation injury to the population:

— direct external irradiation with γ-rays from the passing radioactive cloud;
— internal irradiation from inhaling radioactive aerosols (inhalation hazard);
— contact radiation from radioactive fallout on the skin and clothes;
— total external irradiation of the population with γ-rays from radioactive fallout on the soil and local objects (buildings, constructions etc.);
— internal irradiation from consuming water and local food products contaminated by radioactive substances.

Table 13.1 **International Nuclear Event Scale (INES), used to inform the public about the severity of events at nuclear facilities**

Level	Description of event
Level 0 (deviation)	An event with no safety significance.
Level 1 (anomaly)	An event beyond the authorized operating regime, but not involving significant failures of safety provisions, significant spread of contamination, or overexposure of workers.
Level 2 (incident)	An event involving significant failure of safety provisions, but with sufficient in-depth defence remaining to cope with additional failures; and/or resulting in a dose to a worker exceeding a statutory dose limit; and/or leading to the presence of activity in on-site areas not expected by design and which require corrective action.
Level 3 (serious incident)	A near-accident, where only the last layer of in-depth defence remained operational; and/or involving severe spread of contamination on-site or deterministic effects to a worker; and/or a very small release of radioactive material off-site (i.e. critical group dose of the order of tenths of a mSv).
Level 4 (accident without significant off-site risk)	An accident involving significant damage to the installation (e.g. partial core melt); and/or overexposure of one or more workers that results in a high probability of death; and/or an off-site release with a critical group dose of a few mSv.
Level 5 (accident with off-site risk)	An accident resulting in severe damage to the installation, and/or an off-site release of activity radiologically equivalent to hundreds or thousands of TBq of I^{131}, likely to result in partial implementation of countermeasures covered by emergency plans. Examples: the 1979 accident at Three Mile Island, USA (severe damage to the installation) and the 1957 accident at Windscale, UK (severe damage to the installation and significant off-site release).
Level 6 (serious accident)	An accident involving a significant release of radioactive material, and likely to require full implementation of planned countermeasures, but less severe than a major accident. Example: the 1957 accident at Kyshtym, USSR (now in the Russian Federation)
Level 7 (major accident)	An accident involving a major release of radioactive material with widespread health and environmental effects. Example: the 1986 accident at Chernobyl, USSR (now in Ukraine).

During a major nuclear accident, the following three phases are identified:

— **Early phase**—from the threat of a serious release to the first few hours after the beginning of a release;

— **Intermediate phase**—from the first few hours, to 1–2 days after the start of the release;

— **Recovery phase**—from some weeks to several years after the start of the release.

Information presented in Annex 4 (Tables 1–4) gives a general summary of the actions of IAEA, WHO, other international organizations, and local health authorities in response to nuclear accidents, in compliance with the Convention on Early Notification and the Assistance Convention.

In the event of a nuclear accident, the criteria for implementing countermeasures to protect the population will depend on the phase of the accident. At the early and intermediate phases, decisions should be based on a comparison of the estimated radiation doses (calculated at the start of the accident) and intervention levels of doses given in Tables 1 and 3 of Annex 5. The dose criteria for taking protective countermeasures at the early phase are often crude estimates taken over a short period of time. During the recovery phase, decision-making is based on intervention levels of doses presented in Table 2 of Annex 5. The dose criteria for the relocation of the population refer to the estimated doses of both external and internal radiation during the first year. The dose criteria for implementing restrictions on consuming radionuclide-contaminated food products and drinking-water (Annex 5, Table 4) refer to estimated annual doses of internal radiation from radionuclides consumed in food and water.

13.4 The role of WHO in a radiation emergency

WHO, as the lead United Nations agency for health issues, has the responsibility for shaping, coordinating and initiating health-related emergency assistance programmes at the global level. WHO has established a network of collaborating centers (REMPAN) for promoting radiation emergency medical preparedness and for providing practical assistance and advice to countries in the event of an emergency involving radiation overexposure. The roles of WHO and REMPAN in radiation emergencies are outlined in Table 13.2.

13.5 Mitigation of effects

In general, the first priority is to limit the exposure to radiation that occurs primarily through radioactive fallout, either by evacuation or by sheltering the affected population. Depending on the strength of the explosion or release and the prevailing meteorological conditions (e.g. wind and precipitation), a radius of between 30 and several hundreds of kilometres from the release epicentre should be declared a priority area for action. Sheltering may be considered a preliminary solution before evacuation. Suitable sheltering sites include nuclear shelters, caves, mines and any place with a barrier of solid substances between the radiation and people. Radiation-free air, water and food will be required to diminish the hazard.

Victims of radiation from nuclear explosions should be moved as quickly as possible to an appropriate medical establishment. In some types of incidents, hundreds or even thousands of people may need to be examined for external or internal contamination. Such examinations require specialized equipment. The scope of—and the need for—decontamination will depend on whether there is evidence of body-surface contamination. Contaminated clothing will need to be handled appropriately and disposed of according to accepted procedures. Contaminated individuals will need to be thoroughly showered and be provided with uncontaminated clothing. Any illness should be treated immediately. If there is evidence of internal contamination with radioactive iodine (I^{131}), stable iodine prophylaxis is needed to avoid excessive thyroid radiation doses and, especially in young people, to reduce the risk of thyroid cancer in later life. See Box 13.1 for further information and recommended stable iodine dosages.

Depending on the results of diagnostic investigations, substantial surgical treatment may be required. This can only be provided by competent, trained physicians and nurses operating in sterile treatment facilities.

Table 13.2 **Roles of WHO and REMPAN in a radiation emergency**

Type of accident	Roles of the collaborating centres within REMPAN
A major release of radioactive material from a nuclear reactor	■ provide assistance and advice for the management of exposed individuals ■ provide a team for on-site emergency treatment ■ transfer (if possible and necessary) severely exposed patients to collaborating centres for specialized medical care ■ provide a survey team for rapid external radiation monitoring and/or contamination surveys with appropriate equipment ■ provide facilities and staff for medical investigations and treatment ■ assist in the development of measures necessary to limit health effects ■ provide follow-up medical supervision and treatment
High radioactivity sources leading to severe exposure of some individuals	■ visit the accident site to identify and isolate the source of radiation ■ make an assessment of likely exposure ■ recommend appropriate medical treatment ■ transfer patients to specialized medical facilities (if necessary and requested) ■ assist in developing procedures to strengthen countries' abilities to manage such accidents themselves
Excessive exposure of patients and/or medical staff due to the administration of radiation for medical purposes	■ circulate information relating to such incidents for the benefit of Member States

---

Box 13.1 **Stable iodine prophylaxis**

Exposure to radioisotopes of iodine following an accidental release can result in a significant increase in thyroid cancer, especially in young children. Inhaled and ingested radioactive iodine is preferentially taken up by the thyroid, and young children's thyroids are particularly sensitive to radiation.

Stable iodine blocks the uptake of radioactive iodine by the thyroid. It is available in a number of forms and is most effective when taken as close as possible to the first exposure to radioactive iodine. A single dose will normally protect against inhalation exposure. If a release lasts longer than a day, the preferred response, if practicable, is evacuation. Further doses to protect against radiation exposure from ingesting radioactive food may be required if uncontaminated food supplies are not available. The recommended single doses are:

Age	Recommended dosage[1]
>12 years	100 mg
3–12 years	50 mg
1 month to 3 years	25 mg
<1 month	12.5 mg

[1] equivalent mass of iodine—the iodine dose is usually taken either as potassium iodate or potassium iodide.

When radionuclide contamination spans national boundaries, international and national authorities would normally take the lead role in radiation emergencies. However, local authorities can play a key role in alleviating the health consequences of radiation emergencies (see Box 13.2).

Care must be taken when handling victims who have been externally contaminated by radionuclides, as the radiation that they emit can affect helpers. Their clothes must be changed and they must be bathed. In handling them, especially in the initial stages, helpers should wear thick clothing and gloves.

Many of the workers in nuclear power plants and research institutions are likely to be technically well-qualified and experienced. They will often be an integral part of the emergency response plan with roles in both the monitoring and cleanup efforts that utilize their broad experience.

If it is necessary to evacuate the population in the vicinity of the accident, radiation levels in air, water and food must be monitored. Health authorities must be prepared to provide safe water and food if these have been contaminated.

Prompt, honest and authoritative warning is important to enable people to evacuate or shelter from the radioactive plume (farmers, construction workers, forest workers, and other outdoor workers may be less accessible and more difficult to inform). Monitoring fallout in down-wind regions and countries is essential. The exposure of standing crops and the uptake of radionuclides by farm animals is an important consideration.

Box 13.2 Role of the local authority[1]

Affected individuals will often turn first to the local authority for advice, treatment and reassurance. Preparation and planning for radiation emergencies should not be viewed as the concern of central governments only.

Local authorities that are prepared and have planned for radiation emergencies can assist in solving public-health problems in a number of ways.

Before an emergency they can:

■ inform and train doctors and other front-line professionals to whom the public are likely to turn in an emergency;
■ inform the public about the possibility of an emergency, its probable consequences and possible remedial actions.

During an emergency they can:

■ provide information, guidance and reassurance to the public;
■ provide stable iodine prophylaxis, where appropriate;
■ ensure the availability of immediate medical treatment to those who require it;
■ provide advice on the safety of food and beverages.

After an emergency they can:

■ regulate the production and distribution of food;
■ organize the provision of long-term health care to victims;
■ support medical, psychological and social recovery.

Addressing public anxiety is a difficult and complex task that requires careful consideration. The public must be informed of the nature and extent of any radiation emergency and the likely effects on health. On the other hand, inappropriate and excessive reactions on the part of the authorities may unjustifiably heighten fears and lead to crowding at medical facilities, as individuals seek information and treatment.

[1] Source: World Health Organization (1997b).

Unless uncontaminated fodder and water can be provided to cows, milk may have to be condemned. A programme to monitor the radioactivity of food may need to be initiated, depending on the concentration of radionuclides in the environment (Eheman, 1989).

Depending on the levels of radiation and the nature and quantity of the radioisotopes in the fallout, large-scale evacuation of populations from contaminated areas may be required for long periods of time (World Health Organization, 1996b). The above intervention measures, and other measures as required, should be undertaken in accordance with the intervention levels developed by FAO, IAEA, OECD/NEA, PAHO and WHO (International Atomic Energy Agency, 1996). See Table 1 of Annex 4 for further details. Immediately after exposure to radiation (before screening by specialists), both the alleviation of symptoms and psychological support of victims are very important. It must be remembered that vomiting, the most common initial symptom of a radiation overdose, can also be of psychosomatic origin.

13.6 Inadvertent exposure to radioactive material

Radioactive materials are used for many industrial, research and therapeutic purposes and there is always the possibility that people will be exposed inadvertently. In general, industries and institutions handling radioactive materials have high safety standards and well-established handling procedures, and their workers are generally well protected. The high qualifications of these personnel, and the fact that they are usually well organized, give them the collective strength needed to fight for a safe working environment.

Apart from medical procedures for which a benefit is clearly defined, the most likely sources of significant exposure to radioactive material are discarded or stolen sources whose dangerous properties are not recognized by the perpetrators. Such accidents usually come to light when a radioactive source is found to have been mislaid. Prompt notification of the appropriate authorities and the use of the mass media should make the community aware of the danger. Sometimes the first indication of accidental exposure is the appearance of people with radiation injuries, e.g. radiation burns. When this happens, detailed questionnaires should be used, both to clarify the circumstances leading to the exposure and to trace other possible victims. Compounding the problem is the fact that radiation cannot be perceived by the senses, and that its first symptoms are very unspecific. An account of a radiation accident in Brazil is given in Box 13.3.

The disposal of radioactive wastes is another potential risk. Waste is produced from various steps of the nuclear fuel cycle, in the medical use of radioisotopes, by the military, and from the widespread industrial use of sealed radiation sources. Safety criteria for disposing of such wastes do exist and are quite restrictive. However, most countries

---

Box 13.3 Poverty and radiation exposure in Brazil

In September 1987, metal scavengers dismantled a canister from a radiotherapy machine in an abandoned medical clinic in the city of Goiania, in the State of Goias, Brazil. The canister contained almost 1400 curies of caesium-137. Over the following two weeks, children played with the luminous blue caesium chloride and it was widely distributed throughout the community. A number of the slum dwellers began to immediately exhibit signs of radiation sickness—loss of appetite, nausea, vomiting and diarrhoea. By the time authorities were aware of the situation more than 250 people had been exposed, 104 individuals showed evidence of internal contamination and within 4 weeks four had died.

The cause of the accident was the lack of regulation by the responsible authorities and its severity was exacerbated by the public's lack of knowledge about radiation, the slow response and the lack of resources available.

that produce radioactive wastes still have problems with disposal, especially for intermediate and high-level wastes. High-level waste may have to be safely stored for thousands of years, which requires deep burial of material in corrosion-resistant containers in a geologically stable region. This, and other requirements for a repository, mean that many countries are still addressing the question of disposal. The transport of radioactive material is also a hazardous procedure, and the potential for injury to human health always exists. However, codes of practice for the transport of radioactive materials exist in many countries and more than sixty IAEA member states have adopted the agency's Regulations for Safe Transport of Radioactive Material (Rawl, 1998).

13.7 Further information

For further information on radiation emergencies and health, see: World Health Organization (1984b), World Health Organization (1987b), World Health Organization (1989c), International Atomic Energy Agency (1994), Organization for Economic Co-operation and Development & Nuclear Energy Agency (1994), International Atomic Energy Agency (1995), World Health Organization (1995d), International Atomic Energy Agency (1996), World Health Organization (1997b), and International Federation of Red Cross and Red Crescent Societies (1998).

See also: Web Site www.oes.ca.gov/oeshomep.nsf/all/cep/$file/cep.pdf.

14. Mortuary service and handling of the dead

This chapter is concerned primarily with situations where there are large numbers of deaths following a disaster, requiring organized services for handling the dead. Dead or decayed human bodies do not generally create a serious health hazard, unless they are polluting sources of drinking-water with faecal matter, or are infected with plague or typhus, in which case they may be infested with the fleas or lice that spread these diseases. In most smaller or less acute emergency situations therefore, families may carry out all the necessary activities following a death, where this is customary practice.

14.1 Recovery of the dead

A call for volunteers to carry out search and rescue work can be communicated via the mass media and through contacts with existing community organizations. In addition to providing much-needed assistance, search and rescue activities can also give survivors a sense of purpose and of solidarity, which can later be directed to other relief activities.

Volunteers for search and rescue activities and for removing the dead should ideally be members of an existing community organization; if one does not exist, community members should form an ad hoc organization. This will help representatives of the organization to establish a disciplined system that relies on group cohesion, which will facilitate communications. Professional rescue workers should liaise with the elected representatives of such volunteer groups.

Proximity to the dead is deeply disturbing, as are the odours eventually produced by bodies. Dead bodies should therefore be buried or cremated without delay according to custom, or placed as soon as possible in mortuaries, to which the general population should not have access; here they are exposed solely for purposes of identification by family or friends, and, eventually, for the determination of the cause of death by medical experts. It must be carried out carefully to help families and loved ones deal with their loss.

In the search for survivors following a disaster, it is usually inevitable that search and rescue team members will handle corpses, which can be traumatic. Anyone charged with managing a body recovery team must be aware that high levels of distress are likely in members of such teams, and that the need to recover the bodies must be balanced against this likelihood (Thompson, 1991).

14.2 Organization of the mortuary

The mortuary should be a secure building and should have the following four sections:

— reception room;
— viewing room;
— storage chamber for bodies (not suitable for viewing);
— room for records and for storing personal effects.

The number of deaths in a major disaster may well exceed the normal capacities of the local mortuaries. Many disaster-management plans provide an indication of the number of bodies that local mortuaries can handle, but overlook the fact that these mortuaries are in constant use and will already contain bodies (Clark, Nicholls & Gillespie, 1992). It is therefore better to designate a temporary mortuary site.

Strict sanitary supervision should be maintained at all stages of handling the dead: mortuary personnel should wear gloves and protective working clothes; ideally, bodies should be stored at 4 °C (not frozen); and at the end of a day's work personnel should wash themselves thoroughly with a disinfectant soap. These sanitary provisions are extremely important in epidemics, or in areas where the prevalence of HIV is high and the dead have open wounds.

As a minimum, mortuary equipment should include: stretchers, leather gloves, rubber gloves, overalls, boots, caps, soap and disinfectants, and cotton cloth. A more complete list suited to the needs of mass disasters is given in Box 14.1. A mortuary hoist, picks and shovels or earth-moving machines, and trucks may also be required for transportation and burial purposes.

14.3 Identification of the dead

Early identification of corpses helps to preserve the mental health of the bereaved. Anxiety and uncertainty are replaced by grief, and the process of acceptance of death begins. Prompt identification and disposal ensure that families and friends are not exposed to the offensive by-products of bodily decay.

The identification of dead bodies can be difficult when there are many of them: 1000 unidentified bodies require over 2000 square metres of space to display adequately, and a person walking between the rows of bodies may have to walk some 800 metres. When bodies decay rapidly, handling and identification become very unpleasant, so that it is sometimes preferable to bury the bodies quickly, and to carry out identification later, after disinterment, using forensic anthropological techniques. Rapid burial is not recommended, however, if facilities for conserving bodies, e.g. ice, electricity and embalming fluids, are readily available.

The identification of bodies by people other than family or friends can be a very lengthy process. If the disaster has taken place in an area where people usually carry some form of identification (i.e. credit cards, identity cards, driving licences), a professional team can process 100 bodies per hour. In parts of the world where such items are not carried, the process can obviously take much longer, and rapid burial should therefore be considered.

If it is possible to identify the deceased, a medical examiner should issue a death certificate. An official record of death should be prepared and an identification tag affixed to the body. Personal effects should be returned to the next of kin.

In conflict situations, many deaths may be the result of human rights abuses by one or more of the warring parties. In such situations, it is important to accurately record the cause of death and identify the body, or label the body for later identification, and record the place of burial. This information may be important in an investigation of possible human rights abuses.

14.4 Handling the dead

Burial in individual graves is the method of choice, unless the number of dead is excessively large, or climatic or other constraints make this impossible. Individual graves can be dug manually, providing work, a sense of purpose, and a ritual element for the community affected by the disaster. If the number is too large, or circumstances demand it, trenches can be dug by mechanical means and bodies placed in them head to foot to save space. If it is expected that the bodies will be disinterred, they should be buried 50 centimetres from the surface.

> **Box 14.1 Equipment for mortuary services in major disasters[1]**
>
> Platform ladder for the police photographer.
> Stainless steel postmortem tables or heavy-duty trestle tables covered with plastic sheeting.
> Wheeled trolleys for transporting bodies within the mortuary.
> Accident and emergency trolleys that incorporate an X-ray grid.
> Mortuary hoist or small fork-lift truck.
> Trestle tables and chairs for administrative areas.
> Wall charts to record progress, or large poster boards if there are no walls.
> Tarpaulin or plastic sheeting for the floor, if it is not made of concrete.
> Heavy-gauge black plastic sheeting for temporary screens.
> Refuse bins and bags.
> Cleaning materials—mops, buckets, cloths, soap, towels.
> Disinfectant and deodorizer.
> Protective clothing and heavy-duty rubber gloves.
> Office equipment, including fax, typewriter, computer.
> Property bags and labels.
> Body bags and labels.
> Specialized equipment to be furnished by the pathologist, odontologist, radiographer, etc., as required.
>
> [1] Source: Clark, Nicholls & Gillespie (1992).

Coffins will often be unavailable or of poor quality. It is then advisable to wrap the corpses in plastic sheets; these are resistant to decay, and thus can help to keep the remains separate from the soil.

When locating and planning long-term emergency settlements, an area should be identified for burial. This should be large enough to accommodate the expected number of graves over the life of the settlement, and separate areas for people of different religions. The area should be chosen in consultation with the community concerned, and with attention to ground conditions, groundwater conditions, and distance from water sources.

Although burial is a quick and economical method of body disposal, alternatives can be used if they are more acceptable culturally, and if resources (including time) are available. Such alternatives include cremation, embalming, and certain types of ritual display of the dead. It may be useful to take tissue samples from the deceased for identification purposes. The samples can later be compared with samples from surviving relatives.

14.5 Ceremonial aspects

Disasters have a deeply disruptive effect on communities. Even if their more easily observable consequences are death, wounds, disease, loss of property, etc., the psychological consequences can be equally important and may be longer-lasting. Unfortunately, the techniques for dealing with people suffering from psychological trauma are not as clear-cut as those for dealing with material injuries and a great deal of improvisation will have to be accepted. The community's solidarity networks, rituals and codes are very important in dealing with the psychological impact of disasters and death, and they should be encouraged.

In a disaster, ritualized behaviours normally available to deal with death may be swept aside. The large number of deaths occurring together, the lack of advance warning, the previous good health of so many of the victims, and the clustering of deaths within households can overwhelm normal coping mechanisms, and leave survivors with profound and possibly lifelong trauma. For this reason, the ceremonies of burial or other forms of disposing of the dead should be as formal and as well planned as possible. Many such ceremonies will be religious and involve the entire community or all the family members. Whatever their nature, these ceremonies are essential aspects of the grieving process. Unfortunately, popular beliefs about the health risks of human corpses have sometimes led to the hasty and undignified use of lime or burning to dispose of human remains. Authorities should resist this: ceremonial grieving for the dead is the beginning of recovery in the disaster-recovery cycle.

Relief organizations should cooperate with the authorities in the disaster area to facilitate ceremonial burials. If desired, individual ceremonies can be carried out by families, but collective burial ceremonies may better help society as a whole to deal with the disaster.

14.6 Further information

For further information on:

— mortuary services, see: Clark, Nicholls & Gillespie (1992);
— handling of the dead, see: Thompson (1991), Davis & Lambert (2002), Harvey, Baghri & Reed (2002);
— cultural and social aspects of death in emergencies, see: Wilson & Harrell-Bond (1990).

15. Health promotion and community participation

15.1 Definitions

This chapter presents two aspects of disaster management that are essential to all the technical and management aspects presented in previous chapters: community partici-pation and health promotion. In this book, the following definitions are used:

Community participation

Community participation is the active involvement of people from communities prepar-ing for, or reacting to, disasters. True participation means the involvement of the people concerned in analysis, decision-making, planning, and programme implementation, as well as in all the activities, from search and rescue to reconstruction, that people affected by disasters undertake spontaneously without the involvement of external agencies. While the opportunities for community participation may vary greatly from place to place and at different points in the disaster-management cycle, a participatory approach to disaster-related activities should be promoted to achieve sustainable development.

Health promotion

Health promotion was defined in the Ottawa Charter as "the process of enabling people to increase control over, and to improve, their health. To reach a state of complete phys-ical, mental and social well-being, an individual or group must be able to identify and to realize aspirations, to satisfy needs, and to change or cope with the environment. Health is, therefore, seen as a resource for everyday life, not the objective of living. Health is a positive concept emphasizing social and personal resources, as well as phys-ical capacities. Therefore, health promotion is not just the responsibility of the health sector, but goes beyond healthy life-styles to well-being" (World Health Organization 1986). In the context of disaster management, health promotion involves working with people to prevent, prepare for, and respond to disasters so as to reduce risk, increase resilience and mitigate the impact of disasters on health. Community participation is the basis of successful health promotion.

Health education and hygiene education

Health education is one important activity that is commonly undertaken to promote health. It is the communication of information that enables people to make informed decisions about health-related activities at all stages of the disaster-management cycle. Health education might involve subjects such as the risk of flooding in areas where people are building houses, the location of earthquake shelters, or the areas where safe defecation is possible in a new emergency settlement.

Hygiene education is concerned specifically with communicating on those areas of health that are related to water supply, sanitation, vector-borne disease control, and hygiene practice. Following a disaster, hygieae education is particularly important for reducing the risk of communicable disease and its transmission.

Hygiene promotion

Hygiene promotion follows the same approach as health promotion, in that it is concerned not only with the transmission of information, but with understanding and promoting the capacities of people to improve their own health, chiefly through their ability to: make best use of prevailing environmental-health conditions and existing services and facilities; act to improve environmental-health conditions; and make behavioural changes to reduce certain environmental risks at the household level. Hygiene promotion is concerned with achieving improvements in health through the joint efforts of individuals, families and communities on one hand, and external agencies, health authorities, etc. on the other. It is a process in which environmental-health conditions and hygiene-related behaviours are assessed, and changes in conditions, services and behaviours are achieved. A key feature of hygiene promotion is that it depends for its success on the careful analysis of people's constraints, opportunities and strengths in any situation, to seek solutions to hygiene problems that are realistic and appropriate to people's desires and ways of living. Recent work on hygiene promotion in development and emergency situations has underlined the advantages of hygiene promotion over the more traditional and narrower approach of hygiene education and health education (United Nations Children's Fund, 1999; Ferron, Morgan & O'Reilly, 2000).

In this chapter, the terms hygiene promotion and hygiene education are used broadly to include aspects of health, such as avoiding exposure to all types of hazards, as well as aspects more narrowly defined as relating to hygiene, such as the control of communicable diseases in an emergency.

15.2 Hygiene promotion and community participation in the disaster-management cycle

Vulnerability reduction is achieved not solely by physical measures to mitigate the destructive effects of a hazard. Social measures that help to reduce negative impacts and enhance the resilience of the population are also essential. Safety and health promotion, environmental awareness, and the strengthening of community organization are essential elements in helping people to become less vulnerable to emergencies and disasters.

Moreover, the success of any technical intervention—whether before or after a disaster strikes—depends on the way that it is received and used by the community involved. People must be consulted about their needs and wishes, and be involved in planning as well as in implementation. Their knowledge and capacities must be acknowledged and strengthened as appropriate. Community participation is thus an essential element in emergency-management planning (see Section 3.5.4).

Health promotion and community participation activities are important at all stages of the disaster–management cycle, before and after disaster events, as follows:

- **Emergency prevention and preparedness**: community participation in assessing risks and vulnerability; promoting awareness of environmental hazards and safety consciousness; and strengthening community resilience and organization. Awareness raising and training are essential aspects of disaster mitigation and emergency preparedness.
- **Emergency response and recovery**: community participation in the response phase and in the communication of specific health messages in the immediate aftermath of a disaster; ensuring sustainable and incremental improvements in environmental health.

Emergency prevention and preparedness are rarely followed immediately by an emergency requiring a response. Prevention and preparedness programmes should therefore promote environmental health and support the development needs of communities, regardless of the benefits that they may offer if an emergency occurs. These programmes should be part of the ongoing development activities of communities.

The occurrence of a disaster produces a fundamental change in the way that a community functions. In a relatively short time, the health needs of the people, their capacities to respond, and the community support available to them may change dramatically. Much of the success of emergency management depends on the ability of prevention and preparedness programmes to mobilize people at risk and help develop their awareness and knowledge about managing the hazards they face. The opportunities and needs for community participation and health education in the various phases of emergency management are summarized in Table 15.1.

15.3 Community participation

The involvement of the community is essential for reducing vulnerability to disasters, for facilitating recovery after a disaster has struck, and for stimulating community organization that is the basis for sustainable development.

Both research and practical experience have shown that people are most committed to implementing programmes that they have helped plan. This is as true of disaster-related programmes as of any others. People should be encouraged to take part in identifying the hazards that they face, in assessing their own vulnerability, and in planning ways to increase their preparedness for a disaster. For example, representatives from a community may be invited by emergency-management planners to inspect the area that they inhabit. They may be asked to discuss existing or potential health hazards and to identify vulnerable people and places. This will achieve two very useful objectives:

- Emergency planners will gain very detailed information about local hazards and vulnerability.
- Communities will become more aware of the health risks that they face.

Communities should also be involved in planning environmental-management programmes that seek to reduce the risk of disasters.

The best way for a community to increase its preparedness for, and recovery from, a disaster is to develop strong community organization and leadership with experience in mobilizing its members and coordinating programmes. It is important, therefore, that vulnerable communities are supported with community development programmes *before* a disaster strikes.

However, even where there is no history of strong local organization, community participation should be an essential part of disaster relief and recovery. In an emergency, when rapid action is needed, it is all too easy for the providers of relief to make assumptions about people's priorities. In the immediate aftermath of a disaster, it may indeed be difficult to set up an effective mechanism for consultation and participatory planning. Nonetheless, every effort should be made at least to establish the principle of consultation and participation, which can then be developed over time.

A major disaster can sometimes provide a unique opportunity for reinforcing community organization. People have their own ways of coping with disasters. They are not helpless or passive. Forms of organization emerge spontaneously after a disaster (see Box 15.1), producing new leaders who are able to inspire and mobilize their communities. Building on this new leadership can be a useful way of promoting community involvement in long-term development programmes. However, care must be taken to avoid increasing the influence of leaders who are not motivated by the well-being of the affected community.

Table 15.1 **Opportunities and needs for community participation and hygiene promotion in disaster management**

Disaster-management phase	Community factors	Time factors	Opportunities and needs for community participation	Opportunities and needs for health promotion
Prevention	Baseline situation	No special limitations	Identification of community leaders and groups Identification of health problems Identification of emergency health hazards Study of safety and health beliefs and practices	Preparation of messages based on existing problems and practices and potential emergency health hazards Adaptation of methodologies to actual and potential needs Promoting good health practices in community development and everyday life
Preparedness	Baseline situation	Few, if any, limitations	As above, plus identification of emergency preparedness needs and allocation of responsibilities Training of volunteers and health professionals	Preparation of additional messages geared to emergency health-response strategy
Emergency response	Unstable but adapting	Limited or severely limited	Community cohesion sometimes affected Family units, neighbours, etc. will be essential in search and rescue Heavy reliance on volunteers and trained professionals in the identification of needs and priorities Community participation in assessment of situation and definition of response	Review of actual health situation as modified by the emergency Strong focus on basic emergency health needs Identification of specific messages and communications methods appropriate to the situation Adjustment of health-promotion activities to prevailing environmental health conditions and scarcities, if any
Recovery	Setting into new situation	No special limitations	Community leadership may be strong, loose, evolving, or in turmoil. If necessary, adjustment of community participation plan based on lessons learned in the preceding phase	Use of messages based on problems and practices associated with recovery phase Gradual blending into more stable conditions, focusing of health-education messages on differences from pre-emergency situation, if any Need to deal with psychosocial problems of unsettled situations and uncertain futures
Long-term postemergency situations	From unstable to settled	No special limitations	Identification of new needs for health leadership Building on solidarity of small units (families, tribal groups) to accept responsibilities in protecting environmental health Replacement of traditional channels of communication affected by the emergency	Building a sense of community responsibility in protecting the environment Focus on disaster preparedness and prevention

15.3.1 Principles of community participation

Community participation means the involvement of people from the earliest stages of the development process, as opposed to simply asking their opinion of project proposals that have already been developed, or for their contribution to the implementation of projects imposed from outside.

Participatory approaches have been widely tested in the fields of water, sanitation and hygiene, and experience has shown that involvement of the community can produce wide-ranging benefits. The main principles are:

- Communities can and should determine their own priorities in dealing with the problems that they face.
- The enormous depth and breadth of collective experience and knowledge in a community can be built on to bring about change and improvements.
- When people understand a problem, they will more readily act to solve it.
- People solve their own problems best in a participatory group process.

Community-focused programmes therefore aim to involve all members of a society in a participatory process of: assessing their own knowledge; investigating their own environmental situation; visualizing a different future; analysing constraints to change; planning for change; and implementing change. As shown in Figure 15.1, the success of participatory action depends on a continuous community dialogue, where provisional goals are set and tested, subsequent action is based on analysis, research, and education, and experience is fed back into the process.

Box 15.1 Spontaneous organization by Salvadoran refugees[1]

Refugees from El Salvador, arriving in Honduras in 1981–1982, quickly set up camp committees responsible for ensuring that their concerns were represented before the United Nations High Commissioner for Refugees and the nongovernmental organizations that became involved. In time, subcommittees were formed to deal with specific issues, such as public health, sanitation, hygiene and education.

Refugees who had arrived as illiterate farmers soon acquired effective skills in management, administration and negotiation, and built up a sustainable social structure on which they would build on their return to El Salvador.

[1] Source: Oxfam (1995).

Figure 15.1 **The process of participatory action**

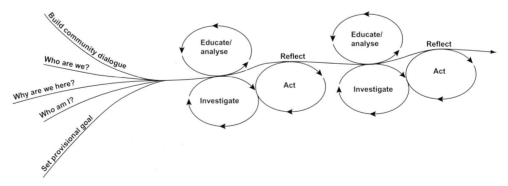

15.3.2 Obstacles to community participation

While past experience has taught the value of community participation, it has also high-lighted the difficulties of mobilizing people. These difficulties are summarized here:

Apathy and disempowerment

There are real difficulties in involving people who are not used to making decisions, who feel powerless, who are apathetic or who are dependent on others. Those in authority may be unwilling to allow people to participate in decision-making. Political, religious and commercial interests may discourage participation.

Conflicts and divisions

Most communities include people from a wide range of social and economic back-grounds, with different needs and interests: rich and poor, young and old, men and women, people from different ethnic or religious groups. A community project designed for the common good may in fact be divisive if it is seen as benefiting one section of the society more than another. Where paid employment is involved, jealousies and conflicts can ensue. There may also be conflict between individual and group interests. For example, in a densely-populated urban slum, discussions might reveal the need to relocate some houses to make fire breaks or drainage channels that would benefit everyone. But the questions "Whose house?" and "How will the owner be compensated?" may give rise to conflicts and divisions.

Poverty

Lack of resources, ill-health and poverty prevent people from participating. Many people work seven days a week for long hours just to be able to feed their families, and may not have the time to participate. As the poorest members of the community, these are often the most vulnerable people and their opinions are most valuable. Special efforts must be made to enable them to participate.

Cynicism

In the past, the word "participation" has often been misused. People have been invited to participate in plans and projects and found later that they were being asked only to "rubber stamp" official plans. Worse, they may have simply been asked to contribute their labour, for example digging trenches for water pipes, a task that would normally be done by municipal authorities in middle-class areas. In the light of such experiences, people's unwillingness to participate is understandable.

15.3.3 Overcoming obstacles and reaching the community

Methods of overcoming obstacles to community participation include the following:

Finding an entry point to the community

It is essential to find an appropriate entry point to the community. This will most often be an existing community-based organization with its roots in the community.

Where a primary health-care system exists, a community-health worker may provide the necessary entry point. Much of what the community-health worker tries to do is highly relevant to risk reduction, especially education on oral rehydration therapy, food and water hygiene, water-supply protection, vector-borne disease control, and disposal of wastes. When the health worker is supported by a community-health committee, this can provide a useful core structure for efforts to prevent or mitigate hazards (such as contamination of drinking-water sources, landslides due to poor building practices, etc.). Care must be taken, however, not to delegate too many additional tasks to community-health workers without providing the necessary extra support in the form of materials, transport and finances.

It is also possible to use existing local health programmes as the starting point. Thus, in Indonesia, a system called local area monitoring has been successful in achieving high childhood immunization coverage. As a result, there were plans for other health programmes, including an environmental health programme, to take advantage of this community-based system (S. Nugroho, personal communication, 1992).

Working with community leaders

A proven method for achieving community participation is to work through individuals who are able to bring people together and promote action. Political and religious leaders must be involved in their official capacity, but selecting other types of leaders may provide a useful balance. Different leaders will need to be identified to reflect the ethnic, caste and religious diversity of the population. Women leaders are particularly important for their ability to represent and articulate women's interests and needs. A method of identifying women leaders is described in Box 15.2.

Once interested leaders have been identified, they may require training, not only in health matters, but also in skills in dealing with people, listening, encouraging and sharing responsibilities and power in emergencies. They must also be supported and their credibility within the community maintained by ensuring that they participate in emergency-planning processes.

It is often important to work with people with strong political, religious and commercial influence, to encourage participation, or at least to overcome obstacles to participation.

Box 15.2 Methods of identifying women leaders

■ Ask a random sample of women to name the three women they would go to for advice about sickness, a family quarrel, money problems, etc.
■ Note the names most often mentioned and then ask these women to name the women they themselves would consult.
■ A shorter list will emerge and the top names can be singled out as leaders.

Ensuring official support for community-led projects

Any community-based programme will need support from health workers and educators. These in turn will need the full support of their managers and of municipal, ministerial and other officials. People's investment of their own time in discussing risk and vulnerability reduction should be seen to produce visible results.

Understanding the socioeconomic make-up of the community

To overcome conflicts of interest, environmental-health personnel must take care to understand the socioeconomic make-up of the community, its divisions, and its past history of self-help community projects (especially if these have failed). For methods of social analysis that can be used to develop an understanding of the socioeconomic make-up of refugee communities, see United Nations High Commissioner for Refugees (1992b).

Making special arrangements to encourage participation

Special arrangements should be made to encourage the participation of all members of the community, for example providing free child care to allow parents of young children to participate.

15.3.4 Community organization in urban and rural areas

Even the poorest and apparently most chaotic village or neighbourhood is organized to a certain extent. Environmental-health workers and disaster-prevention planners need to understand the forms of organization if they are to find appropriate ways to mobilize people to reduce their vulnerability to hazards.

Formal (or political) organizations can be divided into three types: those headed by traditional leaders (chiefs, elders, etc.); those headed by appointed leaders (i.e. selected local representatives); and those headed by elected local representatives.

In addition, there are many kinds of traditional or informal social relations. People may exchange labour and services, there may be patterns of kinship and friendship, and religious groups and special-interest groups may provide a common centre.

In urban areas, informal organizations may include:

— workers' guilds or trades unions, which may unite people practising the same trade or working for the same employer;
— cultural and sports clubs, such as carnival dance clubs or local football clubs;
— political action groups, which often link people in very efficient communications networks.

In rural areas, ties of kinship may be stronger than in urban areas, and tribal or clan elders may have considerable influence. Other examples of informal rural organization include:

— rural industries, such as plantation work or logging, which may create a sense of solidarity among the workers concerned;
— cooperative societies for farmers or other producers: where well-run and successful, these can be a major resource; on the other hand, they will not be useful if they are unpopular because of high service charges, late payments to farmers, or even corruption;
— health establishments and schools: these often provide a social focus in rural areas (the local school head or teacher may enjoy high prestige and be a leader in the community).

Recently-created informal urban settlements in many of the fast-growing cities of the world may present great challenges, as they often lack both the traditional social structures found in rural areas and the formal structures of established urban areas. People in these settlements are also often particularly vulnerable to disasters because of the nature of the land on which they are settled, combined with high levels of poverty.

Environmental-health workers attempting to encourage local participation in a community programme should be aware of the potential usefulness of all these kinds of social organization. They may provide, for example, a forum for the discussion of risk reduction, a source of local knowledge and experience of the hazards faced in an area, and an efficient communications network for disseminating messages and ideas.

In addition, local or international nongovernmental organizations may have ongoing projects in an area that may provide a basis for new work on vulnerability reduction and emergency preparedness. For example, there may be literacy groups, microenterprise support groups, and health and sanitation projects. Before a commitment to collaboration is made, however, it is essential to investigate the history and nature of such projects to understand how effective they are and how they are perceived by the community and the local authorities.

15.4 Hygiene promotion and hygiene education

15.4.1 Perception of risk and predisaster awareness raising

Although most communities have considerable collective understanding of environmental hazards and how to deal with them, some underestimate the risks that they face. Others may be aware of the risks but feel there is little they can do: they underestimate the possibility that risks and/or vulnerability can be reduced, or may simply lack the organizational or physical means to change the situation and may have no alternative. These communities are often those most at risk, because of their poverty, for example, or because of environmental degradation.

Perception of risk may be formed by personal experience, recent local events or folklore. A rich tradition of coping with recurrent risks is often built into cultural practices and passed on informally from generation to generation. However, familiarity with uncommon hazards may be limited, so that people do not recognize their causes and danger signs, or the threats posed to health and the environment.

Public awareness raising and mobilization programmes therefore play an essential part in reducing disaster vulnerability by:

— increasing public awareness of environmental health hazards;
— informing people how disasters can be prevented or how their impact can be reduced;
— increasing people's awareness of the threats to health and safety that may result from a disaster, or that may exist and intensify during an emergency;
— encouraging people to participate in protecting themselves, their environment and their health services from disaster and the effects of disaster.

The promotion of awareness and safety consciousness is not something to be considered only during disasters and emergencies. It should be a routine, long-term, continuing activity that starts with the identification and analysis of risks to specific geographical areas and communities. This analysis is essential for preparedness and prevention activities, and should include information that needs to be communicated to communities at risk (see Sections 3.4 and 3.5). Communities themselves should be involved in the identification and assessment of the risks they face, and the participative approaches described in Section 15.3 should be used to promote community involvement.

Communications activities designed to promote awareness of hazards, risks and appropriate countermeasures may take many forms, such as:

— education in schools for children and adolescents;
— special education programmes for adults, either specifically on disaster preparedness or as an integral part of ongoing health or development programmes;
— public information through the mass media;
— information and mobilization through local organizations and community groups.

A combination of communications methods is usually appropriate.

Programmes for promoting awareness of environmental hazards should be participatory, focused and specific, without being alarmist. The emphasis should be on strengthening existing organizations and activities in the community, and on encouraging people to participate in community activities and to change their own behaviour. To this end, education campaigns should focus on populations in particular settings, such as schools and workplaces, and in the many local organizations already in place, such as cooperatives and women's groups. People should be encouraged to participate in community groups concerned with hazard awareness, disaster prevention and safety. Messages must be specific and deal with the particular hazards to which a population is vulnerable. Care should be taken not to create panic or anxiety. Messages should therefore emphasize mitigation and prevention rather than emergency responses, emphasizing that these activities often produce immediate benefits.

15.4.2 The need for hygiene promotion in emergencies

Following disasters, hygiene promotion may be particularly important because:

- People will expect information about the disaster itself and its aftermath. They will need to know, for example, how they can be reunited with friends and family and where it is safe to stay. In some cases, such as chemical and radiation emergencies, there may be a good deal of suspicion, misinformation and rumour, and it is then essential that people have access to authoritative information.
- There may be many unfamiliar arrangements for water and food supply, excreta disposal, etc., especially when people are forced to evacuate their homes. Rapidly available information about the new arrangements and the importance of complying with them (e.g. the importance of using designated defecation fields) is essential.
- Environmental health staff need to understand rapidly the health risks faced by the affected population and the services required to reduce those risks. They need to know what can be provided by the affected population, how much external assistance will be required, and the best way to organize external assistance to meet the needs and wishes of the affected people.
- Disaster-affected people may face greatly increased risks to their health, and will need to develop adequate responses. For example, under normal circumstances, defecation in fields around houses may be quite customary and safe, but in a crowded camp the same behaviour poses a serious hazard. Water sources may become contaminated as a result of overcrowding, which may also lead to increased transmission and incidence of communicable diseases.

15.4.3 Setting up a hygiene promotion programme in an emergency

A possible plan of action might include the following activities:

- Rapidly establish a team to deal with hygiene promotion and to provide information on environmental health.
- Rapidly assess the health risks to be addressed using information, education and mobilization, and focus on:
  — key health problems, in order of priority and magnitude;
  — physical resources needed and those available (the types of shelter, food, water, sanitation, etc.);
  — human resources available for hygiene promotion activities (health workers, teachers, religious leaders, nongovernmental organizations with available staff, writers, artists, etc.);
  — community characteristics (whether and to what extent there is a sense of community, a pattern of leadership, or local organization, and whether there are cultural traditions regarding health);
  — means of communication and hygiene-education materials available (radio transmitters and receivers, visual material, megaphones, newspapers, printing and copying equipment, and traditional communications channels, such as singing and story-telling).

- Form close liaison with the community. This may be achieved by working through existing community organizations such as women's groups, trade unions, etc., or by establishing community-health committees.
- Choose the subjects to be covered and the type of preventive action to be taken (e.g. promoting hand-washing, ensuring water safety), with a focus on priority issues, rather than a broad range of topics. Actions that can have the greatest impact on reducing morbidity and mortality should be emphasized. Behaviour changes that are promoted should be chosen on the basis of the assessment of health risks, environmental health facilities, and services available in each situation.
- Identify and select trainers, health motivators and leaders from the affected population and from nongovernmental organizations, including children, women and others who can provide peer-group education. It is particularly important to involve women: in many societies women play a major role in water collection and domestic and personal hygiene and they may also be particularly affected by the change in environmental health conditions.
- Develop clear health messages and choose the educational approach and methods to be used. This can be based on pre-prepared messages and communications systems, but must be done in collaboration with selected trainers and community representatives to ensure that the cultural background, traditional practices and perceptions of the target population are taken into account.
- Develop, field-test and use new educational materials, or review existing materials (e.g. posters, leaflets, radio scripts, health talks) and adapt them as necessary.
- Review activities and their immediate impact, and revise and adapt approaches to reflect changes in conditions and health status, if necessary. This may involve interviews, observation and questionnaire surveys to evaluate changes in knowledge, practice and environmental health conditions.

To help meet the needs of particularly vulnerable people among new arrivals at emergency settlements, special measures may be needed to raise their awareness about health risks, hygiene practices, arrangements for water supply and sanitation, and about the support for families and community groups.

Hygiene promotion activities should be coordinated to ensure that messages address priority issues, are consistent and complementary, and that hygiene education is integrated with measures to improve services and facilities.

15.4.4 Participatory approach to hygiene promotion

Hygiene promotion necessarily involves close liaison with the affected population, even in an emergency. To establish successful contacts with the community, it is necessary to:

- Avoid making assumptions about what people already know or do not know about health, hygiene, sanitation, etc. Even the most obvious request or arrangement should be discussed with the community health committee or equivalent representatives, who may themselves need to take soundings from the population.
- Establish rapid procedures for obtaining reactions, ideas and information from communities. Appropriate activities include observing current practices, in-depth interviews with key informants (such as local leaders, teachers, midwives), survey interviews, discussions with focus groups, and various other forms of participatory appraisal techniques.
- Approach people with respect and empathy.
- Build on indigenous knowledge and practices (while explaining how to adapt to emergency conditions in which such practices may become difficult or danger-

ous). This approach may give rise to useful innovations and improvisations by the community.

■ Remember, that in all communities there are people with useful ideas, skills and experience that can be shared with others.

For further information on community liaison, see Pan American Health Organization (1994).

15.4.5 Environmental health messages in emergencies

Following disasters, environmental health is concerned with areas that include water supply and sanitation, waste disposal, vector control, personal hygiene, shelter and food safety. These, in turn, may be subdivided and specific health messages identified, as suggested in Annex 6. It is most important that only a small number of very important messages are chosen for communication, based on an assessment of health risks, to avoid confusing the target audience, and wasting efforts on be havior changes that have little impact on health.

Hygiene messages and communications methods should be chosen in answer to four key questions (United Nations Children's Fund, 1999):

■ Which specific practices are placing health at risk?
■ What could motivate the adoption of safe practices?
■ Who should be targeted by the programme?
■ How can one communicate with these groups effectively?

15.4.6 Communication methods

Communication of health information is most effective when a variety of methods, approaches and materials are used. Broadly speaking, there are three main approaches:

Person-to-person contact

Captive audiences may be found at clinics, feeding centres, food-distribution centres, water-collection points and so on, where health workers and trained volunteers will be able to give advice. In nonemergency periods, health clinics, schools and workplaces may provide similar audiences. Meetings may be called for specific groups, or selected individuals may be brought together for focus group discussions on specific topics, and individual families may also be visited. The influence of existing local groups or social organizations can be very useful in increasing the impact of the information.

This direct approach, particularly if it involves some interaction between health workers and individuals, is most effective in tackling specific issues and encouraging particular changes in behaviour, and in checking that messages are seen as relevant and useful by the people concerned.

Activities suitable for person-to-person exchanges or for small groups include the discussion of personal feelings and experiences, demonstrations, story-telling, role-playing, case studies and educational games (particularly in nonemergency situations).

Teaching aids

Suitable teaching aids include printed materials, posters, films, slides, videos, murals, flannel graphs and flip charts. These are useful for transmitting information and as support to the spoken word, but must be reinforced by interaction and personal contact with members of the target audience.

Using mass communication

Radio, audiocassettes, television, video, newspapers, placards, plays, puppet shows and megaphones are effective means of communicating information quickly to a large number of people and creating awareness of a problem or idea. The relevance and impact of messages, and the effectiveness with which they are communicated, need to be evaluated by discussion with a sample of people.

Following a disaster, mass media may be unavailable or at least severely disrupted. However, radios may be available, and in long-term emergency settlements it may be possible to produce a camp newspaper and to make arrangements with a nearby radio station to broadcast regular programmes on health issues.

15.4.7 Choosing an approach

When deciding on the message and the communications methods to use, it is essential to:

— establish the need for, and relevance of, the hygiene education activity through an assessment that is as participatory as possible, given the nature and urgency of the situation;
— be aware that a hygiene education campaign may be aimed at some people who are not literate: in such circumstances, participatory learning techniques are the most appropriate;
— select and adapt methods to suit the characteristics and interests of the particular target group—young/old, male/female, membership of a religious group, etc. (e.g. fables about animals may be more suitable for children than adults);
— establish procedures at the outset for evaluating the effectiveness of the health promotion campaign, by selecting appropriate indicators for measuring changes in people's health status, behaviour and environment;
— reinforce existing health practices that are beneficial and discourage those that are harmful;
— choose messages that are positive, attractive and based on what people already know, what they want and what they consider to be achievable;
— involve people in the community in the production of their own teaching materials (this is educational in itself and will ensure that such materials are relevant and culturally appropriate);
— use the effectiveness of young people and children in teaching and mobilizing others;
— avoid messages that imply that people are to blame for their own or their children's ill-health: messages and methods must not be judgmental.

15.5 Further information

For further information on:

— community participation, see: Chambers (1983), Chambers, Pacey & Thrupp (1989), World Resources Institute (1990), Cernea (1991), Evans & Appleton (1993), Chambers (1994), Eade & Wright (1994), United Nations High Commissioner for Refugees (1996);
— women and children in emergencies, see: Aarons & Hawes (1979), United Nations Children's Fund (1984), International Federation of Red Cross and Red Crescent Societies (1991), United Nations High Commissioner for Refugees (1991), Wiest (1992), Walker (1994), United Nations Children's Fund (1996);
— gender and social diversity, see: Cernea (1991), Moser (1993), Steady (1993), Eade & Williams (1995);

— hygiene promotion and communication, see: Werner & Bower (1982), Downie, Fyfe & Tannahill (1990), Boot (1991), Bunton & Macdonald, eds. (1992), Boot & Cairncross (1993), Hubley (1993), Bentley et al. (1994), Hermann & Bentley (1994), Eade & Williams (1995), Geefhuysen, Bennet & Lewin (1995), Almedom, Blumenthal & Manderson (1997), United Nations Children's Fund (1999), Ferron, Morgan & O'Reilly (2000), Sphere Project (2000).

16. Human resources

Professional staff and community-based volunteers are required for health-related aspects of disaster management. In each phase of the emergency-management cycle different skills are required for a range of activities, from monitoring and surveillance, through prevention and mitigation, to relief and recovery. Training is essential to ensure that professional staff and volunteers have the skills and awareness necessary for pre- and post-disaster activities.

16.1 Professional staff

The range of activities involved in the complete disaster-management cycle requires a corresponding range of expertise, as follows:

- **Monitoring and surveillance** require specialists in remote sensing, cartography, statistical analysis, and planning. Meteorologists, hydrologists, geologists, volcanologists, epidemiologists and other scientific specialists are also needed.
- **Prevention and mitigation** require staff with expertise similar to those needed for monitoring and surveillance, as well as engineers, architects, and specialists in agriculture, forestry, food storage, water supply and sanitation. Vulnerability reduction calls for the skills of sociologists, economists and experts in social welfare.
- **Relief work** requires staff trained in logistics, communications, administration, nutrition, health, and water supply and sanitation, as well as specialized teams for search and rescue, fire fighting, emergency medicine, and the disposal of toxic or radioactive materials.
- **Recovery**, like any economic and social development, requires experts in the fields of community development, finance, construction, microenterprise development, ecological restoration, etc.

Many of these professional staff are not involved in disaster management in their day-to-day work. This is true, for example, for many technical and managerial staff in the public sector. For such people to be able to contribute effectively in an emergency, it is important to include disaster management in their routine training programmes and academic curricula.

Overseeing the disaster-management cycle should be a national counter-disaster agency with a secretariat of specialists in systems analysis, planning, law and administration. Such a team should be skilled in coordinating and integrating inputs from many sources and should be able to formulate appropriate policies based on the information received about hazards and vulnerability. Coordinators are also necessary at lower levels of government, including municipalities and counties. In addition, trained coordinators, engineers, health specialists, etc., must be available in national and international nongovernmental organizations and intergovernmental agencies.

In conflict-prone areas of the world, the complex emergencies that have developed in recent years require particular skills at all levels. Although this area is outside the scope of this book, there is a growing need for training in the skills demanded of workers in complex emergencies (see Box 16.1).

> **Box 16.1 The challenge of complex emergencies[1]**
>
> All humanitarian practitioners, including those concerned with environmental health, must be trained to deal with the special operational environment created by complex emergencies. Experiences with Kurdish and Rwandan refugees, and humanitarian operations in Angola, Bosnia, Cambodia, Liberia, Mozambique, Somalia and Sudan all underscore the need for new skills. These include skills in: political analysis; negotiation; conflict analysis and resolution; management; propaganda monitoring and humanitarian broadcasting; human rights monitoring and reporting; military liaison; and managing personal and staff security. A broader view of vulnerability is also required that includes an understanding of the roles of politics, ethnicity, gender and class in vulnerability.
>
> [1] Source: Slim (1995).

16.2 Volunteer staff and employed labour

Volunteers make a huge contribution to both vulnerability reduction and emergency response. For example, in the Armenian earthquake of 1988, 90% of people dug out of the rubble were saved by survivors, rather than by professional search-and-rescue teams. In Bangladesh, community-based cyclone warnings are provided by tens of thousands of Red Crescent volunteers.

Effective vulnerability reduction can be a highly social and labour-intensive activity. For example, community participation may be necessary to identify the most vulnerable people, such as disabled or homeless people, because they do not show up on censuses or come to meetings to articulate their needs. Hazard-mitigation programmes, such as reforestation or soil conservation, require a large workforce that has to be provided by the local community.

In an emergency, staff employed for construction, logistics, community outreach and health promotion activities may be recruited on short-term contracts, or seconded from the private or public sector for the period of the emergency. It is important that correct human resources procedures, including recruitment procedures, contracts, job descriptions, disciplinary procedures and benefits are correctly applied. These procedures should be established as far as possible before disaster strikes, so that they may be rapidly applied in an emergency.

Deciding whether to employ volunteers or paid staff for certain activities requires careful thought, as the management and motivation of paid staff and volunteers demand different approaches. Criteria for deciding whether people should be employed as staff or volunteers include the nature of the activity, the origins of the staff (are they from the community concerned?), the need for paid work in the area, the availability of management resources, and relevant policies on community development.

16.3 Training

16.3.1 Training professionals

Disaster training at institutions of higher education

Professional personnel involved in disaster management will have attended institutions of higher education and followed courses from law to engineering. These institutions should be encouraged to integrate modules on the management of emergencies and disasters into existing degree courses and training programmes.

Moreover, for many of these professionals, particularly planners and engineers, disaster prevention should form an important part of their day-to-day work. For this reason, it is important for institutes of higher education to ensure that appropriate emphasis is placed on disaster management. It is recommended that national counter-disaster agencies review curricula, with a view to integrating disaster preparedness and risk reduction into the professional training of, for example, urban planners, sanitary engineers, medical students and nurses.

Municipal officials, emergency service workers, water-supply and sanitation workers, etc., need to attend short courses or refresher courses. The counter-disaster agency should ensure that these are provided at higher educational institutions.

Specialized training courses

Specialized courses for disaster-management professionals are now provided in many countries by universities, regional organizations, nongovernmental organizations and international organizations. A summary of available courses may be found on the Humanitarian Training Inventory (HATI), provided by the United Nations Office for the Coordination of Humanitarian Affairs[1].

16.3.2 Training volunteers

Community-based training for volunteers should take place within the locality, using training materials that are relevant to the specific hazards, vulnerability patterns and resources of the particular area.

Volunteers can be trained, and appropriate training materials produced, in the following ways:

- When using participatory planning techniques to assess local risks, it may be possible simultaneously to create materials concerning local hazards, vulnerabilities, and capacities that can later be used in training.
- Make use of prior experiences with innovative models in large-scale community training. Such models include health-education activities; social mobilization for expanded immunization programmes; and mass adult literacy campaigns and post-literacy follow-up.
- Experience can be drawn from area-based agricultural improvement programmes that use on-farm experiments and demonstrations, master farmers from the community, and group extension. Successful models can provide examples of how community-based risk assessment can be tied to the actual conditions of specific people and places.

Selected community leaders also require training. On-the-job training by supervisors should be combined with regular, short training sessions, using modules for different job functions. These modules should contain learning objectives, and recommend methods and materials for effective learning and teaching.

16.3.3 Integrated training exercises

The functioning of the emergency-response system needs to be tested and evaluated periodically. It is necessary to identify people normally employed in nonemergency-related occupations (e.g. doctors and nurses, police officers, municipal officials) and encourage them to meet from time to time for role-playing exercises designed to test preparedness plans. In this way, they become familiar with each other and understand their individual roles. Such exercises also ensure that plans are appropriate and up-to-date, and that systems are in place.

---

[1] www.reliefweb.int/training/.

The best way to achieve this is through integrated training exercises (ITEs), which bring all the relevant personnel together in realistic test situations. Naturally, rehearsals or drills cannot possibly portray the full reality of a disaster-relief operation. However, rehearsals do re-emphasize points made in training programmes and may reveal weaknesses that would otherwise be overlooked.

When organizing ITEs, the following should be borne in mind:

- Training and exercises should be carried out in a way that not only communicates information, but also builds trust and cooperation among personnel.
- If possible, training activities should simultaneously generate *new* information about hazards, vulnerability and disaster mitigation.
- Large-scale exercises should be carefully planned and explained, so as not to create fear or confusion among the public.
- Training exercises should provide concrete benefits, such as improved sanitation or strengthened infrastructure, so that they are not seen simply as games.

Integrated training for health workers

Hospitals and health-care facilities that are likely to receive casualties during disasters should periodically carry out training exercises. On such occasions, environmental health personnel should be involved as well, in particular to discuss with regular staff what water-supply, sanitation and other hygiene problems are likely to arise under emergency conditions. They should also take the opportunity to inspect the site and buildings, to identify their own vulnerability to environmental hazards.

Primary health-care workers and other community-development workers should meet periodically at a regional centre to practise emergency first aid and review possible measures to reduce risks and improve preparedness in their area.

Integrated training in the community

Training exercises at community level should be organized, involving both the local population and community workers. Because participants may be short of time, such exercises should focus on one element of preparedness at a time. Each exercise should also introduce some practical improvement and aim to achieve an incremental reduction in vulnerability. For example, participants might act out the difficulties to be expected in boiling water in an emergency (shortage of fuel, lack of adequate containers, etc.). On another occasion, the topic might be protecting water supplies from flood waters contaminated by sewage, or the control of mosquito breeding in standing water. In each case, solutions to the problems should be sought and concrete actions taken. In this way, such training does triple duty as environmental health education, community problem-solving, and preparedness training.

Integrated training at national and international levels

Professional support staff from all relevant fields should be called together periodically to enact their roles in an emergency. This can be arranged by the permanent staff of the counter-disaster agency. In the health sector, this would involve forming field teams of environmental health personnel; accessing and testing stored equipment and supplies; and rehearsing damage assessment, emergency health care, and health surveillance. An important part of such exercises should be an evaluation of performance, to reveal weak spots in communication and coordination.

Members of the national counter-disaster agency also need to test their ability to work together efficiently, and to communicate nationally and internationally. For example, test shipments of spare parts could be made to an outlying province, and these tests subjected to critical appraisal.

Early-warning systems should be tested. Those that involve sharing data internationally (e.g. for food security, tropical storms, or tsunamis) tend to be fully automated. Staff should therefore be trained to deal with a breakdown in automatic communication.

Integrated training for the public

Complex problems surround the questions of whether and how to organize large-scale emergency preparedness exercises that involve the public at large. The economic cost of the resulting disruption is often large and the chance of creating confusion and ill-will is high. The evacuation of a major city is a hazard in its own right and should never be "practised", although public education on evacuation routes and warnings is appropriate.

Instead, a more efficient and positive use of people's time and energy may be to conduct periodic safety-awareness events. For example, competitions sponsored by the news media may be held, in which features, such as bad drainage or structurally weak buildings, are sought out and documented by citizens.

16.4 Further information

For further information on human resources, see: Werner & Bower (1982), International Federation of Red Cross and Red Crescent Societies (1997a), Overseas Development Institute/People in Aid (1998), United Nations High Commissioner for Refugees (1999), Davis & Lambert (2002).

References

Aarons A, Hawes H (1979). *Child-to-child.* London, Child-to-Child Programme.

Acheson M (1993). *Interventions in water supply and sanitation.* Geneva, International Federation of Red Cross and Red Crescent Societies.

Ackermann-Liebrich et al. (1997). *Assessing the health consequences of major chemical incidents: epidemiological approaches.* Copenhagen, WHO Regional Office for Europe (Regional Publications European Series, No. 79).

Adams J (1999). *Managing water supply and sanitation in emergencies.* Oxford, Oxfam.

Agarwal B (1990). Social security and the family: coping with seasonality and calamity in rural India. *Journal of Peasant Studies*, 17(3):341–412.

Alexander DE (1993). *Natural disasters.* New York, NY, Chapman & Hall.

Almedom A, Blumenthal U, Manderson L (1997). *Hygiene evaluation procedures: methods and tools for assessing water and sanitation-related hygiene practices.* London, Intermediate Technology Publications / Boston, International Nutrition Foundation for Developing Countries.

American Water Works Association (1984). *Emergency planning for water utility management.* Denver, CO.

Anderson M (1995). Vulnerability to disaster and sustainable development: a general framework for assessing vulnerability. In: Munasinghe M, Clarke C, eds. *Disaster prevention for sustainable development.* Washington, DC, World Bank.

Anderson M, Woodrow P (1989). *Rising from the ashes: development strategies in times of disaster.* Boulder, CO, Westview.

Angotti T (1993). *Metropolis 2000: planning, poverty and politics.* London, Routledge.

Annett H, Rifkin S (1989). *Improving urban health: guidelines for rapid appraisal to assess community health needs.* Liverpool, Department of International Community Health, School of Tropical Medicine.

Appleton J, Save the Children Fund Ethiopia Team (1987). *Drought relief in Ethiopia: planning and management of feeding programmes.* London, Save the Children Fund.

Arlosoroff S, ed. (1998). *Community water supply: the handpump option.* London, Intermediate Technology Publications.

Assar M (1971). *Guide to sanitation in natural disasters.* Geneva, World Health Organization.

Austin LS, ed. (1992). *Responding to disaster: a guide for mental health professionals.* Washington, DC, American Psychiatric Press.

Aysan Y, Oliver P (1987). *Housing and culture after earthquakes: a guide for future policy making in seismic areas.* London, James & James Science Press.

Baker D, Kjellström T, Calderon R, Pasides H (1999). *Environmental epidemiology: a textbook on study methods and public health applications.* Geneva, World Health Organization.

Bari F (1998). Gender and disaster: a case study from Pakistan. In: Enarson E, Morrow BH, eds. *The gendered terrain of disaster.* Westport, CT, Praeger, pp. 125–132.

Bartram J, Ballance R, eds. (1996). *Water quality monitoring: a practical guide to the design and implementation of freshwater quality studies and monitoring programmes.* London, E & FN Spon.

Bates F, ed. (1982). *Recovery, change and development: a longitudinal study of the 1976 Guatemalan earthquake*. Athens, GA, University of Georgia Press.

Bates F, Farrell T, Glittenberg JAK (1979). Some changes in housing characteristics in Guatemala following the February 1976 earthquake and their implications for future earthquake vulnerability. *Mass Emergencies*, 4:121–133.

Beaglehole R, Bonita R, Kjellström (1993). *Basic epidemiology*. Geneva, World Health Organization.

Begum R (1993). Women in environmental disasters: the 1991 cyclone in Bangladesh. *Focus on Gender*, 1(1):34–39.

Belen L (1992). *Meeting the challenges of Mt. Pinatubo: a Red Cross operation*. Manila: Philippine National Red Cross (PNRC).

Benenson A (1995). *Control of communicable diseases in man*, 16th ed. Washington, DC, American Public Health Association.

Bentley M et al. (1994). *The use of structured observations in the study of health behaviour*. The Hague, IRC International Water and Sanitation Centre (Occasional Paper 27).

Berglund M, Elinder C-G, Järup L (2001). *Human exposure assessment: an introduction*. Geneva, World Health Organization.

Berke PR, Kartez J, Wenger D (1993). Recovery after disaster: achieving sustainable development, mitigation and equity. *Disasters*, 17(2):93–109.

Berlage HP (1966). *The southern oscillation and world weather*. The Hague, Koninklijk Nederlands Meteorologisch Instituut.

Birley MH (1991). *Guidelines for forecasting the vector-borne disease implications of water resources development*, 2nd ed. Geneva, World Health Organization (PEEM Guidelines Series, No. 2).

Birley M (1992). *Guidelines for the health impact assessment of development projects*. Manila, Asian Development Bank (Environmental Series, No. 11).

Birley M (1995). *The health impact assessment of development projects*. London, Her Majesty's Stationery Office.

Black M (1994). *Megacities: the coming sanitary crisis*. London, Water Aid.

Blackett I (1990). Low cost sanitation. *Dialogue on Diarrhoea*, 43:7.

Blaikie P et al. (1994). *At risk: natural hazards, people's vulnerability and disasters*. London, Routledge.

Boot MT (1991). *Just stir gently: the way to mix hygiene education with water supply and sanitation*. The Hague, IRC International Water and Sanitation Centre (Technical Paper Series, No. 29).

Boot R, Cairncross S (1993). *Actions speak: the study of hygiene behaviour in water and sanitation projects*. The Hague, IRC International Water and Sanitation Centre.

Bouma MJ et al. (1997). A global assessment of El Niño's disaster burden. *Lancet*, 350, 1435–1438.

Bowen HJ, et al. (2000). Community exposures to chemical incidents: development and evaluation of the first environmental public health surveillance system in Europe. *Journal of Epidemiology and Community Health*, 54(11):870–3.

Bradley D et al. (1992). *A review of environmental health impacts in developing country cities*. Washington, DC, World Bank.

Bryan FL (1992). *Hazard analysis critical control point evaluations: a guide to identifying hazards and assessing risks associated with food preparation and storage*. Geneva, World Health Organization.

Bunton R, Macdonald G, eds. (1992). *Health promotion: disciplines and diversity*. London, Routledge.

Butcher JN et al. (1988). *Psychological interventions with refugees. Report prepared for the Refugee Assistance Program—Mental Health*. Minneapolis, MN, University of Minnesota Hospital, Refugee Assistance Program, National Institute of Mental Health.

Cairncross S, Feachem R (1978). *Small water supplies.* London, Ross Institute (Ross Bulletin, No. 10).

Cairncross S, Feachem R (1993). *Environmental health engineering in the tropics; an introductory text,* 2nd ed. Chichester, Wiley.

Campbell JR, Chung J (1986). *Post-disaster assessment.* Honolulu, East-West Centre (Pacific Disaster Preparedness and Mitigation Manual Series).

Carr M (1984). *Blacksmith, baker, roofing-sheet maker . . . employment for rural women in developing countries.* London, Intermediate Technology Publications.

Carter WN (1991). *Disaster management: a disaster manager's handbook.* Manila, Asian Development Bank.

Catholic Institute for International Relations (1989). *Nicaragua: testing the water.* London.

Centers for Disease Control and Prevention (1992). Famine-affected, refugee, and displaced populations: recommendations for public health issues. *MMWR,* 1992, 41(RR-13): 1–76. Atlanta, GA.

Cernea M, ed. (1988). *Involuntary resettlement in development projects.* Washington, DC, World Bank.

Cernea M, ed. (1991). *Putting people first,* 2nd ed. New York, NY, Oxford University Press and the World Bank.

Chalinder A (1998). *Temporary human settlement planning for displaced populations in emergencies.* London, Overseas Development Institute (Good Practice Review No. 6).

Chambers R (1983). *Rural development: putting the last first.* London, Longman.

Chambers R (1994). Participatory rural appraisal (PRA): challenges, potentials and paradigms. *World Development,* 22 (10):1437–1454.

Chambers R, Pacey A, Thrupp L (1989). *Farmer first: farmer innovation and agricultural research.* London, Intermediate Technology Publications.

Chartier Y, Diskett P, UNHCR (1991). Health update: refugees and displaced communities. *Dialogue on Diarrhoea,* 45:1–6.

Chavasse DC, Yap HH (1997). *Chemical methods for the control of arthropod vectors and pests of public health importance,* 5th ed. Geneva, World Health Organization (unpublished document WHO/CTD/WHOPES/97.2; available on request from World Health Organization, 1211 Geneva 12, Switzerland).

Chen LC, ed. (1973). *Disaster in Bangladesh: health crisis in a developing nation.* London, Oxford University Press.

Christen J (1996). *Dar es Salaam Urban Health Project. Health care waste management in district facilities: situational analysis and system development.* St. Gallen, Switzerland, Swiss Centre for Development Cooperation in Technology and Management (SKAT).

Christensen H (1985). *Refugees and pioneers: history and field study of a Burundian settlement in Tanzania.* Geneva, United Nations Research Institute for Social Development.

Clark DH, Nicholls J, Gillespie F (1992). Planning for mortuary facilities in mass disasters. *Disaster Management,* 4(2):98–102.

Clark L (1988). *The field guide to water wells and boreholes.* London, Wiley. (Geological Society of London Professional Handbook Series).

Clay J, et al. (1988). *The spoils of famine: Ethiopian famine policy and peasant agriculture.* Cambridge, MA, Cultural Survival.

Collins A (1993). Environmental influences on the distribution and the incidence of cholera: a case study in Quelimane, Mozambique. *Disasters,* 17(4):321–340.

Cooper Weil DE et al. (1990). *The impact of development policies on health.* Geneva, World Health Organization.

Cruz W, Repetto R (1992). *The environmental effects of stabilization and structural adjustment programs: the Philippines case.* Washington, DC, World Resources Institute.

Cullis A, Pacey A (1992). *A development dialogue: rainwater harvesting in Turkana.* London, Intermediate Technology Publications.

Cuny FC (1983). *Disasters and development.* New York, NY, Oxford University Press.

Davis I (1975). Disaster housing: a case study in Managua. *Architectural Design*, January, pp. 42–47.

Davis I (1978). *Shelter after disaster*. Headington, Oxford, Oxford Polytechnic Press.

Davis I, ed. (1981). *Disasters and the small dwelling*. London, Pergamon.

Davis I (1986). The planning and maintenance of urban settlements to resist extreme climatic forces. In: Oke TR, ed. *Urban climatology and its applications with special regard to tropical areas*. Geneva, World Meteorological Organization, pp. 277–312 (World Climate Programme Publication 652).

Davis J, Lambert R (2002). *Engineering in emergencies: a practical guide for relief workers*, 2nd ed. London, Intermediate Technology Publications.

de Lepper M, Scholten H, Stern R, eds. (1995). *The added value of geographic information systems in public and environmental health*. Dordrecht, Kluwer.

de M. Monzon F (1990). People's participation in housing construction in Huancayo, Peru. In: Gamser MS, Appleton H, Lewin R, eds. *Tinker, tiller, technical change*. London, Intermediate Technology Publications.

de Ville de Goyet C (1993). Post disaster relief: the supply—management challenge. *Disasters*, 17(2):169–176.

Delmas G, Courvallet M (1994). *Public health engineering in emergency situation*. Paris, Médecins Sans Frontières.

DfID (1995). *Stakeholder participation and analysis*. London, Department for International Development.

Dian Desa (1990). Water purification with *Moringa* seeds. In: Kerr C, ed. *Community health and sanitation*. London, Intermediate Technology Publications, pp. 63–67.

Downie R, Fyfe C, Tannahill A (1990). *Health promotion: models and values*. Oxford, Oxford University Press.

Drabek T (1986). *Human systems response to disaster*. London, Pergamon.

Drèze J, Sen A (1989). *Hunger and public policy*. New York, NY, Oxford University Press.

Dufresne C, Thompson P (1996). Interagency coordination during emergencies. In: *New approaches to new realities: first international emergency settlement conference*. Wisconsin, MA, University of Wisconsin Disaster Management Center, topic 5.

Dymon UJ, Winter NL (1993). Evacuation mapping: the utility of guidelines. *Disasters*, 17(1):12–24.

Dynes RR, DeMarchi B, Pelanda C, eds. (1987). *Sociology of disaster*. Milan, Franco Agneli Libri.

Eade D, Williams S (1995). Health education and the promotion of healthy behaviour. In: *The Oxfam handbook of development and relief*, Vol. 2. Oxford, Oxfam, pp. 767–772.

Eade D, Wright RM, eds. (1994). *Natural connections: perspectives in community-based conversation*. Washington, DC, Island Press.

Eheman CR (1989). Nuclear-reactor incidents. In: Gregg MB, ed. *The public health consequences of disasters*. Atlanta, GA, Centers for Disease Control.

European Commission (1996). *The control of major accident hazards involving dangerous substances*. Brussels (Directive 96/82/EC (known as the Seveso II Directive, Ref: OJL 10/1997)).

Evans P, Appleton B, eds. (1993) *Community management today. The role of communities in the management of improved water supply systems*. The Hague, International Water and Sanitation Centre (Occasional Paper 20).

Feachem R, Cairncross S (1978). *Small excreta disposal systems*. London, Ross Institute (Ross Bulletin No. 8).

Fernandez A (1979). Relationship between disaster assistance and long-term development. *Disasters*, 3:32–36.

Ferron S, Morgan J, O'Reilly M (2000). *Hygiene promotion: a practical manual for relief and development*. London, Intermediate Technology Publications.

Foster HD (1980). *Disaster planning: the preservation of life and property.* New York, NY, Springer-Verlag.

Franceys R, Pickford J, Reed R (1992). *A guide to the development of on-site sanitation.* Geneva, World Health Organization.

Geefhuysen C, Bennett E, Lewin R (1995). *Health information: its collection and use.* Brisbane, Australian Centre for International and Tropical Health and Nutrition.

Gibbs SL (1990). *Women's role in the Red Cross/Red Crescent.* Geneva, International Federation of Red Cross and Red Crescent Societies (Henry Dunant Institute, Studies on Development No. 1).

Goma Epidemiology Group (1995). Public health impact of Rwandan refugee crisis: what happened in Goma, July 1994? *Lancet,* 348:339–344.

Good, J (1996a). Needs and resource assessment. In: *New approaches to new realities: first international emergency settlement conference.* Wisconsin, MA, University of Wisconsin Disaster Management Center, Topic 3.

Good, J (1996b). Site selection, planning and shelter. In: *New approaches to new realities: first international emergency settlement conference.* Wisconsin, MA, University of Wisconsin Disaster Management Center, Topic 13.

Group of Agricultural Pesticides Manufacturers (GIFAP) (1993). *Treatment in case of pesticide poisoning: guide to the treatment of poisoning by chemicals in agriculture and public health.* Geneva.

Haas E, Kates R, Bowden M, eds. (1977). *Reconstruction following disaster.* Cambridge, MA, Massachusetts Institute of Technology Press.

Hagman G, et al. (1984). *Prevention better than cure.* Stockholm, Swedish Red Cross.

Hall N (1990). Water collection from thatched roofs. In: Kerr C, ed. *Community health and sanitation.* London, Intermediate Technology Publications.

Hanna JA (1995). *Disaster planning for health care facilities.* Ottawa, Canadian Hospital Association.

Hansen A, Oliver-Smith A, eds. (1982). *Involuntary migration and resettlement: the problems and responses of dislocated peoples.* Boulder, CO, Westview.

Hardoy J, Satterthwaite D (1981). *Shelter: need and response. Housing, land and settlement policies in seventeen third world nations.* Chichester, Wiley.

Hardoy J, Satterthwaite D (1989). *Squatter citizen: life in the urban third world.* London, Earthscan.

Hardoy J, Cairncross S, Satterthwaite D, eds. (1990). *The poor die young: housing and health in third world cities.* London, Earthscan.

Harrell-Bond BE (1986). *Imposing aid: emergency assistance to refugees.* Oxford, Oxford University Press.

Harvey PA, Baghri S, Reed RA (2002). *Emergency sanitation: assessment and programme design.* Loughborough, Water, Engineering and Development Centre.

Hermann E, Bentley M (1994). *Rapid assessment procedures to improve the household management of diarrhea.* Boston, MA, International Nutrition Foundation for Developing Countries.

Hiemstra W, Reijntjes C, van der Werf EJ, eds. (1992). *Let the farmers judge.* London, Intermediate Technology Publications.

Hope A, Timmek S (1987). *Training for transformation: a handbook for community workers.* Gweru, Zimbabwe, Mambo Press.

House SJ, Reed RA (1997). *Emergency water sources: guidelines for selection and treatment.* Loughborough, Water, Engineering and Development Centre.

Howard J, Spice R (1981). *Plastic sheeting: its use for emergency housing.* Oxford, Oxfam.

Hubley J (1993). *Communicating health: an action guide to health education and health promotion.* London & Basingstoke, Macmillan.

Ignacio LL, Perlas A (1994). *From victims to survivors: psychological intervention in disaster management.* Manila, University of the Philippines.

Ikeda K (1995). Gender differences in human loss and vulnerability in natural disasters: a case study from Bangladesh. *Indian Journal of Gender Studies,* 2(2):171–193.

International Atomic Energy Agency (1994). *Safety guides. Intervention criteria in a nuclear or radiation emergency.* Vienna (Safety Series, No. 109).

International Atomic Energy Agency (1995). *Annual report for 1994.* Vienna (document GOV/2794; available on request from World Health Organization, 1211 Geneva 12, Switzerland).

International Atomic Energy Agency (1996). *International basic safety standards for protection against ionizing radiation and for the safety of radiation sources.* Vienna (Safety Series, No. 115).

International Committee of the Red Cross (2001). *Coping with stress: humanitarian action in conflict zones.* Geneva.

International Federation of Red Cross and Red Crescent Societies (1991). *Working with women in emergency relief and rehabilitation programmes.* Geneva (Field Studies Paper No. 2).

International Federation of Red Cross and Red Crescent Societies (1993a). *World disasters report 1993.* Geneva.

International Federation of Red Cross and Red Crescent Societies (1993b). *A pocket guide to assessing vulnerabilities for programmes of the Red Cross and Red Crescent Societies.* Geneva.

International Federation of Red Cross and Red Crescent Societies (1994). *Vulnerability and capacity assessment guidelines.* Geneva.

International Federation of Red Cross and Red Crescent Societies (1996). *World disasters report 1996.* Geneva.

International Federation of Red Cross and Red Crescent Societies (1997a). *Handbook for delegates.* Geneva.

International Federation of Red Cross and Red Crescent Societies (1997b). *World disasters report 1997.* Oxford, Oxford University Press.

International Federation of Red Cross and Red Crescent Societies (1998). *World disasters report 1998.* Oxford, Oxford University Press.

International Federation of Red Cross and Red Crescent Societies (2000). *World disasters report 2000.* Oxford, Oxford University Press.

International Federation of Red Cross and Red Crescent Societies (2001). *World disasters report 2001.* Oxford, Oxford University Press.

International Federation of Red Cross and Red Crescent Societies, International Committee of the Red Cross (1994). *Code of conduct for the International Red Cross and Red Crescent movement and NGOs in disaster relief.* Geneva.

International Federation of Red Cross and Red Crescent Societies, Johns Hopkins University (2000). *Public health guide for emergencies.* Baltimore, MD, The Johns Hopkins University.

International Institute for Environment and Development (1993). Health and well-being in cities. *Environment and urbanization,* 5(2).

Jacob M (1989). *Safe food handling.* Geneva, World Health Organization.

Jahn SAA (1981). *Traditional water purification in tropical developing countries—existing methods and potential applications.* Eschborn, German Agency for Technical Cooperation (GTZ).

Jiggins J (1986). Women and seasonality: coping with crisis and calamity. *IDS Bulletin,* 17(3):9–18.

Jensen E (1996). Introduction and overview: typology and causes of emergency settlement. In: *New approaches to new realities: first international emergency settlement conference.* Wisconsin, MA, University of Wisconsin Disaster Management Center, topic 1.

Johns W (1987). *Establishing a refugee camp laboratory: a practical guide.* London, Save the Children Fund.

Jordan TD (1984). *A handbook of gravity-flow water systems.* London, Intermediate Technology Publications.

Keifer MC, ed. (1997). Human health effects of pesticides. *Occupational Medicine: State of the Art Reviews,* 12(2).

Kanji N, Kanji N, Manji F (1991). From development to sustained crisis: structural adjustment, equity and health. *Social Science and Medicine,* 33(9):985–993.

Kerr C, ed. (1989). *Community water development.* London, Intermediate Technology Publications.

Kibreab G (1985). *African refugees.* Trenton, NJ, Africa World Press.

Kibreab G (1987). *Refugees and development in Africa.* Trenton, NJ, Red Sea Press.

Kreimer A (1979). Emergency, temporary and permanent housing after disasters in developing countries. *Ekistics,* 46:361–365.

Kreimer A, Munasinghe M, eds. (1991). *Managing natural disasters and the environment.* Washington, DC, World Bank.

Kumar K (1993). *Rapid rural appraisal methods.* Washington, DC, World Bank.

Lee JA (1985). *The environment, public health, and human ecology.* Baltimore, MD, Johns Hopkins University Press.

Lillibridge SR (1997). Industrial disasters. In: Noji EK, ed. *The public health consequences of disasters.* New York, Oxford University Press, pp 354–372.

Lima B (1986). *Primary mental health care of disaster victims in developing countries.* University of Colorado, Natural Hazards Research and Applications Information Centre.

Lloyd B, Helmer R (1991). *Surveillance of drinking water quality in rural areas.* London, Longman.

Lystad M, ed. (1988). *Mental health response to mass emergencies.* New York, NY, Brunner-Mazel.

Manderson L, Valencia L, Thomas B (1992). *Bringing the people in: community participation and the control of tropical diseases.* Geneva, World Health Organization (unpublished document TDR/SER/RP/92/1; available on request from World Health Organization, 1211 Geneva 12, Switzerland).

Martin SF (1992). *Refugee women.* London, Zed Books.

Maskrey A (1989). *Disaster mitigation: a community based approach.* Oxford, Oxfam.

McAuslan P (1985). *Urban land and shelter for the poor.* London, Earthscan and International Institute for Environment and Development.

McMichael AJ (1993). *Planetary overload: global environmental change and the health of the human species.* Cambridge, Cambridge University Press.

McMichael et al. (1996). *Climate change and human health: an assessment prepared by a Task Group on behalf of the World Health Organization, the World Meteorological Organization and the United Nations Environment Programme.* Geneva, World Health Organization (unpublished document WHO/EHE/96.7; available on request from World Health Organization, 1211 Geneva 12, Switzerland).

Médecins Sans Frontières (1997a). *Refugee health: an approach to emergency situations.* London and Basingstoke, MacMillan.

Médecins Sans Frontières (1997b). *Guide of kits and emergency items: decision-maker's guide.* 4th English ed. Brussels, Médecins Sans Frontières.

Mitchell JK (1996). *Megacities and natural disasters.* Tokyo, United Nations University Press.

Moser C (1993). *Gender, planning and development: theory, practice and training.* London, Routledge.

Natural Disasters Organization (1992). *Australian emergency manual: community emergency planning guide,* 2nd ed. Dickson.

Neal DM, Phillips BD (1995). Effective emergency management: reconsidering the bureaucratic approach. *Disasters*, 19(4):327–337.

New Zealand Ministry of Health (1995). *Civil defence and food safety*. Wellington (Food Administration Manual S13).

Nicholls N (1988). Low latitude volcanic eruptions and the El Niño Southern Oscillation. *Journal of Climatology*, 8:91–95.

Noji EK, ed. (1997). *The public health consequences of disasters*. New York, NY, Oxford University Press.

Oliver-Smith A, ed. (1986a). *Natural disasters and cultural responses*. Williamsburg, VA, College of William and Mary (Studies in Third World Societies No. 36).

Oliver-Smith A (1986b). *The martyred city: death and rebirth in the Andes*. Albuquerque, NM, University of New Mexico Press.

Oliver-Smith A (1991). Successes and failures in post-disaster resettlement. *Disasters*, 15(1):12–21.

Oliver-Smith A (1992). Disasters and development. *Environment and Urban Issues*, 20(1):1–3.

Olson KR, Mycroft FJ (1994). Emergency medical response to hazardous materials incidents. In: Olson KR, ed. *Poisoning and drug overdose*, 2nd ed. Norwalk, CT, Appleton & Lange.

Organisation Mondiale de la Santé (1989). *Le personnel de santé et la communauté face aux catastrophes naturelles. [Health workers and the community in natural disasters]*. Geneva.

Organisation for Economic Co-operation and Development (1992). *Guiding principles for chemical accident prevention, preparedness and response*. Paris (document OECD/GD (92)43).

Organisation for Economic Co-operation and Development (1996). *Guidance Concerning Health Aspects of Chemical Accidents*. Paris.

Organisation for Economic Co-operation and Development and Nuclear Energy Agency (1994). *Radiation protection, today and tomorrow*. Paris.

Organisation for Economic Co-operation and Development and United Nations Environment Programme (1994). *Health aspects of chemical accidents*. Paris (document OECD/GD (94)1).

Overseas Development Institute, People in Aid (1998). *Code of best practice in the management and support of aid personnel*. London, Overseas Development Institute.

Oxfam (1990). *Safety in wells: dangers and safety measures for hand dug wells and similar engineering projects*. Oxford, Oxfam.

Oxfam (1995). *The Oxfam handbook of development and relief*. Oxford, Oxfam.

Pacey A, Cullis A (1986). *Rain water harvesting: the collection of rain fall and run-off in rural areas*. Intermediate Technology Publications, London.

Pan American Health Organization (1981). *Emergency health management after natural disaster*. Washington, DC (PAHO Scientific Publication 407, pp 3–6).

Pan American Health Organization (1982). *Environmental health management after natural disaster*. Washington, DC (PAHO Scientific Publication 430).

Pan American Health Organization (1983). *Health services organization in the event of a disaster*. Washington, DC (PAHO Scientific Publication 443).

Pan American Health Organization (1987). *Assessing needs in the health sector after floods and hurricanes*. Washington, DC (PAHO Technical Paper 11).

Pan American Health Organization (1993). *Mitigation of disasters in health facilities: evaluation and reduction of physical and functional vulnerability*. Washington, DC.

Pan American Health Organization (1994). *Communicating with the public in times of disaster: guidelines for disaster managers on preparing and disseminating effective health messages*. Washington, DC.

Pan American Health Organization (1995). *Guidelines for assessing disaster preparedness in the health sector.* Washington, DC.

Pan American Health Organization (1996). *Manual de vigilancia sanitaria—saneamiento en desastres, [Sanitary surveillance manual—sanitation in disasters].* Washington DC.

Pan American Health Organization (1998). *Mitigación de desastres naturales en sistemas de agua potable y alcantarillado sanitario: guías para el análisis de vulnerabilidad. [Mitigation of the effects of natural disasters on drinking-water and sewerage systems: guidelines on the analysis of vulnerability].* Washington, DC.

Pan American Health Organization (2000). *Natural disasters—protecting the public's health.* Washington DC.

Pantelic J (1991). The link between reconstruction and development. In: Kreimer A, Munasinghe M, eds. *Managing natural disasters and the environment.* Washington, DC, World Bank.

Parker D, Mitchell J (1995). Disaster vulnerability of megacities. *Geojournal,* 37(3):295–302.

People in Aid (1997). *The People in Aid code of best practice in the management and support of aid personnel.* London, Overseas Development Institute (Relief and Rehabilitation Network Paper, No. 20).

Perrin P (1996). *War and public health: handbook on war and public health.* Geneva, International Committee of the Red Cross.

Pickford J (1977). Water treatment in developing countries. In: Feachem R, McGarry M, Mara D, eds. *Water, wastes and health in hot climates.* Chichester, Wiley, pp. 162–191.

Pickford J (1995). *Low-cost sanitation: a survey of practical experience.* London, Intermediate Technology Publications.

Pike EG (1987). *Engineering against schistosomiasis/bilharzias.* London, Macmillan.

Pryor L (1982). *Ecological management in natural disasters.* Gland, Switzerland, International Union for the Conservation of Nature Commission on Ecology and League of Red Cross and Red Crescent Societies.

Quarantelli E (1980). *Sociology and social pathology of disasters.* Columbus, OH, Disaster Research Center, Ohio State University.

Quarantelli E (1989). *A review of the literature in disaster recovery research.* Newark, DE, Disaster Research Center, University of Delaware.

Raintree J, ed. (1987). *D&D User's manual: an introduction to agroforestry diagnosis and design.* Nairobi, International Council for Research in Agroforestry.

Rajagopalan S, Shiffman MA (1974). *Guide to simple sanitary measures for the control of enteric diseases.* Geneva, World Health Organization.

Rawl R (1998). Transport Safety. *IAEA Bulletin* 40(2):18–20.

Reed RA (1994). *Sanitation for refugees and similar emergency situations.* Unpublished technical guide prepared for Oxfam GB.

Reed RA, Dean PT (1994). Recommended methods for the disposal of sanitary wastes from temporary field medical facilities. *Disasters,* 18(4):355–367.

Reed RH (1997). Solar inactivation of faecal bacteria in water: the critical role of oxygen. *Letters of Applied Microbiology* 24:276–280.

Richards PJ, Thomson AM (1984). *Basic needs and the urban poor.* London, Croom Helm.

Rivers J (1987). Women and children last. *Disasters,* 6(4):256–267.

Roche C (1994). Operationality in turbulence: the need for change. *Development in Practice,* 4(3):160–172.

Rozendaal JA (1997). *Vector control: methods for use by individuals and communities.* Geneva, World Health Organization.

Rubin C, Barbee D (1985). Disaster recovery and hazard mitigation: bridging the intergovernmental gap. *Public Administration Review,* 45:57–63.

Satterthwaite D et al. (1996). *The environment for children.* London, Earthscan.

Savage-King F (1992). *Helping mothers to breastfeed,* revised ed. Nairobi, African Medical and Research Foundation.

Schultz CR, Okun DA (1984). *Surface water treatment for communities in developing countries.* John Wiley and Sons, Inc., New York.

Scott M (1987). The role of non-governmental organizations in famine relief and prevention. In: Glantz M, ed. *Drought and hunger in Africa.* Cambridge, Cambridge University Press, pp. 349–366.

Scrimshaw SC, Hurtado E (1989). *Rapid assessment procedures for nutrition and primary health care.* Los Angeles, CA, University of California Latin America Center Publications.

Scrimshaw NS, Gleason GR, eds. (1992). *Rapid assessment procedures: qualitative methodologies for planning and evaluation of health-related programmes.* Boston, MA, International Nutrition Foundation for Developing Countries.

Shaw R (1998). *Running water: more technical briefs for health, water and sanitation.* London, Intermediate Technology Publications.

Shook G, Englande AJ (1992). Environmental health criteria for disaster relief and refugee camps. *International Journal of Environmental Health Research,* 2:171–183.

Simmonds S, Vaughan P, Gunn SW, eds. (1983). *Refugee community health care.* Oxford, Oxford University Press.

Skeet M (1977). *Manual for disaster relief work.* Edinburgh, Churchill Livingstone.

Skinner R, Rodell M (1983). *People, poverty and shelter: problems of self-help housing in the Third World.* London, Methuen.

Slim H (1995). The continuing metamorphosis of the humanitarian practitioner: some new colours for an endangered chameleon. *Disasters,* 19(2):110–126.

Smith K (1992). *Environmental hazards: assessing risk and reducing disaster.* London, Routledge.

Sobsey MD (2002). *Managing water in the home: accelerated health gains from improved water supply.* Geneva (unpublished document WHO/SDE/WSH/02.07; available on request from Water, Sanitation and Health Programme, World Health Organization, 1211 Geneva 27, Switzerland).

Sphere Project (2000). *The Sphere Project humanitarian charter and minimum standards in disaster response, first final edition.* Geneva, The Sphere Project.

Steady F, ed. (1993). *Women and children first: environment, poverty and sustainable development.* Rochester, VT, Schenkman.

Sullivan JB, Krieger GR, eds. (1992). *Hazardous materials toxicology.* Baltimore, MD, Williams & Wilkins.

Tabibzadeh I, Rossi-Espagnet A, Maxwell R (1989). *Spotlight on the cities: improving urban health in developing countries.* Geneva, World Health Organization.

The Citizen Disaster Response Centre (1992). *Disasters: the Philippine experience.* Manila.

Thompson J (1991). The management of body recovery after disasters. *Disaster Management,* 3(4):206–210.

Thomson M (1995). *Disease prevention through vector control: guidelines for relief organisations.* Oxford, Oxfam.

Turner J (1982). Issues in self-help and self-managed housing. In: Ward P, ed. *Self-help housing.* London, Alexandrine.

United Kingdom Department for Environment, Food and Rural Affairs (1999). *Environment sampling after a chemical accident.* A collaborative document published by the United Kingdom Department for Environment, Food and Rural Affairs. London, Her Majesty's Stationery Office.

United Nations (1991). *Recommendations on the transport of dangerous goods.* New York, NY.

United Nations (1998). *Security in the field: information for staff members of the United Nations system.* New York, NY.

United Nations Centre for Human Settlements (1989). *Solid waste management in low-income housing projects: the scope for community participation.* Nairobi.

United Nations Children's Fund (1984). *Reaching children and women of the urban poor.* New York, NY (Occasional Paper 3).

United Nations Children's Fund (1986). *Assisting in emergencies: a resource handbook for UNICEF field staff.* New York, NY.

United Nations Children's Fund (1996). *State of the world's children 1996.* New York, NY.

United Nations Children's Fund (1999). *A manual on hygiene promotion.* New York, NY (Water, Environment and Sanitation Series, No. 6).

United Nations Commission on Human Settlements (1996). *An urbanizing world: global report on human settlements 1996.* Oxford, Oxford University Press.

United Nations Department of Humanitarian Affairs (1992). *Glossary: internationally agreed glossary of basic terms related to disaster management,* Geneva (unpublished document DHA/93/36; available on request from United Nations Department of Humanitarian Affairs).

United Nations Development Programme, Inter-Agency Procurement Services Office (1995). *Emergency relief items, compendium of generic specifications. Vol. 1, Telecommunications, shelter and housing, water supply, food, sanitation and hygiene, materials handling, power supply; Vol. 2, Medical supplies and equipment, selected essential drugs, guidelines for drug donations.* New York, NY.

United Nations Environment Programme (1992). *Saving our planet: challenges and hopes. The state of the environment report (1972–1992).* Nairobi (UNEP/GCSS, III/2).

United Nations Environment Programme (1998). *Awareness and preparedness for emergencies at local level (APELL): a process for responding to technological accidents.* Nairobi.

United Nations Environment Programme, International Environmental Technology Centre (1992). *Earthquake waste symposium report.* Osaka.

United Nations High Commissioner for Refugees (1989). *Policy for acceptance, distribution and use of milk products in refugee feeding programmes.* Geneva (UNHCR/IOM/88/89 and UNHCR/FOM/76/89).

United Nations High Commissioner for Refugees (1991). *Sectoral checklist for women and children.* Geneva.

United Nations High Commissioner for Refugees (1992a). *Water manual for refugee situations.* Geneva.

United Nations High Commissioner for Refugees (1992b). *A framework for people oriented planning in refugee situations taking account of women, men and children.* Geneva.

United Nations High Commissioner for Refugees (1996). *Refugee emergencies: a community-based approach.* Geneva.

United Nations High Commissioner for Refugees (1997). *Vector and pest control in refugee situations.* Geneva.

United Nations High Commissioner for Refugees (1999). *Handbook for emergencies,* 2nd ed. Geneva.

United Nations Office of the Disaster Relief Co-ordinator (1982a). *Disaster prevention and mitigation—a compendium of knowledge: sanitation aspects.* New York, NY, United Nations.

United Nations Office of the Disaster Relief Co-ordinator (1982b). *Shelter after disaster.* Geneva.

United Nations Office of the Disaster Relief Co-ordinator (1984). *Disaster prevention and mitigation—a compendium of knowledge: preparedness aspects.* New York, NY, United Nations.

United Nations Office of the Disaster Relief Co-ordinator (1986). *Disaster prevention and mitigation—a compendium of knowledge: social and sociological aspects*. New York, NY, United Nations.

United Nations Office of the Disaster Relief Co-ordinator (1991). *Mitigating natural disasters*. Geneva.

United States Agency for International Development (1998). *Field operations guide for disaster assessment and response*. United States Agency for International Development, Bureau for Humanitarian Response, Office of Foreign Disaster Assistance, Washington, DC.

United States Department of Transportation (1996). *North American emergency response guidebook*. Washington, DC.

United States Environmental Protection Agency (1990). *Hazmat team planning guidance*. Washington, DC (EPA/540/G-90/003).

United States Federal Emergency Management Administration (1994). *Handbook of chemical hazard analysis procedures*. Washington, DC.

van Brabant K (2000). *Operational security management in violent environments*. London, Overseas Development Institute (Good Practice Review 8).

van Leeuwen CJ, Hermens JLM (1995). *Risk assessment of chemicals: an introduction*. Kluwer Academic Publications, Dordrecht, Boston, MA.

van Wijk-Sijbesma C (1985). *Participation of women in water supply and sanitation*. The Hague, International Reference Centre for Community Water Supply and Sanitation (Technical Paper 22).

Voluntary Health Association of India (1993). *Turning disasters into developments*. New Delhi.

von Kotze A, Holloway A (1996). *Reducing risk: participatory learning activities for disaster mitigation in southern Africa*. Durban, International Federation of Red Cross and Red Crescent Societies.

Walker B, ed. (1994). *Women and emergencies*. Oxford, Oxfam.

Walker DJ, ed. (1992). *Food storage manual*. Rome, World Food Programme.

Walker P (1989). *Famine early warning systems: victims and destitution*. London, Earthscan.

Warford JJ (1995). Environment, health and sustainable development: the role of economic instruments and policies. *Bulletin of the World Health Organization*, 73(3):387–395.

Watson RT, Zinyowera MC, Moss RH, eds. (1996). *Climate change 1995: contribution of Working Group II to the second assessment report of the Intergovernmental Panel on Climate Change*. Cambridge, Cambridge University Press.

Watt SB, Wood WE (1979). *Hand dug wells and their construction*. London, Intermediate Technology Publications.

Waugh W (1995). Geographic information systems: the case for disaster management. *Social Science Computer Review*, 13(4):422–431.

Werner D, Bower B (1982). *Helping health workers learn*. Palo Alto, CA, Hesperian Foundation.

White A (1981). *Community participation in water and sanitation*. Rijswijk, Netherlands, International Reference Centre for Community Water Supply (Technical Paper 17).

Whiteside M (1996). Realistic rehabilitation: linking relief and development in Mozambique. *Development in Practice*, 6(2):121–128.

Wilson K, Harrell-Bond B (1990). Dealing with dying. *Refugee Participation Network Newsletter*, No. 9, August 1990. Oxford, Refugee Studies Programme.

Wiest R (1992). *The needs of women and children in disasters and emergencies*. Winnipeg, University of Manitoba Disaster Research Unit.

Winblad U, Kilama W (1985). *Sanitation without water*. London, Macmillan.

Wisner B (1993). Disaster vulnerability: scale, power and daily life. *GeoJournal*, 30(2):127–140.

World Commission on Environment and Development (1987a). *Our common future.* New York, Oxford University Press.

World Commission on Environment and Development (1987b). *Food 2000.* London, Zed Books.

World Health Organization (1980). *Environmental management for vector control. Fourth report of the WHO Expert Committee on Vector Biology and Control.* Geneva (Technical Report Series 649).

World Health Organization (1984a). *The role of food safety in health and development. Report of a Joint FAO/WHO Expert Committee on Food Safety.* Geneva (WHO Technical Report Series, No. 705).

World Health Organization (1984b). *Effects of nuclear war on health and health services; report of the International Committee of Experts in Medical Sciences and Public Health to Implement Resolution WHA34.38.* Geneva.

World Health Organization (1986). *The Ottawa Charter on Health Promotion.* Geneva (WHO/HPR/HEP/95.1).

World Health Organization (1987a). *Improving environmental health conditions in low-income settlements: a community-based approach to identifying needs and priorities.* Geneva (WHO Offset Publication No. 100).

World Health Organization (1987b). *Global pollution and health: results of health-related environmental monitoring.* Geneva (unpublished document; available on request from World Health Organization, 1211 Geneva 12, Switzerland).

World Health Organization (1989a). *Coping with natural disasters: the role of local health personnel and the community.* Geneva.

World Health Organization (1989b). *Health surveillance and management procedures for food-handling personnel: report of a WHO consultation.* WHO Technical Report Series, No. 785. Geneva.

World Health Organization (1989c). *Guideline for iodine prophylaxis following nuclear accidents.* Copenhagen, WHO Regional Office for Europe (Environmental Health Series No. 35).

World Health Organization (1989d). *Rehabilitation following chemical poisonings: a guide for public officials.* Geneva.

World Health Organization (1990). *Emergency preparedness and response: rapid health assessment in chemical emergencies.* Geneva (unpublished document ERO/EPR/90.1.9; available on request from World Health Organization, 1211 Geneva 12, Switzerland).

World Health Organization (1991a). *Environmental health in urban development, Report of an Expert Committee.* Geneva (WHO Technical Report Series, No. 807).

World Health Organization (1991b). *Environmental health management in emergencies.* Alexandria, WHO Regional Office for the Eastern Mediterranean.

World Health Organization (1991c). *Surface water drainage for low-income communities.* Geneva.

World Health Organization (1991d). *The WHO golden rules for safe food preparation.* Alexandria, WHO Regional Office for the Eastern Mediterranean.

World Health Organization (1992a). *Manual for the inspection of imported food.* Geneva.

World Health Organization (1992b). *WHO Commission on Health and Environment. Report of the Panel on Urbanization.* Geneva (unpublished document WHO/EHE/92.5; available on request from World Health Organization, 1211 Geneva 12, Switzerland).

World Health Organization (1993a). *Guidelines for drinking water quality,* 2nd ed. Vol. 1, *Recommendations.* Geneva.

World Health Organization (1993b). *Guidelines for cholera control.* Geneva.

World Health Organization (1993c). *Biomarkers and risk assessment: concepts and principles.* Geneva, International Programme on Chemical Safety / World Health Organization.

World Health Organization (1995a). *Coping with major emergencies—WHO strategy and approaches to humanitarian action.* Geneva (unpublished document WHO/EHA95.1, available on request from Emergency and Humanitarian Action, World Health Organization, 1211 Geneva 12, Switzerland).

World Health Organization (1995b). *Hygiene in food service and mass catering establishments.* Geneva (unpublished document WHO/FNU/FOS/94.5; available on request from Food Safety, World Health Organization, 1211 Geneva 27, Switzerland).

World Health Organization (1995c). *Vector control for malaria and other mosquito-borne disease: the report of a WHO Study Group.* Geneva (WHO Technical Report Series 857).

World Health Organization (1995d). *Fifth Coordination Meeting of WHO Collaborating Centres in Radiation Emergency Medical Preparedness and Assistance.* Geneva (unpublished document WHO/EHG/95.02; available on request from Protection of the Human Environment, World Health Organization, 1211 Geneva 12, Switzerland).

World Health Organization (1996a). *Mental health of refugees.* Geneva.

World Health Organization (1996b). *Health consequences of the Chernobyl accident: results of the IPHECA pilot projects and related national programmes: scientific report.* Geneva (unpublished document WHO/EHG/95.19; available on request from Protection of the Human Environment, World Health Organization, 1211 Geneva 12, Switzerland).

World Health Organization (1997a). *Guidelines for drinking-water quality,* 2nd ed. *Vol. 3, Surveillance and control of community water supplies.* Geneva.

World Health Organization (1997b). *Before, during and after radiation emergencies.* Copenhagen, WHO Regional Office for Europe (Local authorities health and environment briefing pamphlet series, 11).

World Health Organization (1997c). *Yellow tox, world directory of poisons centers.* Geneva, International Programme on Chemical Safety / World Health Organization.

World Health Organization (1998a). *The WHO recommended classification of pesticides by hazard and guidelines for classification 1998–1999.* Geneva, International Programme on Chemical Safety / World Health Organization (Unpublished document WHO/IPCS/98.21).

World Health Organization (1998b). *Poisons Information Monographs.* Geneva, IPCS INTOX Project, International Programme on Chemical Safety / World Health Organization. *http://www.inchem.org.*

World Health Organization (1999a). *Community emergency preparedness: a manual for managers and policy-makers.* Geneva.

World Health Organization (1999b). *Rapid health assessment protocols for emergencies.* Geneva.

World Health Organization (1999c). *Safe management of wastes from health-care activities.* Geneva.

World Health Organization (1999d). *Public health and chemical incidents. Guidance for national regional policy makers in the public/environmental health roles.* Geneva, International Programme on Chemical Safety / World Health Organization.

World Health Organization (2000a). *Global Water Supply and Sanitation Assessment 2000 Report.* Geneva.

World Health Organization (2000b). *The management of nutrition in major emergencies.* Geneva.

World Health Organization, United Nations Environment Programme (1991). *Manual on water and sanitation for health in refugee camps.* Geneva.

World Resources Institute (1990). *Participatory rural appraisal handbook.* Washington, DC.

Websites

AlertNet (the Reuters Foundation): (www.alertnet.org).

Asian Disaster Preparedness Centre: (www.adpc.ait.ac.th).

BBC News: (www.bbc.co.uk/hi/english/world).

Center for International Emergency, Disaster and Refugee Studies: (www.jhsph.edu/refugee).

Centers for Disease Control and Prevention (CDC): (www.cdc.gov).

Centre for Research on the Epidemiology of Disasters (CRED): (www.cred.be).

Disaster Relief Organisation: (www.disasterrelief.org).

Disasters: The Journal of Disaster Studies, Policy and Management: (www.odi.org.uk/publications/index.html).

EM-DAT: The OFDA/CRED International Disaster Database: (www.cred.be/emdat).

Emergency Nutrition Network Online: (www.ennonline.net).

Humanitarian Affairs Review: (www.humanitarian-review.org).

Humanitarian Practice Network: (www.odihpn.org).

Humanitarian Resources Network, Emerging Infectious Diseases Network (EIDNet): (www.humanitarian.net/eidnet).

Humanitarian Times: (www.humanitariantimes.com).

Intermediate Technology Development Group Ltd.: (www.itdg.org).

International Committee for the Red Cross (ICRC): (www.icrc.org).

International Federation of Red Cross and Red Crescent Societies (IFRC): (www.ifrc.org).

International Journal of Mass Emergencies and Disasters: (www.usc.edu/dept/sppd/ijmed).

International Organisation for Migration: (www.iom.int).

Internet Disaster Information Network: (www.disaster.net).

Journal of Humanitarian Assistance: (www.jha.ac).

Journal of Refugee Studies: (www3.oup.co.uk/refuge).

Médecins Sans Frontières (MSF): (www.msf.org).

National Disaster Prevention Center (CENAPRED): (www.cenapred.unam.mx).

National Research Institute for Earth Science and Disaster Prevention (NIED): (www.bosai.go.jp).

Natural Disaster Management in India: (www.ndmindia.nic.in).

Natural Hazards Disasters Network: (www.jiscmail.ac.uk/lists/natural-hazards-disasters.html).

Oxfam: (www.oxfam.org).

Pacific Disaster: (www.pdc.org).

Pan American Health Organisation: (www.paho.org).

Sanitation Connection: (www.sanicon.net).

South Eastern Europe Reconstruction Site: (www.seerecon.org).

Sphere Project Humanitarian Charter and Minimum Standards in Disaster Response: (www.sphereproject.org).

United Nations Children's Fund: (www.unicef.org).

United Nations Development Programme: (www.undp.org).

United Nations Disaster Assessment and Coordination team (UNDAC): (www.reliefweb.int/undac).

United Nations Environment Programme: (www.unep.org).

United Nations High Commissioner for Refugees: (www.unhcr.ch).

United Nations Mine Action Service: (www.un.org/Depts/dpko/mine).

United Nations Office for the Coordination of Humanitarian Affairs (OCHA): (www.reliefweb.int).

United Nations website locator: (www.unsystem.org).

University of Wisconsin Disaster Management Center: (http://epdweb.engr.wisc.edu/dmc).

US Environmental Protection Agency: (www.epa.gov).

USAID/OFDA Field Operations Guide (FOG): (www.usaid.gov/ofda/fog).

Working Group on Humanitarian and Emergency Assistance (WGHEA): (www.nrc.ch).

World Bank: (www.worldbank.org).

World Health Organization: (www.who.int).

ANNEX 1

WHO model of country-level emergency planning

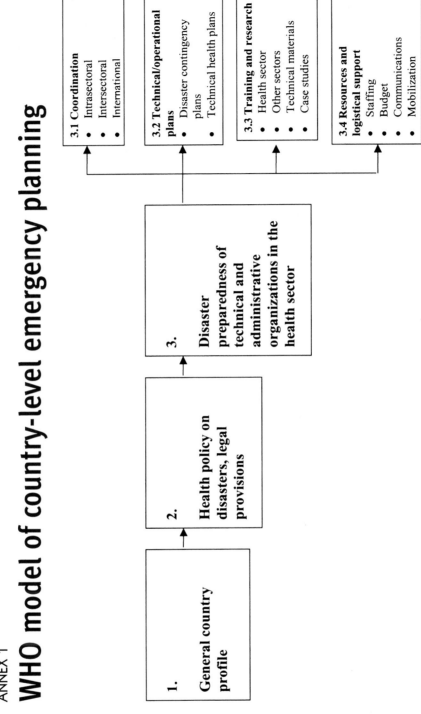

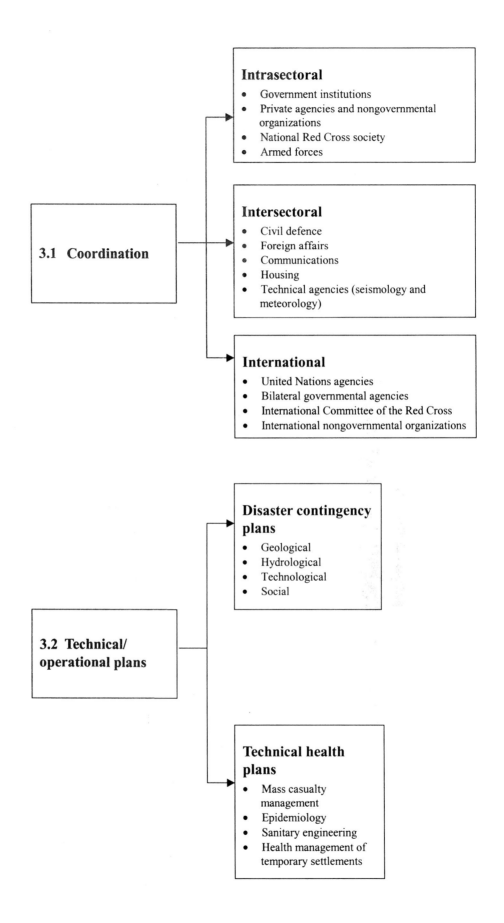

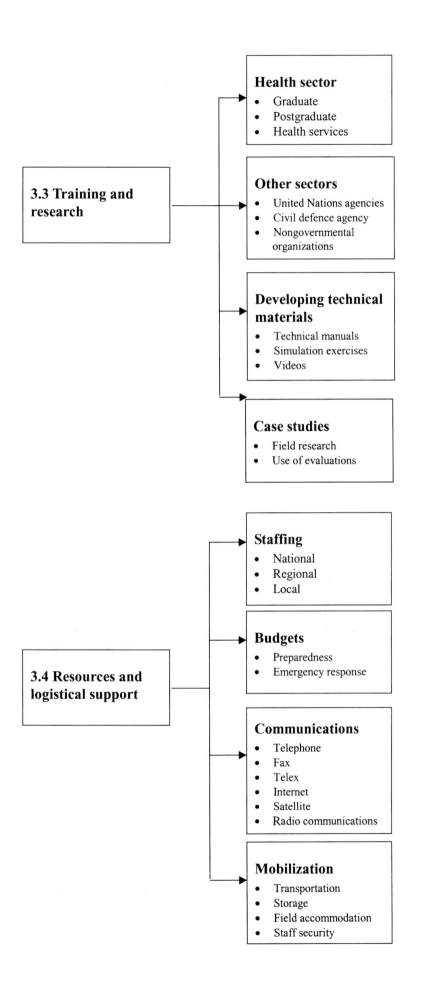

3.3 Training and research

Health sector
- Graduate
- Postgraduate
- Health services

Other sectors
- United Nations agencies
- Civil defence agency
- Nongovernmental organizations

Developing technical materials
- Technical manuals
- Simulation exercises
- Videos

Case studies
- Field research
- Use of evaluations

3.4 Resources and logistical support

Staffing
- National
- Regional
- Local

Budgets
- Preparedness
- Emergency response

Communications
- Telephone
- Fax
- Telex
- Internet
- Satellite
- Radio communications

Mobilization
- Transportation
- Storage
- Field accommodation
- Staff security

ANNEX 2

Equipment and supplies for environmental health activities in disasters and emergencies

Essential items of equipment and supplies include the following (to be modified according to local conditions).

- Equipment for personnel:
  - water-storage and water-treatment equipment;
  - tents, tarpaulins;
  - first-aid kits and personal health items;
  - stoves and fuel;
  - cooking and eating utensils;
  - food;
  - sleeping bags, blankets;
  - portable radio receiver;
  - waterproof bags;
  - detailed local information and statistics;
  - identity cards, travel warrants and any other official documents that may be required by authorities;
  - rain protection;
  - flashlights;
  - telecommunications equipment;
  - extra batteries for hand-portable communications and facilities for charging from vehicles;
  - public address equipment.
- Equipment for emergency water supply, particularly for displaced populations:
  - packaged water-storage/water-treatment kit;
  - pumps and piping;
  - fuel storage for pumps;
  - treatment chemicals;
  - water-quality testing kits;
  - tapstands and self-closing taps;
  - basic pipe-fitting tools;
  - water collection and storage containers.
- Equipment for emergency sanitation:
  - picks, shovels, rakes, hoes;
  - plastic sheeting, poles and nails;
  - tractors with trailers and spreaders;
  - tractors with loaders and excavator attachments;
  - cement mixers;
  - moulds and vibrators for making squatting plates;
  - cement, calcium chloride, steel reinforcing bars, sand, aggregate.
- Materials, tools and supplies needed for repairing and operating damaged urban water and sanitation networks:
  - accurate maps of networks, location of facilities;

— equipment for locating pipes;
— equipment for detecting leaks;
— equipment for quick coupling and patching of pipes;
— assorted sizes and types of water pipe;
— pipe-laying tools;
— pipe-fitting tools;
— jointing materials;
— excavation equipment;
— valves;
— hose pipes;
— welding equipment;
— protective clothing;
— boots;
— heavy-duty gloves;
— well-head fittings and pumps;
— fuel tanks;
— generators;
— tanks for water distribution;
— pipes with valves and fittings;
— sludge pumps;
— sewage pipes with jointing material;
— chemicals for water treatment.
■ Equipment for vector control:
— this should follow local practice. See Chapter 10 for details.
■ Items used in monitoring and surveillance:
— maps;
— baseline statistical data;
— calculators;
— dictation equipment;
— photographic equipment;
— blood-collection equipment;
— equipment for carrying specimens and water samples;
— chlorine test equipment;
— water-quality test equipment;
— tape measures;
— compass and hand-held GPS equipment;
— hand level;
— insect-collection equipment;
— pens, notebooks, data collection forms, clipboards;
— water-pressure gauge;
— graph paper;
— mapping pins;
— portable computer with modem and communications, and mapping software.
■ Laboratory equipment and materials:
These should be in accordance with national guidelines. Emergency stocks of
reagents for cholera diagnosis should be held where cholera outbreaks are
expected. For further details, see Johns (1987).
■ Administrative and office items:
— paper;
— pens, pencils;
— computers, printers, typewriters;
— filing equipment;

— photocopiers;
— batteries;
— lighting and generators.

More specialized equipment may occasionally be needed, especially in larger, damaged urban areas, and may include:
— large mobile chlorinators;
— mobile water-treatment equipment;
— large water and sewage pumps;
— large power generators;
— bulldozers and graders;
— well-digging/repair equipment;
— drilling rigs;
— welding equipment for emergency repairs to tools, equipment and vehicles.

ANNEX 3

Accidental pesticide poisoning

Diagnosis

Pesticide poisoning may mimic several other conditions, and it is essential to make the appropriate diagnosis. At first sight, it may mimic symptoms of syndromes, such as those associated with gastroenterological and other infectious diseases, that are common in tropical countries.

Diagnosis is based on history of exposure, clinical features and analytical support. IMPORTANT POINTS TO BE ESTABLISHED ARE AS FOLLOWS:

- *Has the patient been exposed to a pesticide?*
  If so, when did it occur and under what circumstances (accidental, occupational or intentional)?
- *If so, what was the pesticide, and to which chemical group does it belong?*
  If the container or name of the pesticide has arrived with the patient, this information may be available through a poisons centre or other organization.[1] The label may also include a brief indication of the treatment (but beware of container reuse).
- *By what route has the patient absorbed the pesticide: dermal, ocular, inhalatory, ingestion or combined?*
- *For how long was the patient exposed, and when did exposure cease?*
  Time elapsed since exposure? Duration of exposure? Has exposure in fact ceased? Is the patient still wearing contaminated clothing? Was the patient decontaminated?
- *What was the time between exposure and the onset of symptoms?*
- *What signs and symptoms are observed?*

Treatment

Treatment of any pesticide poisoning depends on the history of exposure, the level of exposure, the clinical status of the patient and the chemical concerned.

Treatment must never be delayed, pending the result of laboratory tests.

In areas where pesticides are used heavily, stocks of suitable antidotes should be readily available.

Supportive therapy is basically the same as for any form of poisoning; vasoactive drugs should be used with caution.

Consider the possibility of transportation (and the conditions of transportation) to an appropriate health facility. The following is a suggested sequence of treatment in a well-established medical centre:

- CHECK VITAL SIGNS AND APPLY RESUSCITATIVE MEASURES IF REQUIRED.

---

[1] For addresses, see: World Health Organization (1997c); also on http://www.intox.org.

- IF ANTIDOTE(S) ARE REQUIRED GIVE THEM AS SOON AS POSSIBLE, AND STOP FURTHER ABSORPTION OF THE POISON (e.g. REMOVE WET CLOTHING, DECONTAMINATE SKIN, USE ADSORBENTS SUCH AS ACTIVATED CHARCOAL, OR EMPTY THE STOMACH).
- CONSIDER ENHANCEMENT OF ELIMINATION.
- MONITOR PROGRESS OF PATIENT FREQUENTLY OVER FIRST FEW HOURS, AND REGULARLY FOR DAYS, AS REQUIRED.
- WHEN UNSURE, ALWAYS CHECK WITH THE NEAREST POISONS CENTRE.

ANNEX 4

International and national actions in response to a radiation emergency

Information in Tables 1–4 summarizes the actions of the World Health Organization, the International Atomic Energy Authority, other international organizations, and local health authorities in response to a nuclear accident, in compliance with the Convention on Early Notification and the Assistance Convention.

Table 1. **International response during the early phase of an accident[1]**

IAEA	WHO/HQ	Regional offices	Other international organizations
1. Establish direct telephone links with the accident State and States that might be affected.	1. Develop communication with Regional Offices and Member States. This includes developing links with the Ministries of Health of the accident country, of the affected States and of those that may be affected.	1. If information about an accident was obtained from an accident country or an affected country, inform WHO/HQ.	**FAO**—Collect and assess information from IAEA, the accident country or affected countries, on possible food contamination. Disseminate relevant information.
2. Identify States within a 1000 km radius from the release location that might be affected.	2. Request that the accident State, IAEA and WMO provide computer modelling maps of the radioactive cloud.	2. Establish communications with WHO/HQ, the Ministries of Health in accident and affected countries, and with WHO/REMPAN members in the Region.	**WMO**—Information on the direction of any released radioactive material should be issued regularly by designated WMO centres, for transmission to States and international organizations.
3. Contact affected States and provide them with special numbers for contacting the IEAE.	3. Request ICRP and IRPA assist in evaluating health consequences.	3. Undertake actions according to emergency plan. **UNEP**—Provide environmental and natural resources information through GEMS, GRID and GERMON, for analysis.	**UNOCHA**—Assist in coordinating the mobilization of resources to overcome
4. States outside the 1000 km zone will also be rapidly informed of the release, but not on a priority basis.	4. Request that REMPAN and GERMON members provide WHO with information on their readiness to assist (upon request) the accident country and affected States. The information should specify the type of assistance available (e.g. workforce, finance).	4. Regularly inform WHO/HQ about any progress in the development of the situation.	

Table 1. (Continued)

IAEA	WHO/HQ	Regional offices	Other international organizations
	5. Contact Regional Offices to mobilize resources (including financial) for the accident countries and affected States. 6. Follow-up on the accident development and, if necessary, convene expert group meeting to obtain recommendations.		consequences of the accident. **United Nations International Emergency Network** -Assist in distributing relevant information after a radiation emergency.

[1] *Abbreviations: FAO = United Nations Food and Agriculture Organization; GEMS = Global Environment Monitoring System; GERMON = Global Environmental Radiation Monitoring Network; GRID = Global Resource Information Database; IAEA = International Atomic Energy Agency; ICRP = International Commission on Radiological Protection; IRPA = International Radiation Protection Association; REMPAN = Network for Radiation Emergency Medical Preparedness and Assistance; UNEP = United Nations Environment Programme; UNOCHA = United Nations Office for the Coordination of Humanitarian Affairs; WMO = World Meteorological Organization.*

Table 2. National and local response priorities

National and Local level	1. First medical care to radiation victims. 2. The accident State and affected States provide IAEA and FAO with information on food and drinking-water contamination. 3. If necessary, implement the following countermeasures: sheltering, radioprotective prophylaxis, iodine prophylaxis, body protection, evacuation, personal decontamination. (See Annex 5). 4. If necessary, request assistance of international community.

Table 3. International and local response during the intermediate phase of an accident

IAEA	WHO/HQ in cooperation with WHO/ROs		Local level
	No request for assistance	**Request[1]**	
1. Transmit requests for assistance and relevant information. 2. Offer to coordinate assistance efforts to States requesting support. 3. Provide the resources for	1. Monitor and study the situation. 2. Communicate between WHO/HQ, WHO/ROs, Ministries of Health of the affected countries, and information exchanges, etc. 3. Maintain REMPAN & GERMON in operational readiness.	1. Acknowledge receipt of the request. Notify the requesting State directly or through IAEA if it is in a position to render the requested assistance and of the terms of such assistance. 2. Within the limits of WHO/HQ and WHO/RO's capability, identify and notify the IAEA of experts, equipment and materials that could be available for provisional assistance.	1. Specify the scope and type of assistance required. 2. Provide the assisting party with information that allows it to determine the extent to which it is able to meet the request. 3. Unless otherwise agreed: provide overall direction, control, coordination and supervision of the assistance; in consultation with the requesting State, designate a person to a

Table 3. **(Continued)**

IAEA	WHO/HQ in cooperation with WHO/ROs		Local level
	No request for assistance	Request[1]	
an initial assessment of the accident or emergency.	4. Mobilize resources.	3. Inform IAEA and other State Parties (directly or through IAEA) of WHO-competent authorities and points of contact.	supervisory role, who should cooperate with the appropriate authority of the requesting State.
4. Develop appropriate monitoring programmes, procedures and standards.	5. Request additional information from the accident country, affected countries, IAEA and other relevant organizations.	4. Request information in compliance with the checklist.	4. Provide local facilities and services for administering the assistance.
5. Send radiological and emergency teams to the site of the accident.	6. If necessary, convene a meeting of experts to obtain recommendations.	5. Request additional information, if the information is seen at WHO/HQ as insufficient.	5. Ensure the protection of personnel, equipment and materials brought into its territory by, or on behalf of, the assisting party.
		6. Inform the country about the type of assistance to be sought by WHO from its REMPAN Collaborating Centres.	6. Ensure the return of the equipment and materials to the assisting party.
		7. Describe the Collaborating Centres that will be approached.	7. Inform WHO about the termination of assistance.
		8. Ask the selected Collaborating Centre for available assistance.	8. *Applicable countermeasures*: sheltering; radioprotective prophylaxis; body protection; decontamination of areas; evacuation.
		9. Establish link between the requested country and assisting centre(s), inform REMPAN of the outcome of the request.	9. *Applicable or essential countermeasures*: evacuation; personal decontamination; relocation; food control.
		10. Keep all REMPAN centres informed about the details of the accident and progress in its management.	

[1] *May come directly from the accident or affected countries, via IAEA, or other international intergovernmental organizations*

Table 4. **International and local actions during the recovery phase of an accident**

International level	Local level
1. Actions depend on the requests of the accident countries or affected countries. They may relate to providing humanitarian assistance to the accident country or affected countries, or to facilitating medical and epidemiological follow-up.	1. *Applicable countermeasures*: personal decontamination; relocation; control of access. 2. *Applicable or essential countermeasures*: food control; decontamination of areas.

ANNEX 5

Selected information from the International Basic Safety Standards for Protection against Ionizing Radiation and for the Safety of Radiation Sources[1]

The management of accident situations outlined in the standards are based on principles of the International Commission on Radiological Protection (ICRP) for planning and deciding interventions to cope with a radiological emergency. These principles are:

- All possible efforts should be made to prevent serious deterministic health effects.
- The intervention should be justified, in the sense that introduction of the protective measure should achieve more good than harm.
- The levels at which the intervention is introduced and later withdrawn should be optimized, so that the protective measure(s) will produce a maximum net benefit.

The main criterion for deciding on intervention is the mean individual dose that is expected to be avoided by the intervention.

Dose levels at which intervention is expected to be undertaken under any circumstances (be justified) are given in Tables 1 and 2.

Table 1. **Acute exposure levels for intervention**

Organ or tissue	Projected absorbed dose (Gy) to the organ or tissue in less than 2 days
Whole body (bone marrow)	1
Lung	6
Skin	3
Thyroid	5
Lens of the eye	2
Gonads	3

Note: Doses greater than about 0.1 Gy (over less than two days) could have deterministic effects on a foetus, which should be taken into account when justifying and optimizing interventions for immediate protective action.

Table 2. **Chronic exposure dose rates for intervention**

Organ or tissue	Equivalent dose rate (Sv.a^{-1})
Gonads	0.2
Lens of the eye	0.4

[1] Jointly sponsored by FAO, IAEA, OECD/NEA, PAHO, WHO, Vienna 1996 (International Atomic Energy Agency, 1996).

Intervention levels in emergency exposure situations are expressed in terms of avertable dose, i.e. a protective action is indicated if the dose that can be averted is greater than the corresponding dose for the intervention level. Standard dose values have been developed by IAEA, and these can help set dose levels for emergency exposures (Table 3).

The recommended generic action levels for foodstuffs are presented in Table 4. Table 4 is based on, and consistent with, the Codex Alimentarius Commission's guideline levels for radionuclides in food moving in international trade following accidental contamination, but it is limited to the nuclides usually considered relevant to emergency exposure situations.

Optimized generic avertable doses recommended for temporary relocation and permanent resettlement interventions are given in Table 5. The avertable dose levels apply to situations where alternative food supplies are readily available. If food supplies are scarce, higher avertable doses may apply.

Table 3. **Recommended generic intervention levels for urgent protective measures**

Protective action	Generic intervention level (dose avertable by the protective action)
Sheltering	10 mSv in a period of no more than two days
Temporary evacuation	50 mSv in a period of no more than one week
Iodine prophylaxis	100 mSv (absorbed dose due to radioiodine)[1]

[1] For children, WHO recommends 10 mSv.

Table 4. **Generic action levels for foodstuffs**

Radionuclides	Food for general consumption (kBq/kg))	Milk and infant foods, drinking-water (kBq/kg)
Cs-134, Cs-137, Ru-103, Ru-106, Sr-89	1000	1000
I-131	1000	100
Sr-90	100	100
Am-241, Pu-238, Pu-239	10	1

Table 5. **Recommended generic avertable doses for temporary relocation and permanent resettlement interventions**

Action	Avertable dose
Initiating temporary relocation	30 mSv in a month
Terminating temporary relocation	10 mSv in a month
Permanent relocation	1 Sv in a lifetime

ANNEX 6
Checklist of hygiene practices that protect health in emergencies and disasters

The following is an extensive list of hygiene practices that protect health in disasters and emergencies. The list may be used as an aid to assessing hygiene practices and risks, and as a means of focusing hygiene messages on a few practices that influence health in a particular situation.

People's ability to achieve these protective actions depends on the availability of material resources, such as adequate clean water, soap, toilets, etc., and personal resources, such as time and energy.

Water safety	
At the source	■ Water for drinking is collected from the cleanest possible source.
	■ If necessary, a distinction is made between water for drinking and water for other uses, such as bathing, laundry, watering animals.
	■ Water sources are protected from faecal contamination by fencing (to keep animals away), and by siting latrines or defecation fields at least 10–30 metres away, depending on ground conditions.
Collection, storage and use of water at household level	■ Water is collected and stored in clean, covered containers.
	■ Water is taken from the storage container with a clean, long-handled dipper or through a tap placed slightly above the bottom container.
	■ Efforts are made not to waste water.
Use of water	■ If there is a risk that water is not safe, it is filtered and/or chlorinated or boiled[1]
	■ Water for making food or drinks for young children is boiled.

Excreta disposal	
Use of designated places for defecation	■ Defecation is avoided near water sources and water-treatment plants, uphill of camps and water sources, in fields destined for crops, along public roads, near communal buildings such as clinics, near food-storage facilities.
	■ Defecation is done in latrines, trenches, defecation fields, etc.
	■ People avoid going barefoot to defecate.
	■ Children do not visit a defecation area alone.
	■ New arrivals at emergency settlements are aware of the arrangements for defecation and the importance of complying with them.
Children's sanitation	■ Uncontrolled defecation by children is stopped. (The faeces of young children are more harmful than those of adults).
	■ The stools of young children or babies are wrapped in leaves or paper and buried or put in a latrine.
	■ Young children are helped to defecate into an easily-cleaned container that can be emptied into a toilet and washed out.
	■ Children are cleaned promptly after defecation and have their hands washed.
	■ People who clean children wash their own hands thoroughly afterwards.

Waste disposal

Solid waste
- Refuse is not scattered about. (This encourages insect breeding and attracts rats which can be a nuisance and transmit disease).
- In the immediate post-disaster period, if organized refuse collection has not been set up, household solid waste is buried by families.
- Once collection arrangements have been made, refuse is placed in the bins provided.
- Filled bins are not left in food-preparation areas.
- Bins are kept securely covered to prevent scavenging by children or animals.
- Manure from livestock is collected and disposed of as safely.

Liquid waste
- Standing pools of polluted wastewater (from washing, food preparation, wasted tap water) are not allowed to form. (They encourage mosquito breeding, which is a health hazard).
- Children are prevented from playing in or near hazardous pools of water.
- Arrangements for disposing of liquid waste, such as using soakage pits, are understood and followed.

Vector control

Personal protection against disease vectors
- Household refuse is removed regularly to avoid build-up of houseflies and rat infestations.
- Foodstuffs are kept in rodent-proof stores or containers.
- Cooked foods, which may have been contaminated by houseflies, are properly reheated to a boil.
- Clothes are laundered frequently and insecticidal shampoos are used to prevent lice.
- In areas where mosquitoes are a problem, bed nets or bedroom screens are used, if available.

Personal hygiene

Water for washing
- If possible, plenty of water is used for washing.
- Clothing is laundered regularly.
- The most readily-available water is used for personal and domestic hygiene.

Hand-washing
- All family members wash their hands regularly: after defecating; after cleaning a child who has defecated and disposing of the stool; before preparing food; before eating; before feeding a child.
- Adults or older children wash the hands of young children.

Shelter

At the disaster site
- Where people are trying to house themselves in the ruins of their previous homes, they take steps to avoid risks from the lack of structural integrity of their buildings.
- If their homes are definitely unsafe, people move.

In longer-term emergency settlements
- People take part in residents' committees to voice their views about the setting up and running of a camp.
- Residents participate in cleaning the settlement.
- Children do not enter dangerous areas of the settlement and, if necessary, volunteers guard unsafe areas.

Food safety

Dealing with contaminated food
- Food that has been contaminated as a result of a disaster is disposed of or, if there is a food shortage, cleaned thoroughly (possibly by submerging in an antiseptic solution) and cooked for an extended period.
- Contaminated fruit is always peeled.
- Perishable food that has spoiled is salvaged by cutting out bad bits, prolonged washing and prolonged cooking (but milk, eggs, meat and fish that have not been stored properly are discarded).

Food handling and preparation	■ Surroundings are kept clean; waste is disposed of properly; and food is stored in closed containers to avoid contamination by insects and vermin.
	■ Food is prepared in a clean place, using clean pots and utensils.
	■ Uncooked food is washed in clean water before it is eaten.
	■ Cooked food is eaten while still hot, and previously prepared food is thoroughly reheated.
	■ Kept foods are covered.
Feeding babies	■ Children up to 6 months of age are breastfed.
	■ Weaning foods are clean and nutritious.
	■ Drinks are given with a cup and spoon rather than a bottle.
	■ People wash their hands before preparing weaning food and feeding a baby.

[1] To make water safe for drinking, it should be brought to a vigorous rolling boil. If boiling or chlorination are not possible at household level, then low-turbidity water may be disinfected by exposing it to bright sunlight for at least one day (Reed 1997).